Health Care Finance, Economics, and Policy for Nurses

Betty Rambur, PhD, RN, FAAN, is the Routhier Endowed Chair for Practice and a professor of nursing at the University of Rhode Island. She was formerly a professor of nursing and health policy at the University of Vermont and from 2000 to 2009 served there as an academic dean. In this role, she led the 2002 merger of the School of Nursing and the School of Allied Health Science to establish the College of Nursing and Health Sciences.

These experiences build on Dr. Rambur's substantive leadership history in health policy and payment reform. From 1991 to 1995 she led North Dakota's 33-member, statewide public/private health financing and delivery reform effort that led to omnibus legislation. In 2013, Dr. Rambur was appointed to Vermont's Green Mountain Care Board by Governor Peter Shumlin and served in this role until 2017. The five-member Green Mountain Care board is a quasi-judicial body. It oversees Vermont's financing, payment, and delivery reform and holds broad regulatory, innovation, and evaluation authority. In May 2020, Dr. Rambur was appointed to the Medicare Payment Advisory Commission by the U.S. Comptroller General, Director of the U.S. Government Accountability Office. MedPAC* is an influential, nonpartisan group of policy experts who advise the U.S. Congress on Medicare payment and policy. She was reappointed to this role in 2003. She has also served on numerous advisory and governing boards, including the boards of trustees of an academic medical center and an independent community hospital.

A registered nurse, Dr. Rambur received her MS and PhD in nursing from Rush University, Family Nurse Practitioner Certificate from the University of North Dakota, and baccalaureate degree from University of Mary, Bismarck, North Dakota, where she also served as the nursing departmental chair from 1991 to 2000. Her program of research focuses on health services, payment and delivery reform, workforce, and ethics and has produced over 70 published articles, seven invited book chapters, two textbooks, and numerous invited presentations on health policy and leadership development. Her particular interests include population health, reducing disparities and overtreatment, health care cost containment, value-informed nursing practice, and reconceptualized models of care, including primary care nursing. Dr. Rambur's professional passion is to translate complex economic and policy issues into easily applicable practical wisdom. An accomplished scholar, teacher, and academic administrator, her research has been honored by Sigma Theta Tau International. In 2013 she received the prestigious Sloan Consortium Excellence in Online Teaching and Learning Award. Dr. Rambur was named a Lois Capps Policy Luminary by the American Association of Colleges of Nursing in 2024. Her teaching expertise includes the organization, finance, and policy of health care and payment reform. She lives in North Kingstown, Rhode Island.

---

*The orientation detailed in this text is that of the author and does not necessarily represent MedPAC or other affiliations of the author.

Health Care Finance, Economics, and Policy for Nurses

A Foundational Guide

Third Edition

Betty Rambur, PhD, RN, FAAN

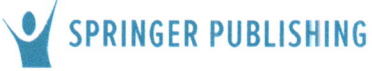

Copyright © 2025 Springer Publishing Company, LLC
All rights reserved.

First Springer Publishing edition 978-0-8261-2322-0 (2015); subsequent edition 2021

No part of this publication may be reproduced, stored in a retrieval system, or transmitted in any form or by any means, electronic, mechanical, photocopying, recording, or otherwise, without the prior permission of Springer Publishing Company, LLC, or authorization through payment of the appropriate fees to the Copyright Clearance Center, Inc., 222 Rosewood Drive, Danvers, MA 01923, 978-750-8400, fax 978-646-8600, info@copyright.com or at www.copyright.com.

Springer Publishing Company, LLC
902 Carnegie Center, Princeton, NJ 08540
www.springerpub.com
connect.springerpub.com

Acquisitions Editor: Joseph Morita
Compositor: S4Carlisle Publishing Services
Production Manager: Kris Parrish

ISBN: 978-0-8261-7235-8
e-book ISBN: 978-0-8261-7236-5
DOI: 10.1891/9780826172365

SUPPLEMENTS:

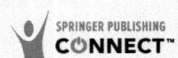 A robust set of instructor resources designed to supplement this text is located at http://connect.springerpub.com/content/book/978-0-8261-7236-5. Qualifying instructors may request access by emailing **textbook@springerpub.com**.

Instructor Materials:
LMS Common Cartridge—All Instructor Resources ISBN: 978-0-8261-7258-7
Instructor Manual ISBN: 978-0-8261-7238-9
Instructor Test Bank ISBN: 978-0-8261-7227-3
Instructor PowerPoints ISBN: 978-0-8261-7237-2
Mapping to AACN Essentials ISBN: 978-0-8261-4319-8
Transition Guide to the Third Edition ISBN: 978-0-8261-4678-6

24 25 26 27 / 5 4 3 2 1

The author and the publisher of this Work have made every effort to use reliable and current sources to provide information that is accurate and compatible with the standards generally accepted at the time of publication. Nevertheless, the authors and publisher are not responsible for any errors or omissions or any consequence from application of the information in this book and make no warranty, expressed or implied, with respect to the content of this publication. Because science and knowledge are continually advancing, readers therefore should always consult current research and specific institutional policies before performing any clinical procedure and should carefully check the manufacturer's package insert before delivering medication. The author and publisher shall not be liable for any special, consequential, or exemplary damages resulting, in whole or in part, from readers' use of, or reliance on, the information contained in this book. The publisher has no responsibility for the persistence or accuracy of URLs for external or third-party internet websites referred to in this publication and does not guarantee that any content on such websites is, or will remain, accurate or appropriate. Similarly, Springer Publishing recognizes that cultural and social language preferences may change and that there may be disagreement on what is considered appropriate terminology within the context of the content. We strive for inclusivity and representation in all our content but must rely on the author's knowledge and interpretation of what is appropriate for the subject matter at the time of writing.

Library of Congress Cataloging-in-Publication Data

Names: Rambur, Betty, author.
Title: Health care finance, economics, and policy for nurses : a
 foundational guide / Betty Rambur.
Description: Third edition. | New York : Springer Publishing Company,
 [2025] | Includes bibliographical references and index. |
Identifiers: LCCN 2024039077 (print) | LCCN 2024039078 (ebook) | ISBN
 9780826172358 (paperback) | ISBN 9780826172365 (ebook)
Subjects: MESH: Healthcare Financing | Decision Making | Health Care Costs
 | Health Policy | United States | Nurses Instruction
Classification: LCC RT86.7 (print) | LCC RT86.7 (ebook) | NLM W 74 AA1 |
 DDC 362.17/30681—dc23/eng/20240916
LC record available at https://lccn.loc.gov/2024039077
LC ebook record available at https://lccn.loc.gov/2024039078

Contact sales@springerpub.com to receive discount rates on bulk purchases.

Publisher's Note: New and used products purchased from third-party sellers are not guaranteed for quality, authenticity, or access to any included digital components.

Printed in the United States of America by Gasch Printing.

To Mikey and Vivian, with the hope that readers of this text can help shape a safe and sustainable health care system for you and your generation.

Contents

Foreword: Reach for Your Roots   Olga Yakusheva, PhD, FAAN(h)   ix
A Note From the Author   xiii
How to Use This Text: A Note to Faculty   xv
Acknowledgments   xxi
Instructor Resources   xxiii

SECTION I: THE CONTEXT OF HEALTH CARE IN THE UNITED STATES

1. How the Money Works: Nurses, Economics, Finance, and Reimbursement   3
2. A Story of Unintended Consequences: How Economic and Policy Solutions Create New Challenges   25
3. Navigating the Health Care Landscape Shaped by the Patient Protection and Affordable Care Act of 2010, Subsequent Federal Legislation and Judicial Action   45
4. Payment Reform: Improving Care Delivery by Changing Who Is Reimbursed, How, and for What   79

SECTION II: HEALTH CARE ECONOMICS: A PRAGMATIC OVERVIEW

5. How Health Care Markets Differ From Other Markets . . . and Why It Matters   109
6. Health Care Outcomes, Cost, Safety, and Value: The Critical Role of Information in Health Care Markets, Decision-Making, and Payments   133
7. Market Entry, Exit, and Antitrust Law—Why It Matters to Nurses   167

SECTION III: ETHICS AND ECONOMICS IN AN AGE OF REFORM: DEMOGRAPHIC SHIFTS, POLITICAL TENSIONS, AND RECOGNITION OF INCREASINGLY SCARCE RESOURCES

8. What Is Ethinomics?   189
9. Models to Guide Ethical Decision-Making   205

SECTION IV: PULLING IT ALL TOGETHER: USING YOUR KNOWLEDGE OF HEALTH FINANCE, ECONOMICS, AND ETHICS TO IMPROVE HEALTH AND HEALTH CARE

10. Governance and Organizational Type   229

11. Building Skills for Board Membership   251

12. Applying Health Economics to Improve Health Care Through Federal and State Policy Formation   269

13. Lessons From the COVID-19 Pandemic and a Look to the Future   293

14. The Health Care Workforce: What Nurses Need to Know   305

SECTION V: EPILOGUE

15. Reflections on Living and Leading in a Changing Nursing World   333

16. Quiz Answers   337

Appendix A: Medicare Eligibility   343
Appendix B: Key Concepts in Health Finance, Economics, Policy, and Ethics: Level Setting Pre-Survey   345
Appendix C: The Policy Analysis Process   349
Glossary   351
Index   357

Foreword: Reach for Your Roots

Did you ever think that our great-great-grandmothers, who were nurses 100 years ago, could have been more financially and professionally independent than nurses today? In the 1930s, both physicians and nurses ran their own independent companies. Families would hire nurses and pay them directly for care, just like they paid physicians for house calls. It was not until the early to mid-20th century that the expansion of the U.S. public health and hospital systems drew private nurses into hospitals. Seeing the improved quality of patient care and the revenue potential from nursing services, hospitals began hiring nurses on staff and billing for nursing services—every patient bill back then had a separate line for nursing services. Nurses possessed business knowledge and acumen to know how much money they were bringing and how it should be used to provide the best possible care for patients and families.

Fast-forward 100 years to this day, and you will find that nursing care is no longer billed separately—instead, it is wrapped into the hospital room rate along with sheets, electricity, and Jell-O. Clinical nurses of today are largely disenfranchised from the business of health care and health care policy. Did you know that nurses are the only health care professionals who cannot bill for their services? That's right—when it comes to the organizational revenue management cycle, nurses are invisible, much like hotel cleaning personnel included in your nightly rate. Unlike nurses a century ago, today's clinical nurses no longer have insight into the revenue they generate for organizations, and they have minimal influence on budget allocations toward nursing. As a new or veteran nurse, you will likely find yourself in situations where you may not have what you need to give your patients the care they deserve—again and again.

So why do nurses need to know economics, finance, and policy? Nurses understand that adequate staffing, education, professional development, and a safe, rewarding work environment are key ingredients for providing high-quality, equitable patient care. Nursing is a profession deeply rooted in compassion and clinical expertise. However, the evolving health care landscape and the growing focus on value and cost reduction necessitate that nurses expand their skill set beyond traditional clinical responsibilities. Being a good nurse today requires an understanding of economics, policy, and reimbursement to navigate the complexities of modern health care and ensure the delivery of high-quality patient care. Section I of this book provides an excellent foundation for this noble quest.

Understanding health care economics—the subject of Section II of this book—will enable you to make value-informed decisions and advocate for interventions that provide the greatest patient benefit at the lowest cost.

This is particularly important in today's value-based environment, where many patients, especially among minoritized and economically vulnerable groups, cannot afford the health care they need. Understanding the functioning of health care organizations, markets, and systems will enable you to make an informed organizational business case for your proposed interventions, aligning patient needs with organizational financial considerations that might stand in the way. Much like motivational interviewing is designed to enhance a patient's intrinsic motivation for behavioral change, the ability to speak the language of business and economics is a must for having your voice heard by the organization and health care system. Moreover, a grasp of health economics can help nurses understand broader trends in health care funding and expenditure, preparing you to contribute to discussions on health care reform and sustainability.

Of course, as a nurse, your primary responsibility will always be to the patient—few want their nurse to prioritize quarterly returns over patient care! The pragmatism of health care economics must be balanced with health ethics. "Ethinomics"—the focus of Section III—is a term that combines "ethics" and "economics." Ethinomics is important to nurses because it underscores the ethical dimensions of health care economics, guiding nurses to advocate for equitable, just, and sustainable health care practices. As a nurse, you will frequently encounter ethical dilemmas involving resource allocation, patient care priorities, and systemic inequities. Reading this section will enable you to make more informed and morally sound decisions, ensuring that patient care is not only clinically effective and economically sound but also ethically and socially responsible.

On an even broader scale, having a deep understanding of health care economics and ethics will situate you perfectly for navigating complex policy landscapes—the focus of Section IV. The COVID-19 pandemic delivered a severe blow to the nursing profession, but let's face it, issues like understaffing, burnout, turnover, and workplace violence have negatively impacted the profession for decades, if not an entire century. Expanding the scope of practice for advanced nursing providers has been one of the most significant recent legislative wins—yet nurse engagement in policy is as old as nursing itself. Florence Nightingale, often hailed as the founder of modern nursing, was much more than a compassionate nurse—she was also a pioneering economist and a formidable social reformist pushing for policies the improved living conditions for the poor, health care access, and overall public well-being. Fast-forwarding to today, from maternal and infant health, to contraception, to nurse staffing guidelines and reimbursement reform, much more needs to be done. By engaging in health policy at all levels, you too can help shape legislation and regulations that directly impact the profession, empowering nurses to advocate for laws that improve patient care, increase access to services, and enhance workplace safety.

Together, the inclusion of economics, ethinomics, and policy in the nursing profession is not just beneficial but essential. As health care continues to evolve, the role of the nurse must expand beyond the bedside, embracing elements of resource management, ethical advocacy, and policy acumen—just like our great-great-grandmothers used to. Ultimately, this comprehensive approach will lead to improved patient outcomes and a more effective and equitable health care system.

The book you are holding in your hands is the ultimate guide to the complexity of our health care system, your role within it, and your influence upon it. May the wisdom shared in these pages inspire you, challenge your assumptions, and equip you with the tools you need to navigate the complex role of a nurse in today's health care economy with confidence and clarity. Happy reading, and enjoy the journey ahead.

Olga Yakusheva, PhD, FAAN(h)
Professor, Johns Hopkins School of Nursing,
Johns Hopkins Business of Health Initiative
Baltimore, Maryland

A Note From the Author

As this book goes to press, the nation's health care system woes remain largely unchecked. These include high costs, uneven quality, and overtreatment of some even as others lack basic care. Burnout among health professionals is high in the nation that spends substantially more on health care than any other around the globe. What can and should be done? More importantly, what can you do?

The need for a contemporary generation of leaders, with fresh ideas and effective actions, is clear. Consideration of the U.S. health care system underscores the desperate need for the readers of this text to better understand health care financing, economics, and policy and then use that knowledge to shape a safer, financially sustainable world with a workforce prepared and willing to do the difficult work of caring for others. Elimination of waste and inefficiency in our health system and redirection of those funds toward public health surveillance and addressing upstream social determinants of health is an ethical obligation for contemporary health care professionals. Understanding the underlying financial, economic, and political structures that shape our world is essential for leveraging effective change toward these ends. Absent such applied understanding, good ideas remain just that, ideas without agency toward action.

WHAT IS THE RESPONSIBILITY OF AN INDIVIDUAL NURSE?

Professionals hold power in society as part of a social contract, an authority derived from a duty to serve something larger than their own needs and interests. Police, for example, carry guns and have intimate access to people's lives as part of a social contract, that is, the duty "to serve and protect." Clergy are privy to peoples' joys, angst, and anguish not because they are inherently special, but instead because of their social contract to support spiritual health and healing. When the contract is broken, for example, by abusive police or predatory clergy, the social and emotional toll is profound, even devastating. Trust erodes, with resulting anger, anxiety, or despair.

Nurses, too, have a social contract, a duty to foster health and healing. And—as the nation's most trusted professional—a particular obligation at times of strife and struggle. As witnessed during the COVID-19 pandemic, legions of nurses selflessly served on the frontlines, often at great risk to themselves. This element of the social contract is clearly understood, tangible, and demonstrated by nurses. Yet the upstream, administrative, leadership, and policy weaving of conditions to support health and healing may be less tangible to nurses who perceive nurses' roles as primarily personal and intimate. This text is focused on changing this narrative among nurses, to support nurses' broad engagement in the social contract and the people we serve. It is my fervent hope that this text, rather than offering easy answers, raises profound, uncomfortable questions that propel you to action in whatever form and format life brings you. It is my hope that you become involved in policy and politics in deep and meaningful ways and use your knowledge of health finance and economics to help shape a more virtuous, just society. Every action and inaction matters. The time is now. So let's get started.

How to Use This Text: A Note to Faculty

Nurses are steeped in many tenets designed to guide their professional decisions and ensure they act in an ethical manner worthy of societal trust. One such tenet—*advocate for your patients*—seems simple enough on the surface. But is it?

To consider this, students might be charged to ponder the following questions:

Does advocating for your patient mean you support *Medicare for All* or, instead, strengthening the *Patient Protection and Affordable Care Act*, more commonly known *Obamacare*? Or, still another option, repealing the law all together? What does it mean when perspectives on this issue differ by region of the country and political affiliation?

Does advocating for your patient mean you support insurance rating bands of 1:3 as advocated by AARP or the 1:5 bands that would provide lower-cost insurance to younger people?

Does advocating for your patient mean striving for universal health screenings or, instead, do you advocate for selective screenings and elimination of some due to concerns that your patient will be overtreated, receive unnecessary care, and risk health care–related harm?

Does being an advocate for your patient mean arguing for first dollar coverage—no cost sharing—for health care insurance to enhance access? Or, instead, are you concerned about excessive health care costs stemming from *moral hazard*? This well-documented phenomenon recognizes that people use more services, including those with little or no value, when they have no financial *skin in the game*. So, does advocating for your patient mean championing *more*, or instead, *less* secondary to concerns about overuse and explosive health care costs?

Reasonable people can look at these situations and the host of others that pack the health care landscape and come to very different, reasoned conclusions. Too often, however, polarized rhetoric gets in the way. Complex issues are fractured into soundbites, and the resulting microfocus obscures the kaleidoscope of interacting forces and phenomena. As a result of the microfocus (or simply being carried by the rhetoric of others), too many people have strong opinions about issues with which they have little detailed understanding, Or, as humorist Josh Billings is reported to have said: *The trouble with a great many of us is "we know so many things that just ain't so."* Moreover, the tentacles of interacting forces and phenomena not only reach backward and forward in time but also throughout all segments of society. Thus, informed understanding requires a disciplined tracing that reliance on soundbites or simple solutions truncates.

The nation needs more from its most trusted group of professionals, nurses. The nation needs nurses with nuanced skill in the complex, interacting arena of finances, economics, quality and outcome measurement, payment, and ethics. It is the palette from which health care delivery emerges.

BUT WHY THIS TEXT?

There are many health care policy texts directed toward nurses. Why is this one different? What does it offer you, the faculty member knighted to carry forward the essential responsibility of enhancing civic responsibility and leadership among nurses?

This text is designed to prepare students at all levels with foundational material that can support a lifetime of informed, impactful advocacy. Unlike many nursing health policy texts, it is not a series of essays written by different authors. Instead, it presents a single story that incorporates finance, economics, policy, ethics, civic responsibility, emerging technologies like artificial intelligence, and preparation for leadership in organizations and on boards of trustees. Making friends with economics, finance, and payment in an easy-to-read, understandable, applicable manner is one goal of this text. This is essential if nurses are to have impact. Great ideas without an idea of how to finance them will remain thought bubbles.

For undergraduate students, this text can serve as a standalone reference, potentially augmented or punctuated with current events that illustrate the issues detailed in the text as they emerge. Because this text incorporates emerging innovations, it is useful not only in courses focused on finance, policy, and ethics but also *Contemporary Issues* courses, *Leadership* courses, and *Capstone* courses. Social media applications are a useful tool to enhance undergraduates' civic engagement with contemporary issues. One successful strategy used by the author is outlined elsewhere (Mercadante & Rambur, 2020).

At the graduate level many students, again, have only a superficial understanding of the interlacing issues of health care finance, economics, and policy. This text can provide that foundation and be augmented with current materials from the many health policy and industry journals, for example, *Heath Affairs, Health Affairs Forefront, Modern Healthcare, Milbank Quarterly, New England Journal of Medicine,* and *JAMA*—including their *Less Is More* series and their new health policy channel, *JAMA Health Forum,* to name but a few. These journals are highly useful adjuncts to nursing literature, presenting a view that includes yet expands beyond just nursing.

HOW TO START, GIVEN THAT GRADUATE STUDENTS MAY BE AT VERY DIFFERENT KNOWLEDGE LEVELS

The author has found it useful to anonymously survey graduate students with a pretest to direct the course at the proper level of depth (see Appendix C for suggested survey questions that you can draw from). Although the author has occasionally had students with great depth in one area—for example, a former vice president of a major nonprofit health insurance company; another with a PhD in ethics who had studied with the great virtue ethicist,

Edmund Pellegrino; a lobbyist for a major consumer organization; and a state Medicaid director, these have been the exceptions, not the rule. And even in these deeply educated individuals, areas outside their usual domains were unfamiliar to them, as are the underlying interactions that created the health system of today. And in both practicing physicians and nurses, the author has found that relatively few are aware of the system that pays them beyond superficial aspects. This text is designed to address these gaps. Finally, review of this text can spawn a wealth of ideas for DNP projects and PhD dissertations.

TEXT ORGANIZATION

Clearly, to be an effective and ethical advocate, a firm understanding of the details of the underlying policies and practice and their antecedents and consequences is essential. From where does the money that forms nurses' compensation emerge and how? This is discussed in Chapter 1. Negative unintended consequences of policies and practices have shaped much of the see-saw evolution of U.S. health care. These are detailed in Chapter 2.

The Patient Protection and Affordable Care Act of 2010 (ACA) has been the focus of much public debate. Most Americans, however, have too little knowledge of the details of the law to analyze it in an informed fashion. This edition has a full chapter (Chapter 3) devoted to a description of this 900-page law as well as details of recent key laws with health and health care dimensions. Table 3.1 outlines the various components of the ACA, including rationale and modifications since the law passed in 2010. The intent is that students can scrutinize the breadth of the law in a single view. Notably, this complex law is far broader than the often-maligned individual mandate and the widely supported allowance that children may stay on their parent's health insurance until age 26. Moreover, the associated administrative rules evolve, for example, the April 2024 rule change that allows states to include adult dental care as a defined *essential benefit*. A firm grasp of the details of the law is essential for students' informed decision-making on aspects to support, aspects to modify, and aspects to eliminate, as well as the overall rationale for inclusion of various elements in the law in the first place.

Payment reform—the move away from fee-or-service with increasing accountability for not only outcomes of care but also cost of care, termed value-based care—will necessarily be an increasing part of the health care landscape. Nurses who can argue and illustrate the value of their work, both outcomes *and* cost, not only provide a great service to this nation, they also hold sizable career advantages over those who cannot. In the author's experience, however, the relationships among concepts like financial risk sharing versus risk bearing, cost shifting, payer mix, value-based care, and nursing practice are elusive to many and awkwardly held by others. Moreover, too few nurses have a firm understanding of the major laws that shape payment, and thus in turn shape care. This, despite the fact that they are immersed in the quality metrics associated with payment in their work settings. Without knowledge of the rationale for payment-related metrics, nurses too easily become tools of the status quo rather than the dynamic innovators we have the potential—perhaps even the responsibility—to be.

Thus, firmly grounded in deep understanding of the facts of financing (Chapter 1), evolution of the system (Chapter 2), the ACA and selected subsequent laws (Chapter 3), health economics inclusive of basic principles, innovations such as the Internet of Things and artificial intelligence, considerations and concerns related to mergers and acquisitions (Chapters 5–7), and ethics (Chapters 8–9), the student has foundational knowledge. Then, and only then, can they decide for themselves what aligns with their assessment of *right, moral, informed action*. A policy analysis framework is described in Appendix D and can be useful to guide graduate students' further policy analysis efforts.

EXECUTIVE ACTION AND ONGOING DEVELOPMENT

Chapters 10 and 11 provide a primer on organizational governance and financial terms and are useful both for those who report to boards and those seeking to serve on a board . . . or needing prompting to do so! Chapter 12 details the state and federal policy formation process. It also describes ways to build on knowledge gained, to enhance involvement in policy and politics, and to accelerate the student's personal leadership trajectory. Chapter 13 outlines lessons from COVID-19 and echoing concerns, and Chapter 14 details the current state of the health care workforce and antecedents and consequences of the nation's ongoing underinvestment in nursing.

WHAT ABOUT THE POLITICAL PROCESS?

In 2017 Litvinov noted that only 25% of U.S. students reach the "proficient" standard on the National Assessment of Educational Progress Civics Assessment, as "civics offerings were slashed as the curriculum narrowed" (para. 5). STEM education increasingly replaced fundamental courses in civics that laced primary education in earlier decades. Too little has changed in the ensuing years. Ward (2022), for example, details the gaps and lack of quality in civics education and its broad impact on society. Moreover, the United States has had unprecedented declines in civics proficiency, with more than 30% of eighth graders performing below basic proficiency in 2022 (Sparks, 2023). Many adults, even well-educated ones, have had little exposure to branches of government, the variety of ways laws are enacted, and the powerful role of administrative rule-making and executive orders detailed in Chapter 12.

An educational approach the author has found to be highly effective is to complete a class assessment of foundational civics knowledge in the first few days of class. Clark's Political Astuteness Inventory (1984, 2008), for example, can offer a solid floor to scaffold more complex knowledge. This classic tool continues to be used in nursing research, often with discouraging findings, for example, that RNs' political astuteness was only at the beginner level (Doherty, 2021). Similarly, O'Hanlon Curry and Fitzpatrick (2024) found that nurse leaders also had only beginner-level astuteness and recommended formal preparation.

If knowledge among your students is similarly scant, starting with Chapter 12 rather than Chapter 1 can offer a useful course design approach, particularly if the timing for your course aligns with an election cycle. In conducting similar assessments over decades, the author has found that this knowledge is indeed meager among many students, both undergraduate and graduate, with the exception of the few who have studied political science or government or been involved in political action. Astonishingly, in the author's queries, many graduate students have had little participation in the political process, and too many have never voted, while some undergraduates are just now aging in to voting awareness and eligibility.

Those students who do have a foundation in civic responsibility can offer supports for others. It is useful to approach this task of student supporting student by highlighting the nonpartisan dimension of the assignment, underscoring the need for a culture of generous listening. Then, those who wish to become involved with a party can be directed to campus *College Democrats, College Republicans*, etc., or nonpartisan groups like *Ignite,* which has a mission of unleashing the political power of young women to prepare them for a range of political actions, including running for office. Most campuses have an array of policy-directed student clubs. In summary, although the text was designed to be used in sequence, with one chapter for each week of a standard semester, if students' political acumen is low and it is an election year, starting with Chapter 12 works well.

It is also helpful to understand students' news source, if any. TikTok or their personal social network is often a source of information. If so, it can be helpful for you to illustrate the Media Bias Chart (Fox-Ramirez, 2024; updated twice a year and available for a free download at https://adfontesmedia.com/gallery/). This interactive chart illustrates not only veracity (y axis) but also left- and right-leaning bias (x axis). An engaging exercise is to have students compare and contrast the content and tone of the reporting from diverse news outlets and then select one they will follow over the semester, each reporting back to the full class at regular intervals.

CONCLUSION AND A REQUEST

In 1993, I was one of seven nurses representing the American Nurses Association in a meeting with then President Bill Clinton to discuss health reform. As I was waiting in the security line, a man who was not associated with our group asked me the following question: *Oh,* he said, *do you have the "typical nurse disease"? What is that?* I responded. *All kinds of good ideas,* he said, *with no idea how to pay for them.* At that moment, I resolved NOT to be that person, the one with good ideas but no idea how to fund them. I resolved to study these issues deeply over a protracted period of time. I also resolved that no one would ever lay a similar charge against my students. Eventually, that intention became the genesis of this text, as I consistently found deep gaps in students' foundational grasp of finance, economics, and the other issues discussed in the text.

As faculty, we collectively create the crucible of learning for our students. Please join me in the effort to ensure that nurses are widely viewed as not only having good ideas but as also possessing the savvy to execute those ideas. Together, let's ensure that the nurse in the White House security line waiting to meet the president in 2030 is recognized as *a typical nurse*—profound and impactful. Or, better yet, perhaps that nurse can be president! Let's light the flame. Together, let's ensure that nurses understand that caring for people and politics are interlaced realities . . . and interesting ones at that!

REFERENCES

Clark, P. E. (1984). Political astuteness inventory. In M. J. D. Clark (Eds.), *Community nursing: Health care today and tomorrow.* (pp. 168–189). Appleton and Lange.

Clark, P. E. (2008). Political astuteness inventory. In M. J. Clark (Eds.), *Community assessment reference guide for community health nursing* (pp. 1–2). Pearson Education.

Doherty, G. (2021). *The political astuteness of New Mexico registered nurses.* Unpublished dissertation. https://scholarworks.waldenu.edu/cgi/viewcontent.cgi?article=11909&context=dissertations

Fox-Ramirez, E. (2024, January 1). *Ad Fontes media releases new media bias chart.* https://adfontesmedia.com/media-bias-chart-jan-2024/

Litvinov, A. (2017, March 16). Forgotten purposes: Civics education in public schools. *NEA Today.* http://neatoday.org/2017/03/16/civics-education-public-schools/

Mercadante, A., & Rambur, B. (2020) Facilitating health policy civic engagement among undergraduate students using collaborative social technology. *Journal of Nursing Education, 59*(3), 163–165.

O'Hanlon Curry & Fitzpatrick, J. (2024) The level of political astuteness in nursing leaders: A baseline assessment. *JONA: The Journal of Nursing Administration, 54*(3), 172–176, https://doi.org/10.1097/NNA.0000000000001403

Sparks, S. (2023, November 28). It's not just U.S. students. Civics scores have dropped around the world. *Education Week.* https://www.edweek.org/policy-politics/its-not-just-u-s-students-civics-scores-have-dropped-around-the-world/2023/11

Ward, S. (2022, May). Lack of quality civic education in public schools in the United States. *Ballard Brief.* https://scholarsarchive.byu.edu/ballardbrief/vol2022/iss2/8

Acknowledgments

Many health policy leaders and thinkers have shaped my thinking and this text. I am grateful for all I have learned from and with you. I am particularly grateful to those who helped launch my work in payment reform at The North Dakota Health Task Force and continued with Vermont's Green Mountain Care Board. You have been wonderful friends and mentors. The brilliance of my fellow commissioners and the staff of the Medicare Payment Advisory Commission has been a pure gift. Special thanks to Gina Upchurch for her masterful assistance with Medicare Advantage. To Dawn Philibert, Nancy Mathews, and Ann Pugh, fellow policy enthusiasts, I am grateful for our robust, wide-ranging discussions, even—or perhaps most especially—when we disagree! Mary Val Palumbo, thanks for always having just one more idea for us to investigate and disseminate; it has been great traveling the world with you. Elizabeth Howlett, thank you for your assistance dissecting the complex federal laws in this text.

Springer Publishing has been a dream to work with. Thanks to Elizabeth Nieginski, who opened the door for the first edition of this text, and the ongoing steady hand of Joe Morita, Brenna Croker, and Kris Parrish throughout the process. Special thanks to Lisa McCoy for careful copyediting, Mary Dyana's composition team at S4Carlisle, and Manjula Devi's team at KGL for careful attention to needed permissions.

I am immensely grateful and blessed to be supported by the Routhier Foundation and to occupy an endowed faculty position that bears the name of the Routhier family at the University of Rhode Island. To the Routhier Foundation and family, thank you for giving me the opportunity to assemble and share my ideas with students, colleagues, and the future of the nursing profession.

And finally, a very special thanks to my husband, Don DeHayes, whose constant support and always thoughtful critique helped shape this text.

Betty Rambur, PhD, RN, FAAN
Routhier Endowed Chair for Practice
The University of Rhode Island
Kingston, Rhode Island

Instructor Resources

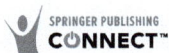 A robust set of instructor resources designed to supplement this text is located at http://connect.springerpub.com/content/book/978-0-8261-7236-5. Qualifying instructors may request access by emailing textbook@springerpub.com.

- LMS Common Cartridge—All Instructor Resources
- Instructor Manual:
  - Classroom Activities
  - Sample Syllabi
- Instructor Test Bank
- Instructor PowerPoint Presentations
- Mapping to AACN *Essentials: Core Competencies for Professional Nursing Practice*
- Transition Guide: Second Edition to Third Edition

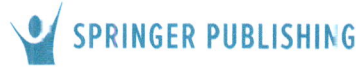

Visit https://connect.springerpub.com/ and look for the "**Show Supplementary**" button on the **book homepage**.

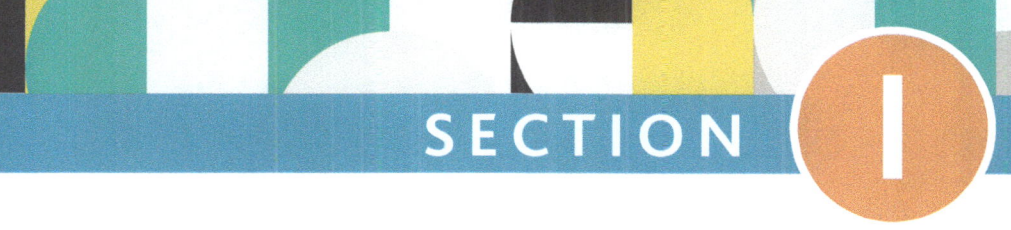

SECTION I

The Context of Health Care in the United States

SECTION I, comprising Chapters 1 to 4, provides foundational background that is essential to successfully navigate contemporary health care. Chapter 1 describes the basics of health finance and economics, rather like an alphabet that is necessary for reading and writing in the health care landscape. Similar to learning a new alphabet, it can be a bit tedious. Be patient. These terms and ideas are a language of power and influence that you will need to maximize your career opportunities.

Chapter 2 details the evolution of the U.S. health care system. Knowledge of this history is essential to understanding many contemporary issues and vexing problems, including persistent cost, quality and access problems, and troubling workforce issues. Although decades of effort have attempted to redress these issues, many reform strategies attempt to address unintended consequences of previous health care policies and accidents of history. Then, in turn, they create their own unintended consequences.

Chapter 3 details the Patient Protection and Affordable Care Act of 2010 and subsequent health care laws that impact nurses and their patients, inclusive of controversies, considerations, and Supreme Court actions.

Chapter 4 pulls this information together to illustrate the ways payment policies—the way nurses, physicians, hospitals, home health care agencies, and other organizations are paid—shapes your daily work life and how you can use this knowledge to influence positive change. So, let us begin with Chapter 1 and sort out foundational concepts like financing, economics, reimbursement, cost shifting and payer mix. Remember, each of these directly shapes your professional income and opportunities. As such, they are worth serious consideration.

CHAPTER 1

How the Money Works: Nurses, Economics, Finance, and Reimbursement

CHAPTER 1 introduces health economics and its influence on contemporary nursing and health care. Following completion of this chapter, you will be able to:

- Define health economics and differentiate it from related concepts such as health financing and reimbursement.
- Describe how health care is paid for in the United States.
- Illustrate elements related to payment for health care services, such as third-party payers, commercial insurance, cost shifting, and the importance of payer mix.

> *1964: Mary Jane is excited to be in the sixth grade. Her first day of middle school was magnificent. As her mother putters in the kitchen to make her after-school snack, Mary Jane settles in to read her history text. "America is the land of endless opportunity and unlimited natural resources," announces the text's opening statement. Reading these lines, Mary Jane smiles, thinking, "How wonderful it is to live in a world in which there are no limits!"*

This, of course, was never true.

> *2025: Will is excited to be in the sixth grade. Knowing that his mother will not be home from work for several hours, he grabs a snack as he opens the portal to his integrated humanities e-text. Glancing through the headings, he sees that many issues of the day are woven into the chapters: global climate change, job displacement due to automation and artificial intelligence, income inequality, race relations, pandemics, immigration, gun violence, and unsustainable industries that range from U.S. business practices to health care. The book suggests that new ways of thinking are needed to solve these problems, many of which are rooted in issues of scarce, maldistributed resources. Pondering, Will hopes he is up to this challenge.*

Nurses care about their patients. Some nurses, who like Mary Jane were imprinted with the myth of endless abundance, believe that there should be no limits on what is done for patients. Indeed, earlier generations of nurses, physicians, and other providers were socialized to believe that it is unethical to even consider the cost of care when making treatment decisions. A "more is better" philosophy prevailed.

Contemporary nurses know better. They know that resources both within and beyond health care are not unlimited. They know that choices among alternatives will be, and need to be, made. What nurses often lack are the tools to help them think about ethical and practical ways in which scarce resources are managed, allocated, and used to maximize value and outcomes. This competency is an essential element of contemporary nursing practice because the societal transition from a world of certainty and perceived abundance to one of multiplicity and scarcity illustrated in the opening scenarios characterizes today's health care delivery. Health care is too expensive, is fragmented, and too often is an emporium of confusion for health care professionals and those seeking access alike (see Figure 1.1). It is characterized by irregular quality, error, access gaps, and profound distribution inequities. Moreover, the COVID-19 pandemic underscored the shortsightedness of ignoring the public health infrastructure and health disparities, a topic we will return to in Chapter 13. Unfortunately, many health professionals have been educated as if the world they will be working in is Mary Jane's world of 1964.

Luckily, there is a whole discipline—complete with theories, research, and practical applications—that provides foundational nursing knowledge in the contemporary era. This discipline is economics. The overarching field of economics is concerned with the question of how goods and services are produced, organized, and delivered to maximize efficiency and value. The emphasis on value is important. Value is defined as a quotient of outcomes divided by cost. Thus, a fundamental question is this: Are the outcomes, both short- and long-term, worth the cost? Economics is not necessarily concerned with *more*, but with *better*, a concern that nurses share as a core value.

THEORETICAL ECONOMIC APPROACHES

There are different theoretical approaches to economics. One approach most nurses have been exposed to since elementary school is *classic free market* or *laissez-faire economics*, which contends that less governmental intervention maximizes value. Conversely, Keynesian economics suggests a stronger role for government, particularly in times when the economy is strained. Both of these models assume rational, logical decision-making. Newer models of economics question if human behavior is altogether that logical and instead acknowledge the role of emotions in decision-making. This approach is called *behavioral economics*. All of these orientations are useful to nurses. However, the economics conceptualization that is most useful to nursing care is *health economics*, yet another approach that focuses on the unique aspects of health care markets. Health economics is a relatively new discipline. It emerged as a distinct field following the 1963 publication of a manuscript by Nobel Prize–winning economist Kenneth Arrow titled *Uncertainty and the Welfare Economics of Medical Care* (Arrow, 1963). Others built on Arrow's seminal work and furthered understanding of the ways health economics shapes health care.

HEALTH ECONOMICS

Why Study Health Economics?

The models and theories of health economics—and the research they have spawned—are useful to nurses. Like a mirror or guidepost, understanding health economics helps the nurse make sense of the often convoluted, paradoxical, and invisible yet pervasive ways economics shapes the organization, financing, and delivery of health care as well as your salary and career opportunities. Moreover, many of the policy decisions at institutional, state, and federal levels relate to economic incentives and how the money flows through the system. Thus, to serve patients and help shape a world in which the holistic, patient-/family-/community-centric vision of the profession of nursing can become a reality, nurses need a confident command of economic terms and ideas and need to be able to apply them in the practice setting.

Yet for many of us nurses, the interpersonal aspect of the nursing role—taking care of people and building relationships—is precisely what drew us to the nursing profession in the first place. Economics, with complex mathematical formulas, nuanced theories, and interfaces with system-level finances, can seem far removed from the working knowledge, concerns, and everyday work life of the nurse. Nevertheless, the field of economics and the profession of nursing share key interests.

What Sorts of Things Do Economists Think About?

Some of the most pressing issues of economics are also issues nurses face every day. For example (adapted from Kernick, 2003):

- What do we do when there is a greater need than resources with which to meet this need?
- From what perspective should these competing demands be viewed: that of individuals, society at large, businesses, or health professionals? Or is there a way that these can be considered simultaneously?
- What is value, and how do we maximize it?
- What is the influence of health care on health?

These are not abstract considerations. See Box 1.1 for a familiar, boots-on-the-ground example of the first bullet: a greater need than resources.

The latter question, the influence of health care on health, is of also particular importance to nurses as well as society at large, as it relates to *social determinants of health* (SDHs) such as educational level and family/neighborhood socioeconomics inclusive of schools, safety, healthy food access, and green tree canopies (Box 1.2).

SOCIAL DETERMINANTS OF HEALTH

Although nearly 18 cents of every dollar spent in the United States goes to health care, health care contributes only marginally to health. As illustrated in Figure 1.1, there is a substantial misalignment between where the United States spends its health care dollars and what impacts health. Although the exact figures vary by source, the overall pattern consistently finds that medical care receives nearly 90% of national health expenditures, yet makes a small contribution to health. An interpretation of The Network for Excellence in Health Innovations reports that this 90% of total expenditures contributes a mere 6% to health status. In the same vein, healthy behaviors contribute roughly 37% but receive a mere 9%

BOX 1.1

Working in an acute care setting, one of your patients is decompensating. This requires you to focus attention on that one patient, largely to the exclusion of others. Such "missed care" is associated with poorer outcomes for the other assigned patients (Kalánková et al, 2020). Missed care, in turn, fosters nurse workplace dissatisfaction and fuels turnover. As nurses resign, they may not be quickly replaced or are replace by those with less experience, which can again lead to more missed care.

BOX 1.2

WHAT DO GREEN TREE CANOPIES HAVE TO DO WITH HEALTH EQUITY?

Miller (2023) notes that the absence of trees is not just aesthetic but impacts a range of health issues. The lack of trees creates urban heat islands, whereby asphalt not only absorbs but also amplifies the heat. Thus, heat-related illnesses increase. The lack of open spaces can negatively impact outside exercise and socializing, which also impacts health. The poorest communities have 41% less tree cover than the most wealthy (Poon, 2021).

of national health expenditures. There are also many interactive effects (Galea, 2016); see Figure 1.1). It can be difficult or impossible to live a life characterized by healthy behaviors in a dangerous physical or social environment. The best overall predictors of health status are factors such as socioeconomic status and educational attainment. So, in the aggregate, the healthiest among us are educated Americans with good jobs who live in safe neighborhoods. This creates a paradoxical tension; when more public and private money is put into health care, fewer resources are available for job creation and education, which in turn means an entire population may have fewer opportunities for the education, employment, and lifestyle that are associated with better health. Thus, how money is distributed ultimately impacts the health of a population *upstream*—that is, before the manifestation of illness—through SDH (see Box 1.3 for the World Health Organization's definition of *SDH*). Health economics concerns itself with these issues because it considers and analyzes the manner in which scarce resources are allocated in light of alternative ways to allocate resources that impact determinants. It also considers how resource allocation impacts human behavior.

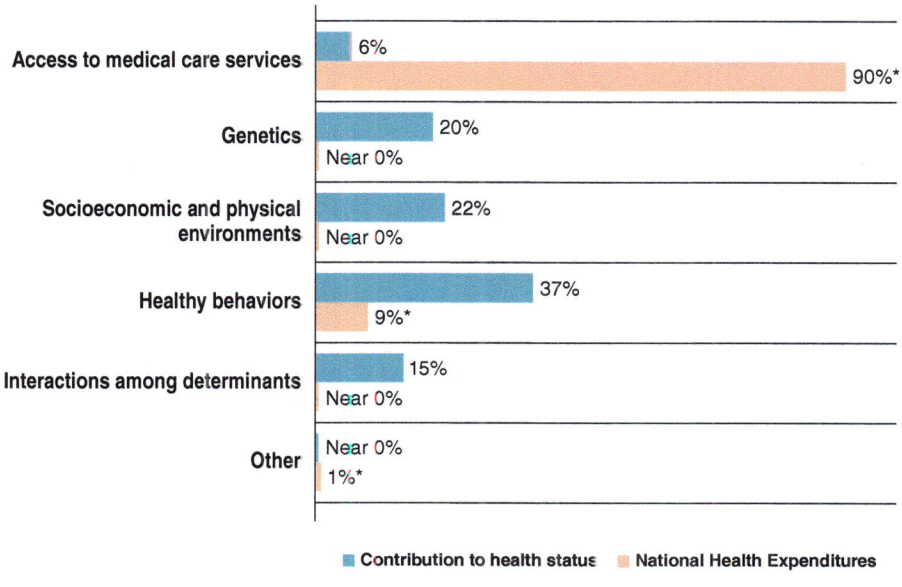

FIGURE 1.1: Determinants of health and their interactions.

Note: The spending mismatch: Health determinants versus health expenditures.

Source: Adapted from Galea, S. (2016). 18 charts that make the case for public health. https://www.bu.edu/sph/news/articles/2016/18-charts-that-make-the-case-for-public-health/

BOX 1.3

WHAT ARE SOCIAL DETERMINANTS OF HEALTH?

The World Health Organization (n.d.) defines SDH as follows:

"Social determinants of health (SDH) are the non-medical factors that influence health outcomes. They are the conditions in which people are born, grow, live, work, and age and the wider set of forces and systems shaping the conditions of daily life. These forces and systems include economic policies and systems, development agendas, social norms, social policies and political systems. The SDH have an important influence on health inequities—the unfair and avoidable differences in health status seen within and between countries. In countries at all levels of income, health and illness follow a social gradient: the lower the socioeconomic position, the worse the health" (para 1–2). In the U.S., state and federal regulators have developed parameters to drive health systems to address health disparities, yet health inequity exists in all U.S. states, including those states that have health systems that function at a higher level than others (Hartnett, 2024; Radley et al., 2024).

HOW ECONOMICS DIFFERS FROM FINANCING AND REIMBURSEMENT

Financing: What Does It Mean?

Thus, *economics*, broadly defined, is concerned with the production, distribution, and consumption of services. As Wallach notes: "At its heart, economics is about the allocation of limited resources—whether on a personal, national, or global scale. It involves figuring out how people make choices in conditions of scarcity when they must weigh competing priorities, consciously or not. . . . Every decision involves tradeoffs: every tradeoff has an impact" (2022, para 9). Economics differs from *financing*, which refers to the obtaining of funds. Financial literacy is necessary to navigate daily life, and most nurses have a working knowledge of both of these concepts, despite not having identified them within their workplace or their professional knowledge. Here is an everyday example of the concept of financing. Please be careful to differentiate this concept from that of economics.

> *Justine has just completed college. Eager to rent an apartment, she checks the average monthly cost of housing and utilities in her region and estimates transportation and food costs. She realizes that she will need to clear at least $5,000/month if she lives alone, but with three roommates, that figure drops to $2,800/month. Justine decides that the latter is more feasible; she will need to find a way to finance $2,800/month.*

As this general example illustrates, financing refers to how the resource comes to what is often called *the agent*—Justine in this example. In health care, the parallel to the agent to whom the resources are gathered is the *payer*, a concept that will be discussed shortly. Justine may have several options for financing her costs. She may find a job—certainly something most parents wish for. She may instead ask for her parents to finance all or part of her monthly expenses. Or perhaps she is an heiress and can live off the interest of a trust fund. In any case, her expenses must first be financed. Note also that financing refers to how the money is obtained, but not what it is used for.

How Is Health Care Financed in the United States?

The U.S. health care system also has several different mechanisms by which funds for health services are obtained. These U.S. health financing options include *out-of-pocket* money at the point of service from those who use health care, *taxes*, and *insurance premiums* (see Figure 1.2). Each of these is discussed in greater detail, but for now it is important to simply distinguish the difference between health financing and health economics: Health economics is a broad term that refers to overarching questions about the allocation of scarce resources, whereas financing is a narrow term that relates to how the money for services is generated in the first place.

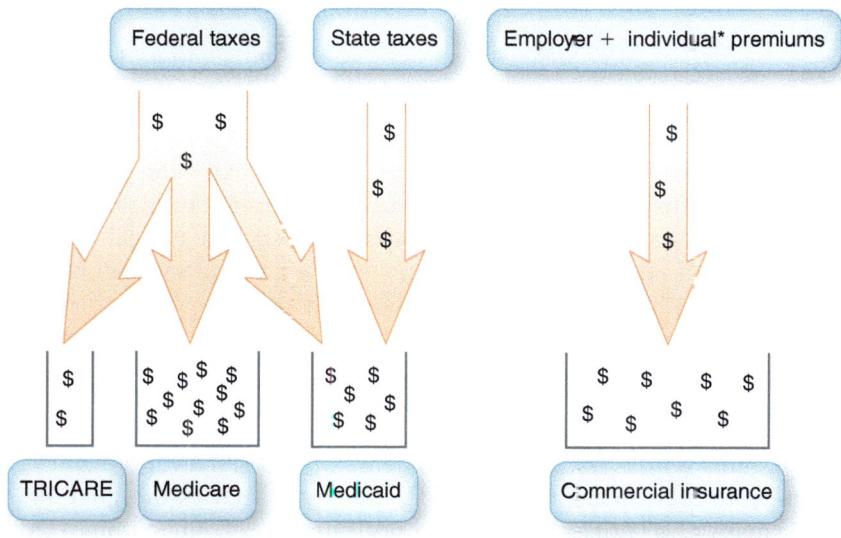

*Individuals also pay out of pocket

FIGURE 1.2: Financing of health care in the United States.

REIMBURSEMENT: HOW ARE HEALTH CARE PROVIDERS PAID?

These two concepts, economics and financing, differ still from another key concept: *reimbursement*. Reimbursement refers to the money paid to providers of care for services delivered and is discussed later in this chapter as well as throughout this text. To summarize, financing refers to how the financial resources (money) for health services are raised, and reimbursement refers to what and how providers are paid for providing those services. You can think about this as money going into a bucket (financing) and money later being poured back out to pay for services used (reimbursement). Those providing reimbursement, that is, those paying providers for the delivery of health services, are aptly called *payers*. As used in health care, the term *payers* includes *commercial insurance companies* and state and federal governments, termed *governmental payers*, but not individuals paying out of pocket at the time of receiving a health care service. This is an important concept and is developed in more depth in the following section.

Who Is a Payer?

> Joey has just started a part-time job while he works on his BS in nursing. He is pleased to have a position in the billing department of University Hospital. There is a big learning curve, however, as he is confused about the different payers. The supervisor tells Joey that "payer mix" is very important to the hospital's financial status. Just beginning to understand who a payer is, Joey now begins to wonder what "payer mix" means, what a good mix or a bad mix is, and how that is managed or controlled.

Although payers reimburse providers for the health care services they provide, the process is different than for other goods and services because the payer is an intermediary between the user of the services—the patient—and the provider of the services, such as the doctor, hospital, nurse practitioner, or home health agency. Although nurses provide services, typically the term *provider* references those who are reimbursed by a payer, such as doctors and hospitals. This rather odd situation is largely the result of the historical evolution of employer-based health insurance and is detailed in Chapter 2.

Payer Mix

Unlike nations with a "single-payer system" in which a level of health care is covered through financing from a single payer such as the government through taxes, the United States has a multipayer system. Within a multipayer system, payer mix refers to the combination of different payers any one provider may be reimbursed by and the proportion of each payer to the overall revenue of the provider. The multipayer financing mechanism thus creates the option for a provider to be reimbursed by different payers, who reimburse at different rates. These payers can be considered *insurers*, so let us look more carefully at what the term insurance coverage really means.

INSURANCE COVERAGE

Commercial Insurance

Commercial insurance is insurance that an individual or business can purchase. Common examples include state-level programs like Blue Cross and Blue Shield and national companies like Aetna, to mention just two. In the United States, these commercial insurance companies can be *nonprofit* or *for-profit*; for-profit companies have the expressed mission of returning financial dividends to stockholders in the company. Nonprofit companies also intend to make a profit (termed margin), but these must be retained by the organization to support self-preservation, growth, or new initiatives. In the case of a nonprofit company, this extra revenue is termed a *positive margin* resulting in a *surplus* rather than a profit. Unlike for-profit companies, nonprofit companies do not have shareholders. Finally, having more expenses than revenue represents a *negative margin*. The Patient Protection and Affordable Care Act (ACA) of 2010 set new limits on the amount of revenue the company can retain rather than putting into care services. This will be detailed in Chapter 3.

Governmental or Tax-Funded Insurance Coverage

Medicare and Medicaid are tax-funded insurance coverage programs. They are federal programs but with many differences. Medicare is overseen at a national level, meaning states have little say in how Medicare operates within the state unless they obtain a waiver. Medicaid is a federal program administered at a state level. Both have specific inclusion criteria. Medicare is a system of national health insurance providing coverage for those older than 65 and people of any age with end-stage renal disease or amyotrophic lateral sclerosis. Medicaid is a program for poor and some disabled individuals. Medicare is primarily financed via general revenue, payroll taxes and beneficiaries' premiums, whereas Medicaid is a mix of state and federal taxes, with relatively poorer states receiving a larger federal match than richer states (see https://www.kff.org/medicaid/state-indicator/federal-matching-rate-and-multiplier to see your state's Federal Medical Assistant Percentage and multiplier. Note: No state has a multiplier of less than 1, meaning each state received at least a 100% federal match for each state dollar they put in Medicaid). Unless a state receives a waiver, the overall terms and conditions of Medicaid must be met.

There are four categories of Medicare (see Box 1.4) with complex eligibility and financing (see Appendix A). These eligibility criteria have received public scrutiny since several 2020 Democratic presidential hopefuls called for a widening of eligibility in *Medicare for All*, *Medicare for All Who Want It*, or a lowering of the age eligibility, topics that we will return to in Chapter 2.

Together, Medicare, Medicaid, the Children's Health Insurance Program (CHIP), and the ACA subsidies accounted for 25% of the federal budget, $1.4 trillion, in 2022 (Centers on Budget and Policy Priorities, 2023; see Figure 1.3).

The greatest proportion of the budget goes toward Social Security, major health programs (Medicare, Medicaid, the CHIPS, and ACA subsidies), and defense. The mismatch between federal revenue generation and spending, in the view of the author, is alarming. In 2023, the nation took in 4.6 trillion in taxes and spent 6.21 trillion (creating more national debt), and 1.19 trillion federal tax dollars were directed toward health care programs. The nation's growing national debt will impact future generations as well as our own. Given the magnitude of the discrepancy between revenue generation and expenses and the large role federal health programs play in this financial equation, Keckley (2024) calls for hospitals to rethink their future. He underscores other pressing matters facing the nation that also require financial

BOX 1.4

TYPES OF MEDICARE

There are four categories of Medicare. They are termed Part A, Part B, Part C, and Part D.

Medicare Part A pays for hospital care and is financed by taxes on employers and employees that are held in the Hospital Insurance Trust Fund. In March 2023, it was projected that the Hospital Health Insurance Trust Fund would be depleted in 2031. Despite this grim prediction, it is an extended timeline from the earlier projection of 2028 calculated the year before. Depletion of the Trust Fund would result in markedly decreased reimbursement to providers who treat Medicare patients, fewer covered benefits for Medicare beneficiaries, higher beneficiary cost sharing when using services, reduced Social Security benefits (to pay to be a Medicare beneficiary), or some combination of these (Centers for Medicare and Medicaid Services [CMS], 2023). This is key background knowledge for payment reform discussed in Chapter 4.

Medicare Part B pays for professional services such as physician care and is financed by general tax revenue and beneficiary premiums. This beneficiary premium is an ongoing monthly sum eligible people pay to have Part B insurance coverage. Since its inception, Medicare Part B was prohibited from reimbursing nurses, an ongoing challenge discussed in later chapters.

Medicare Part C (Medicare Advantage) is Medicare obtained through a private health insurance company; for example, Blue Cross and Blue Shield, United, or Aetna. This growing sector will be discussed in greater detail in Chapter 5.

Finally, **Medicare Part D** covers prescription drug costs and is financed like Part B plus some state funds.

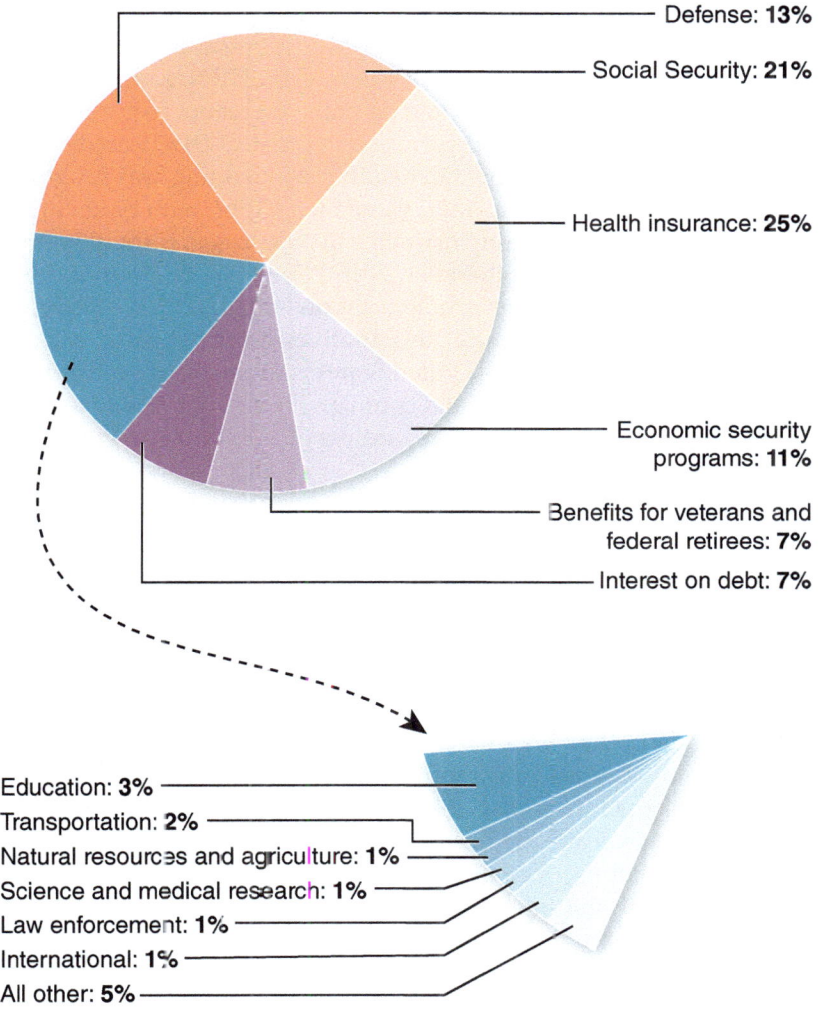

- Defense: **13%**
- Social Security: **21%**
- Health insurance: **25%**
- Economic security programs: **11%**
- Benefits for veterans and federal retirees: **7%**
- Interest on debt: **7%**
- Education: **3%**
- Transportation: **2%**
- Natural resources and agriculture: **1%**
- Science and medical research: **1%**
- Law enforcement: **1%**
- International: **1%**
- All other: **5%**

Note: Percentages do not add to 100 percent due to rounding.

FIGURE 1.3: Most of the budget goes toward defense, Social Security, and major health programs.

Source: Reproduced with permission from the Center on Budget and Policy Priorities. http://cbpp.org/most-of-budget-goes-toward-defense-social-security-and-major-health-programs-0.

investment, including "the fragile geopolitical landscape involving relationships with China, Russia and Middle East" (para 3). The nurse's' role in decreasing unnecessary expenditures, termed value-informed nursing practice, is detailed throughout this text.

In summary, given these percentages, it is easy to see that our government is heavily involved in (a) financing health care and (b) playing a major role as a payer. Thus, the next time you hear someone say "Government has no place in health care," you can sagely respond now that you know that our government is deeply involved in U.S. health care as a financier through taxes and as a payer through Medicare, Medicaid, CHIP, and TRICARE, the program for military dependents and military members using health care services not available through other means. A pre–COVID-19 analysis of the U.S. governmental portion of overall health care spending was roughly 63% and was projected to be 67% in 2024. Canada, a nation with national health insurance that guarantees health insurance to all citizens, is roughly 70% tax funded (Himmelstein & Woolhandler, 2016). Some conclude that this U.S. figure represents too much government involvement, and Medicare, Medicaid, and other tax-supported health initiatives must be scaled back. Conversely, others conclude that the United States is more than two-thirds of the way to a publicly funded system and could go the rest of the way to national health insurance for all Americans, regardless of age. What do you think?

Payer Mix and Cost Shifting

Each of these payers reimburses providers at different levels. Medicare theoretically reimburses *at cost*, whereas Medicaid reimburses below the cost of service provision. This "underpayment" is then shifted to the cost of commercial insurance. So, too, those without insurance who receive care—termed *charity care*—as well as those whose insurance does not fully cover the cost of care and they are unable to pay—termed *bad debt*—are added to the charges paid by those with commercial insurance. This phenomenon of higher reimbursement from commercial insurance to offset the lower reimbursement from Medicare, Medicaid, and charity care/bad debt has the curious name of *cost shifting*, even though it is not cost that it shifts, but charges. Understanding cost shifting can be difficult for the lay public because it seems illogical that one payer would reimburse so differently than another for the exact same service. There is dramatic variability throughout the nation as well. See Figure 1.4 for a hypothetical illustration of cost shifting. Details about your region's hospital charges can be found at https://www.rand.org/pubs/research_reports/RR3033.html and specific hospitals can be found here https://dashboard.sagetransparency.org Rand Corporation (2024) reports that commercial insurance payments continue to rise above Medicare, with commercial insurance prices paid to inpatient and outpatient hospitals rising to 254% of what Medicare would have paid in the most recent year available for analysis. Although there is dramatic variability among payers and in different regions of the nation, recall that Medicare is designed to reimburse at cost, a perspective energetically opposed by the American Hospital Association.

In addition to variability among payers, the numbers and proportions of individuals on Medicaid vary from state to state. This is because states have jurisdiction over the level of poverty at which an individual is eligible for Medicaid coverage. One state may start to cover individuals at 133% of the poverty level, for example, meaning that according to the *Federal Poverty Level (FPL) Guidelines*, the person would need to make $20,029.80 or less annually to be eligible for Medicaid. Another state may be more generous, allowing a person to make up to 300% of the FPL. or up to $45,180.00,[1] and still be eligible for Medicaid benefits. This difference impacts the proportion of Medicaid-supported patients the delivery setting will see and treat. This proportion matters: No organization can consistently lose money (negative operating margin), pay its employees (including nurses), and ultimately stay in business. If Medicaid is a primary payer for a large number of patients in a given clinic, for example, that clinic may need to seek and treat a larger number of patients with commercial insurance, which pays at a higher rate than Medicaid *and* Medicare for the same services, and thus balance the clinic's budget. It is also the reason payer mix is so important to any provider. A setting with more commercially insured patients and fewer Medicaid-insured patients will have a more robust financial situation than one with the obverse situation. Why should you, as a nurse, care about this? Your financial compensation—salary and benefits—depends on the financial viability of the organization you work for. Now that you have been introduced to this dynamic, let's take a deeper dive into insurance and how it works.

Explanation: Medicare reimbursement is theoretically set at the cost of care; however, since the 2013 federal budget sequester and other cuts, it is less than the deemed actual cost, sometimes called "Medicare lite" reimbursement. Medicaid generally reimburses providers less than Medicare for the same

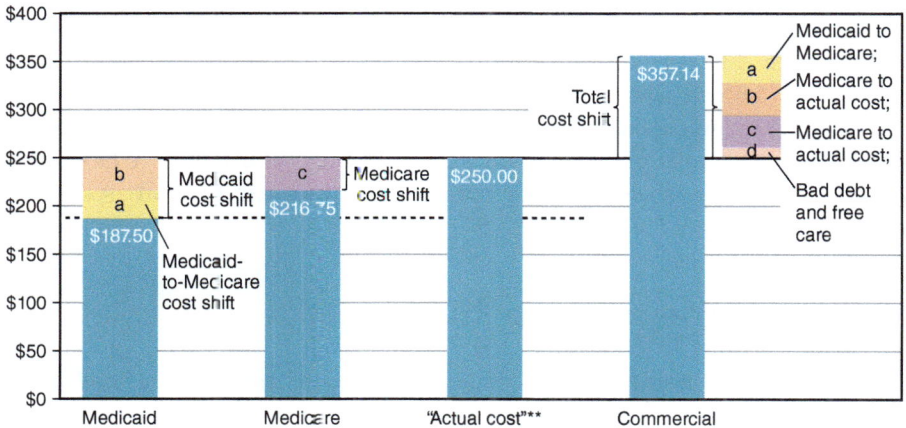

FIGURE 1.4: Illustration of cost shifting in a hypothetical procedure with an "actual cost" of $250.

services, and thus substantially less than the deemed actual cost. All of these "underpayments," including uncompensated care in the form of bad debt and charity care, are shifted to commercial insurance charges, meaning that those with commercial insurance pay more for the same service because they are compensating for underpayment by Medicare and Medicaid. This diagram also illustrates the importance of *payer mix*, given the financial incentive to see commercial insurance patients and limit Medicaid. "Actual cost," however, is actually very difficult to determine. (See Evans, 2018, for further discussion and an illustration of what one organization did about it.) The issues of the lack of price transparency and price variability represent serious health financing problems in the United States and will be discussed in later chapters. Although cost shifting is commonly voiced as a perplexing challenge in U.S. health care financing, some suggest that it is instead an enabled pricing myth (Colorado Health Institute, 2019) that supports current health care costs and prices and demands compensatory increased reimbursement from commercial payers (Potter, 2015).

Finally, although this concept may seem strange to readers, it exists in many industries, including higher education. Imagine, for example, a university in which the average cost per student credit hour is $750. The cost of educating a nurse in this institution is $1,450 per credit hour. Conversely, the cost of educating a political science student is $370. All students pay the same tuition, and the cost of educating the nursing student is shifted to the political science student who—in essence—subsidizes the cost of nursing education.

The COVID-19 pandemic provided an ideal and, of course, unfortunate opportunity to test cost shifting as either sound economic theory or a myth. Analysis by Glied (2021) noted that commercial insurance reimbursed hospitals 250% to 400% more for COVID-19 admissions than governmental insurers, similar to reimbursement spreads for other maladies. She concludes that the higher reimbursement from commercial payers does not create an equal health care experience for those who are, for example, on Medicaid or uninsured. Instead, she notes: ". . . the extra revenue derived from private patients also provides hospitals with the slack that enables them to maintain greater inventories of protective equipment, larger staffs, and more flexibility in the use of their assets" (p. 2). What does all this mean for you as a nurse and as an employee?

INSURANCE, OR THE WELL CARRY THE SICK

Oscar is furious. He was hoping for a big raise this year, and things seemed on track. Now this! Big Company Human Resources just issued an announcement that the cost of health insurance is going up more than expected next year, a whopping 9%. Although a 2% across-the-board salary increase and a 3% merit pool for employees had been budgeted—and Oscar expected to benefit from both of these—the increased cost of commercial health insurance is going to eat away all of that 5% pool. In addition, employees will see an increase in their contribution to health insurance and more cost sharing in the form of co-payments and deductibles. As a result, employees like Oscar who obtain their health insurance through their workplace will see a corresponding net decrease in their take-home pay. Seething, Oscar mutters, "Those insurance companies are just so greedy."

Jamal is the chief executive officer of Statewide Insurance Company. Reviewing the financials for the past year, he notes that there had been a dramatic increase in the use of health care by the employees in Big Company. Not only were more employees using health care, they were using very expensive health care. "I wonder if the employees realize that their use of healthcare in the previous year is a major contributing factor to the rate hike this year."

Perhaps because insurance costs are always on the rise, insurance companies are often on the receiving end of a great deal of negative public attention. Yet in nonprofit insurance companies ("nonprofit" meaning companies that are not designed to make profits to return to shareholders), insurance premiums—the amount members pay each month to be insured—reflect health care use by the members (termed *medical trend*), overhead to manage associated administrative costs, and a solvency pool or sort of safety net savings account in case there is an unexpectedly high number of claims. The latter are termed *reserves*.

Thus, insurance is a form of financial *risk sharing* in which funds are redistributed from those who are not using health services to those who are (see Figure 1.5). In health care, the *well carry the sick*, with those who use few services financially covering much of the cost of services for those who use many. Typically, an individual does not know when or if they will need health services, and it is therefore an uncertain financial risk. By design, insurance spreads the financial risk out among the members of the insurance group. The insured group is typically called an *insurance pool*.

A Simple Example to Illustrate How Insurance Works

To illustrate, imagine two scenarios. In the first, you are uninsured. You are in a small accident, and the cost of your care is $1,000. You are responsible to pay the full $1,000 to those who treated you. These providers of health care may be hospitals, physicians, nurse practitioners, or others, such as physical therapists. In the second scenario, you again have an accident resulting in a $1,000 charge, but this time you are in an insurance group of 1,000 people. Now the risk is shared by everyone, and, hypothetically, each person's contribution to your care is a mere $1. Health insurance, although a bit more complicated, works exactly like this in concept, except that the payment from each member

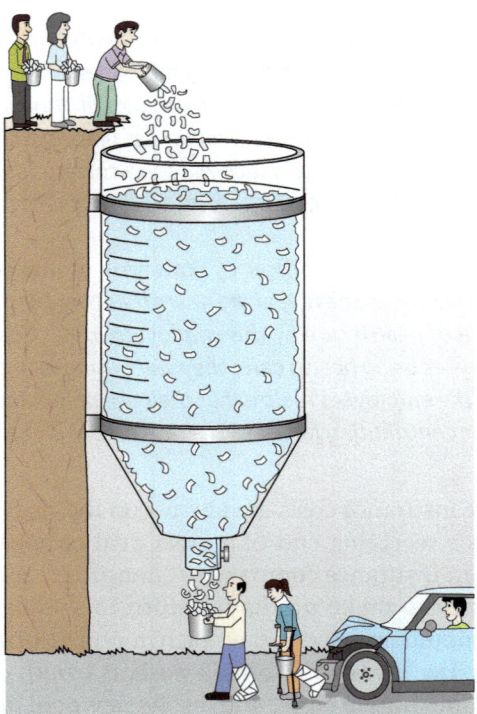

FIGURE 1.5: How insurance works.

of the group does not happen individually at the time of your accident. Instead, it happens in the form of a monthly *premium*, with the term *premium* referring to the amount each member pays to the insurance company each month. (Conceptually, the premium is analogous to the monthly gym membership; you pay the set amount each month whether you use any services or not.) The insurance company then, in turn, doles out reimbursement for services to providers. If there is a great deal of use of health care services or a few members are receiving a great deal of very high-cost services, the insurance premium for the whole group will go up the next year. The insurance company uses the cost experience of the group to determine the likely amount of money needed in the next year. The cost experiences of the group include both the *medical trend* and the *pharmaceutical trend*. In short, insurance premiums mirror the underlying cost of care for individuals within the group insurance plan.

What Factors Impact Cost Within a Risk-Sharing Arrangement?

The size and nature of the group that is sharing risk matter. In a large group, there are simply more people among whom risk may be spread. Again, by way of illustration, imagine a hypothetical group in which there are only three people. In this small group, there are not many people among whom the costs of care can be spread. Therefore, in general, a large insurance group, such as employers with many workers, will be able to have lower monthly premiums, more covered services, or both because there are more people to spread out this uncertain risk.

The health status, age, and other aspects of members of the pool also impact the cost of care for individuals in the insurance group and so ultimately also impact the cost of their insurance premiums. This concept is familiar. Here are examples from automobile insurance:

> Moira is glad to be alive! Driving through a rural area of Kentucky, her car suddenly skidded off the road into a tree. Although she was fine, her car was totaled. Three days later, although still relieved that she escaped unharmed, she ponders: "I wonder how much my insurance rates will go up."

This is an example of what is called *experience rating*, where your individual history directly impacts the cost of your insurance. It can also impact you because you are a member of a high-risk group.

> Moira's 15-year-old son, Josh, has just received his driver's permit. She is well aware that her insurance premium will go up when she puts Josh on her car insurance policy. Novice drivers have more accidents, and, overall, young men have more accidents than young women. Josh, no matter how responsible he is, fits the profile of these high-risk, high-cost insurees. Moira knows that insuring Josh will bring a dramatic increase in her monthly premiums.

Experience rating is one approach to health care risk appraisal. The second is *community rating*. In experience rating, ill individuals pay higher premiums than well individuals. In community rating, ill groups pay higher premiums than well groups. Health insurance plans using experience rating will charge higher insurance costs for older, sicker individuals than for individuals who are younger and well. Similarly, individuals who are in high-risk occupations would have higher premiums. Unlike experience rating, community rating redistributes charges evenly throughout the group being insured. Community rating charges all individuals in the same group the same premium cost, regardless of their age, gender, occupation, or other factors that impact health. Thus, cost increases for an individual reflect the group experience over the previous year.

Which is better: experience rating or community rating? Although on the surface it may seem logical that those who are well have less expensive premiums than those who are not, experience rating results in more expensive premiums for those who most need health care. Recall that the foundational premise of health care insurance is that it redistributes funds by human need; community rating does this more consistently than experience rating (Bodenheimer et al., 2024). Community rating evens out the insurance charges throughout the group, meaning that some well people will have higher costs than they would in experience rating, as they are carrying the cost of others. At some point, however, it likely will be their turn, and others will carry the cost of their care. Some states have passed laws to ensure that only community rating or modified community rating will be allowed within the state. The ACA also shaped relevant insurance coverage rules, which will be detailed in Chapter 4.

In summary, health economics considers issues of value and efficiency, whereas financing considers how funds are gathered. One mechanism by which health care is financed is health insurance. In this, the United States includes commercial payers as well as governmental payers, all of which reimburse providers at different levels. As illustrated in the contrast between Will and Mary Jane in the opening scenarios, contemporary nurses face a complicated world. Many of the troubling elements of the current health care system are the result of the unintended consequences of solutions adopted to address health system shortcomings. It is like an economic Whac-A-Mole game: One problem solved immediately creates another unsolved one. These unintended consequences are a driver of the evolution of the health care system to its present form. This is the focus of Chapter 2.

End-of-Chapter Resources

THOUGHT QUESTIONS

1. What is health economics? How is it similar to and different from other branches of economics? How does it differ from health financing?
2. Who pays for health care in the United States? How?
3. What is the role of government in the financing of U.S. health care?
4. What is the best way to finance health care? Why?
5. What are the pros and cons of risk-rated insurance and community-rated insurance? Which is better and why?
6. Define the following key terms:
   Behavioral economics
   Classic free market
   Commercial insurance
   Community rating
   Experience rating
   Governmental payers
   Health economics
   Health care financing
   Keynesian economics

Laissez-faire economics
Medical trend
Payer
Payer mix
Premium
Profit
Reimbursement
Reserves
Social determinants of health
Surplus

EXERCISES

1. You are asked to present to Nursing Grand Rounds. The organizers share that nurses seem to be confused about how insurance rates are determined as well as the concept of payer mix. Develop your talk to address these concerns.
2. Develop a short presentation to describe how U.S. health care is financed.

QUIZ

True or False

1. In health care, financing and reimbursement refer to the same thing.
2. Health economics is a distinct branch in the field of economics.
3. The best overall predictor of health status of a population is access to health care.
4. Commercial insurance companies in the United States are always nonprofit organizations.
5. There is no difference in the amount of reimbursement providers receive from different payers.
6. In *experience rating*, insurance companies charge ill individuals more for health insurance than well individuals.
7. In health care, a payer mix of 80% Medicare will reimburse providers more than a payer mix of 80% commercial insurance.
8. Nonprofit insurance companies have shareholders and an organizational mission that includes returning dividends to shareholders.
9. The cost experiences of an insurance pool largely determine the next year's premium increase.
10. The cost experience of an insurance pool includes both the medical trend and the pharmaceutical trend.

Multiple Choice

11. In the United States, health care is financed via
    A. Taxes
    B. Insurance premiums
    C. Patients, as an out-of-pocket expense
    D. All of the above
12. Medicare
    A. Is a publicly financed health care coverage for most Americans 65 years of age and older
    B. Is financed through a combination of state and federal taxes
    C. Both A and B
    D. Neither A nor B
13. The term *payer mix* refers to the proportion of reimbursement a provider receives from commercial insurance, Medicare, and Medicaid. Payer mix is important because
    A. Organizations are reimbursed by Medicare at higher rates than all other payers
    B. It provides a financial incentive for providers to treat patients who are on Medicaid
    C. Both A and B
    D. Neither A nor B
14. Which of the following payer mixes would provide the most reimbursement?
    A. 60% Medicaid, 20% uninsured, 5% commercial insurance, 15% Medicare
    B. 60% commercial insurance, 20% Medicare, 5% uninsured, 15% Medicaid
    C. 60% Medicare, 20% uninsured, 5% commercial insurance, 15% Medicaid
    D. All would provide the same level of reimbursement
15. Which of the following payer mixes would provide the least reimbursement?
    A. 60% Medicaid, 20% uninsured, 5% commercial insurance, 15% Medicare
    B. 60% commercial insurance, 20% Medicare, 5% uninsured, 15% Medicaid
    C. 60% Medicare, 20% uninsured, 5% commercial insurance, 15% Medicaid
    D. All would provide the same level of reimbursement

NOTE

1. The 2024 federal poverty guidelines for a family size of one who resides in the contiguous U.S. states.

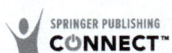

A robust set of instructor resources designed to supplement this text is located at http://connect.springerpub.com/content/book/978-0-8261-7236-5. Qualifying instructors may request access by emailing textbook@springerpub.com.

REFERENCES

Arrow, K. (1963). Uncertainty and the welfare economics of medical care. *The American Economic Review*, 53(5), 941–973.

Bodenheimer, T., Grumbach, K., & Willard-Grace, R. (2024). *Understanding health policy: A clinical approach* (9th ed). McGraw Hill/Lang.

Centers for Medicare and Medicaid Services. (2023). *Trustees report and trust funds.* https://www.cms.gov/OACT/TR

Center on Budget and Policy Priorities. (2023, September 28). *Policy basics: Where do our federal tax dollars go?* https://www.cbpp.org/research/federal-budget/policy-basics-where-do-our-federal-tax-dollars-go

Colorado Health Institute. (2019). *The cost shift myth.* Author. https://www.coloradohealthinstitute.org/sites/default/files/file_attachments/Cost%20Shift%20Report.pdf

Evans, M. (2018, August 21). What does knee surgery cost? Few know, and that's a problem. *The Wall Street Journal.* https://www.wsj.com/articles/what-does-knee-surgery-cost-few-know-and-thats-a-problem-1534865358

Galea, S. (2016). *18 charts that make the case for public health.* https://www.bu.edu/sph/news/articles/2016/18-charts-that-make-the-case-for-public-health/

Glied, S. (2021). COVID-19 overturned the theory of medical cost shifting by hospitals. *JAMA Health Forum*, 2(6), e212128. https://doi.org/10.1001/jamahealthforum.2021.2128

Harnett, K. (2024, April 18). Racial health disparities persist even in top-performing states. *Modern Healthcare.* https://www.modernhealthcare.com/providers/racial-health-disparities-commonwealth-fund-report

Himmelstein, D., & Woolhandler, S. (2016). The current and projected taxpayer shares of U.S. health costs. *American Journal of Public Health*, 106, 449–452. https://doi.org/10.2105/AJPH.2015.302997

Kalánková, D., Kirwan, M., Bartoníčková, D., Cubelo, F., Žiaková, K., & Kurucová, R. (2020). Missed, rationed or unfinished nursing care: A scoping review of patient outcomes. *Journal of Nursing Management*, 28(8), 1783–1797. https://doi.org/10.1111/jonm.12978

Keckley, P. (2024, April 15). *8 Reasons hospitals must re-think their future.* The Keckley Report. https://paulkeckley.com/the-keckley-report/2024/4/15/8-reasons-hospitals-must-re-think-their-future/

Kernick, D. (2003). Introduction to health economics for the medical practitioner. *Postgraduate Medical Journal*, 79, 147–150. https://doi.org/10.1136/pmj.79.929.147

Miller, N. (2023, September 6). Tree equity and tree's impact on surface temperatures, human health: A research roundup. *The Journalist's Resource.* https://journalistsresource.org/home/tree-health-equity/

Poon, L. (2021, June 25). *The U.S. neighbourhoods with the greatest tree inequity, mapped.* Bloomberg. https://www.bloomberg.com/news/articles/2021-06-25/mapping-the-unequal-distribution-of-trees

Potter, W. (2015). *The enduring myth of cost shifting.* The Center for Public Integrity. www.publicintegrity.org/2015/03/30/17009/enduring-myth-cost-shifting

Radley, D. C., Shah, A., Collins, S. R., Powe, N. R., & Zephyrin, L. C. (2024, April). *Advancing racial equity in US health care: The Commonwealth Fund 2024 State Health Disparities Report.* The Commonwealth Fund. https://doi.org/10.26099/vw02-fa96

Rand Corporation. (2024, May 13). *Private health plans during 2022 paid hospitals 254 percent of what Medicare would pay.* https://www.rand.org/news/press/2024/05/13.html

World Health Organization. (n.d.). *What are social determinants of health?* https://www.who.int/health-topics/social-determinants-of-health#tab=tab_1

CHAPTER 2

A Story of Unintended Consequences: How Economic and Policy Solutions Create New Challenges

CHAPTER 2 details the evolution of the U.S. employer-based fee-for-service system and the rise of tax-funded financing via Medicare and Medicaid. Origins that fostered the many nursing workforce challenges seen today are described and will be detailed in Chapter 14. Chapter 2 also briefly reviews selected elements of the Patient Protection and Affordable Care Act (ACA) of 2010, with subsequent changes to it, and other key laws related to transparency and other contemporary issues detailed in Chapter 3. Chapter 2 also illustrates some financing proposals that were voiced during recent presidential campaigns and continue to be debated. Finally, Chapter 2 details changes rapidly introduced in response to the economic and care delivery upheavals associated with COVID-19.

Following completion of this chapter, you will be able to:

- Detail the historic context that gave rise to contemporary health care financing mechanisms and the biomedical orientation to care.
- Discuss early payment reform models such as prospective payment and health maintenance organizations (HMOs).
- Describe the financing approach of the ACA and subsequent changes to it.
- Detail contemporary policy debates such as Medicare for All, Medicare for All Who Want It, and other public options.
- Describe the fundamental flaws in traditional U.S. health care financing that were powerfully revealed during the COVID-19 pandemic.

Carolyn is excited to visit her great-grandfather in the assisted living facility. Born in 1930, he is full of tales of the Old West. Papa John, as Carolyn calls him, beams with pride when she shares that she has just graduated with her baccalaureate degree and is practicing as an RN. Thinking about health care, Papa John begins to muse on the epidemic of 1918. He shares that his older brother, Nick, nearly died of what Papa thinks was diphtheria but perhaps was the flu pandemic. The country doctor could do nothing

> for Nick, and finally, with Nick near death, his mother called on Florence, the village "wise woman." Florence crushed herbs to create a compound and, with a sheet of paper rolled to a cone, blew the compound into Nick's mouth. Later that night, Nick's fever broke, and by morning he was well. Papa John shares that his mother always credited the village wise woman with saving her son's life. Carolyn, who just received her first paycheck, wonders about compensation for services rendered. "Papa John," she asks, "did you pay Florence anything?" "Of course," Papa proudly responds. "Every fall we would give her a chicken!" Carolyn ponders the barter system and concludes that she and her classmates are very happy to be paid with money, not chickens.[1]

> Shanice is a nurse practitioner in a primary care clinic in a major urban area. She is mostly satisfied with her job but is hoping for a substantial raise in salary following her upcoming annual review. In preparation, she decides to talk to the clinic business manager about her salary hopes. The business manager firmly states that the availability of funds for a raise will depend on four factors: (a) the clinic's achievement of quality metrics for those patients within the pay-for-performance system; (b) rates negotiated with the insurance company for those patients in the independent provider arrangement; (c) changing the ratio of Medicaid to private-pay patients, so that the clinic sees fewer Medicaid patients and more private-pay patients; and (d) decreasing the cost of care for patients in the Accountable Care Organization. "Is it really this complicated," Shanice wonders, "or is the business manager just trying to put me off?"

Most U.S. nurses entered professional life at a time when employer-based insurance represented the most common private financing mechanism and fee-for-service was the primary mechanism for reimbursing providers. Similarly, Medicaid and Medicare, also using fee-for-service reimbursement mechanisms, have been publicly funded fixtures in health care since 1965. Together, these predominant models seem "normal" or just how health care costs are managed. Thus, it is often a surprise to discover that this commonplace situation is almost a fluke of history, studded with unintended consequences and fixes.

As Carolyn learned from her great-grandfather, health care had a very different profile in the early 1900s. Infections and injuries were common causes of death, and little—other than easing suffering and hoping for the best—could be done to help those in need. Like the wise woman serving Papa John's brother, providers of care were often not paid at all or were compensated within some sort of barter system. Imagine, for a moment, if in your practice as an RN, you were compensated with what people were able to give you when they could, like the yearly chicken that the village wise woman received.

THE INFLUENCE OF THE FLEXNER REPORT

Several forces of history changed the course of U.S. health care from the world described in the opening vignette and set the stage for the medical industrial complex of today. The first of these is the Flexner Report, which reformed medical education.

In the early 1900s, education for physicians was loosely organized. There were many for-profit schools, with no uniform standards for students' education and training. At the urging of the American Medical Association and in response to concerns about the quality and consistency of care, the Carnegie Foundation hired Abraham Flexner, an educational reformer, to study medical education in the United States and Canada. Flexner concluded that the problems in medical education resulted from having too many schools preparing physicians and the lack of uniformity in that education. Flexner was influenced by the "hyper-rational world of German medicine" (Duffy, 2011, p. 276) and by the biomedical model he saw at Johns Hopkins and its curricular approach that focused on laboratory sciences and research. As Duffy notes, Flexner rated schools in comparison to Johns Hopkins as follows:

> Schools were assigned to one of three categories on the basis of his evaluation: A first group consisted of those that compared favorably with Hopkins; a second tier was comprised of those schools considered substandard but which could be salvaged by supplying financial assistance to correct the deficiencies; and a third group was rated of such poor quality that closure was indicated. The latter was the fate of one-third of American medical schools in the aftermath of the report. (p. 272)

Schools with fewer financial resources and less developed science departments had a difficult time meeting the criteria, and many of these served students of color and women. Barkin et al. (2010) note that the Flexner criteria for medical education forced the closure of most of the schools serving Black and female medical students, and opportunities for women and students of color evaporated; in the years following the Flexner Report, there was an increase in both the numbers and proportions of White male medical students and a decrease in students with other salient identity markers, with a near elimination of women from the physician workforce between the years 1920 and 1970.

A more careful review of the Flexner Report suggests that closure of schools serving women and people of color was not merely an unintended consequence. Flexner considered only two institutions serving Black students: Meharry in Philadelphia and Howard in Washington, DC, as the exceptions to the need for closure. However, he also emphasized that the Black physician's role was to keep Black people sufficiently healthy so as to not contaminate White people. Moreover, he stressed that Black physicians should focus on hygiene, unlike the White physician's focus on surgery (Laws, 2021). This clearly racist agenda also included a socioeconomic agenda.

Specifically, medical education following the Johns Hopkins model also became longer and more expensive (Harley, 2006). A review by Prislin et al. (2010) of the consequences of the Flexner Report states that the socioeconomic schism in admission to medical school was sustained, given that 75% of U.S. medical students were from the two upper-income quintiles, that is, upper class or upper middle class, at the time of his analysis. This economic divide continues. Shahriar et al. (2022), for example, found that 50% of medical students were in the top one-fifth of family incomes and nearly a quarter were in the top 5%, in both cases, regardless of race or ethnicity. They suggest that a focus on family income will be key to creating a more diverse physician workforce.

The Flexner Report also spurred physician specialization rather than the primary care orientation common in other countries that have high-performing, less expensive health care systems. Flexner's model was focused on a biological and physiological orientation, creating a shift away from and eventual closure of preparation programs for what we now call "complementary and alternative medicine"–oriented hospitals, colleges, and teaching programs. Indeed, following the Flexner Report, 80% of the programs in homeopathy, naturopathy, eclectic therapy, physical theory, osteopathy, and chiropractic care closed (Stahnisch & Verhoef, 2012). Notably, today, such orientations are termed "complementary" or "alternative" in contrast to what we now see as "traditional" care, which is care within the Flexner model. But as the opening scenario illustrated, there was no complementary, alternative, or standard medical care at the time. There were only sick individuals and those who wanted to treat them using the skills and information of their training. Thinking back to Carolyn's great-grandfather, it appears that the village wise woman may have been more successful in treating Nick than the medical doctor was, and we do not know how either of them was trained. In summary, after the Flexner Report, medical education became less diverse and more controlled, as it transitioned from a for-profit apprenticeship model to one that is university based with carefully selected students (Prislin et al., 2010). On the flip side, it excluded many and created a scientific orientation that Duffy concludes was not balanced by similar excellence in caring.

WHAT ABOUT NURSES?

Physicians also carved out a broad and exclusive scope of practice for themselves, with echoes to the present day with, for example, the American Medical Association's continued opposition to expanded nursing scope of practice. Nurses, if educated at all, were trained in hospitals with entry-level responsibilities similar to those of a maid. Later, hospital-based training programs for nurses were designed to ensure a fleet of physician-led, free labor to the facility. Graduation of nurses was a by-product of training, not the main aim. Instead the main intention was service to the institution (Ervin, 2021). To this day, hospitals bundle nurses' professional work into room charges, creating perverse incentives to keep nurse staffing as low as possible because nursing care represents a "labor cost," unlike the "revenue generation" of physician care (Yakusheva & Rambur, 2023). These current workforce issues will be discussed in depth in Chapter 14. For now, let's focus on the history that led us to this place. Consider Abigale's story, a young woman preparing as a nurse:

> 1915. Abigale, orphaned at age 13, has just completed her nursing training at Saint Alexius Hospital. The founding sisters could be tough, but she learned a great deal. "With any luck at all," Abigale muses, "I'll get a job working for a nice, wealthy family. Maybe they will even have a room for me!"

After graduation, most nurses worked as private duty nurses at minimal wages, even though only families with resources could afford to hire a nurse in the first place. Nursing education did not bring social status or financial independence. Thus, the changes shaped by the Flexner Report set the stage for medicine, but not nursing, to be a regulated, organized, and well-compensated profession. The Flexner Report set in motion a cascade of effects that continues to influence health and health care more than 100 years later, an example of the power of policy to create lasting change.

EARLY HOSPITALS

Just as the profession of medicine of 100 years ago was very different from that of today, so too were the hospitals. Sultz and Young (2011) note:

> Hospitals in early America served quite different purposes from those of today. They were founded to shelter older adults, the dying, orphans, and vagrants, and to protect the inhabitants of a community from the contagiously sick and the dangerously insane. (p. 70)

Hospitals were dirty, overcrowded, and contaminated, and those with other options would not choose hospital care over the care that could be provided in their own homes. Over time, however, religious orders saw the opportunities to serve vulnerable individuals, and religious nursing groups played an important role in the development of hospitals (Sultz & Young, 2011). Some of these orders, for example, the Order of Saint Benedict (n.d.), included "care of the sick" as a central tenet in their guiding *Rule of Saint Benedict* and organized elements of their monastic life around such care, including the establishment of hospitals.

THE INTRODUCTION OF EMPLOYER-BASED HEALTH INSURANCE

Nevertheless, despite some advances in hospital care, many potential patients remained uninterested in or were unable to pay for hospital services. As a result, many hospitals were not able to consistently attract patients. In response, Baylor University Hospital had a brilliant and, for that time, somewhat radical idea on how to attract "customers" in the form of patients capable of paying for care. In 1929, they began to offer 1,500 Dallas schoolteachers up to 21 days of hospital care for $6 a year per person. As the Great Depression intensified and people had even less money for anything at all, much less something like hospital care, hospital-centered prepaid insurance plans, requiring the use of a particular hospital, grew. In turn, these prepaid hospital plans became the basis of the American Hospital Association's establishment of Blue Cross, which differed in that it allowed patients a choice of hospitals. Initially opposed by physicians, the opportunity for guaranteed income became of interest to physician groups as the Great Depression took effect and people could not afford to see a doctor—or at least not able to pay for that visit. The first Blue Shield plan was set up by the California Medical Association in 1939, and similar plans quickly spread across the nation. It is important to note that Blue Cross, established by the American Hospital Association, financially enabled and thus encouraged the use of hospital care, while Blue Shield financially enabled and thus encouraged the use of physician care, all within the biomedical model of care heralded by the Flexner Report. In retrospect, what is notable in these plans is the lack of incentives for quality, cost control, or appropriate utilization. The reason? These organizations emerged to address a different problem, that is, ways to ensure that hospitals and physicians were paid (Bodenheimer & Grumbach, 2020; Starr, 1982).

SOCIAL REFORM ADDRESSING UNINTENDED CONSEQUENCES OF EMPLOYER-BASED INSURANCE

The model of employer-based insurance that started with Dallas teachers grew rapidly because of another historical event: World War II. During World War II, employers were constrained by wage and price controls and so instead looked to *fringe benefits* as a strategy to recruit and retain workers. Employer-based health insurance represents one such fringe benefit. Yet employer-based insurance has one dramatic unintended consequence: It leaves out those who are not employed. These include retired individuals, those with a disability or other challenges precluding work, those who are self-employed (like artists), and the partners or children of parents who are not working or do not have family health insurance. By the 1960s, the group most likely to be living in poverty was older adults, with nearly three-fourths of U.S. older adults living below the poverty line (DeLew, 2000).

In the social climate of the 1960s, it is not surprising that a sweeping corrective action was undertaken, reflecting testimony such as this:

> I am one of your old retired teachers that has been forgotten. I am 80 years old and for 10 years I have been living on a bare nothing, two meals a day, one egg, a soup, because I want to be independent. . . . And I worked so hard that I have pernicious anemia, $9.95 for a little bottle of liquid for shots, wholesale, I couldn't pay for it. (Stevens, as cited in DeLew, 2000, p. 76)

As a corrective action, Medicare, a publicly funded fee-for-service insurance overseen by the federal government for those 65 and older, was established in 1965 as an amendment to the original Social Security Act. Also similarly established in 1965 was Medicaid, a publicly funded fee-for-service federal program administered by states for low-income individuals, families with children, and most disabled and blind individuals younger than 65. At the time, President Lyndon Johnson's "Great Society" was a social reform movement that aimed to eliminate poverty. It was within this social milieu that Medicare and Medicaid were signed into law on July 30, 1965, as amendments to the Social Security Act, attempting to correct the gaps that emerged under employer-based insurance models. Notably, President Franklin D. Roosevelt had decided not to include health insurance in the original Social Security Act because of fierce opposition from physicians. Roosevelt feared that such inclusion would mean the demise of the entire Social Security program he was trying to establish. President Johnson presented the first two Medicare cards to former President Truman (Roosevelt's vice president) and Mrs. Truman and at the ceremony noted: "We marvel not simply at the passage of this bill, but what we marvel at is that it took so many years to pass" (Harris, as cited in DeLew, 2000, p. 75). In summary, Medicare, now a staple of the American health care system, was a hard-won, long-in-the-making reform. Financing for those of any age with a diagnosis of end-stage renal disease was added in 1972, and amyotrophic lateral sclerosis (Lou Gehrig's disease) was added as an automatic qualifying condition in 2001. This has raised questions among some about why. Why these diseases? Why should only those 65 and older have national health insurance? This will be discussed in the last section of this chapter.

PUBLIC FUNDING FUELS HEALTH INDUSTRY GROWTH

Public financing for those 65 and older, the poor, and those whose disabilities precluded employment heralded a new era in the American health care system. For the first time, there was a guaranteed revenue stream to treat those who, in aggregate, were guaranteed to be ill or seek health care services. Before the advent of these health care financing approaches, these individuals had a substantial incentive to avoid seeking treatment because they were solely responsible for paying for those services. Medicare and Medicaid removed the financial disincentives for these large groups of people in the society—the older adults, the poor, and the disabled—to seek treatment. In the same vein, under fee-for-service reimbursement, physicians and hospitals had no financial disincentive to limit treatment, both necessary and unnecessary. Thus fueled, the health care industry began its explosive growth. Physician income, which prior to 1965 tracked the annual inflation growth rate, skyrocketed. The money in the system also fueled the growth of specialty services and progressively more technologically enhanced services in hospitals (e.g., intensive care units and cardiac monitoring) and, with it, new roles for nurses as well as the growth of roles for other providers. These emerging roles, then called "allied health" roles—presumably because they were "allied" with medicine and its social, political, and financial power—became *unbundled* from other services. In the early 1970s, for example, nurses debrided wounds and provided complex ambulation for hospitalized patients. These services were bundled in room charge fees, much like the maid services that marked nursing's early hospital history. Soon, however, such services came to be provided by physical therapists for an additional charge, or "fee-for-service." These professions then also had the financial fuel to grow their services in both complexity and volume. In summary, when fully insured, patients have little incentive to limit the different services they seek and receive, a phenomenon economists term *moral hazard*. Hospitals, specialty services, and "allied health" grew, and some services once provided by nurses were unbundled from nursing care and supplied by other providers. Nursing specialization also grew in response to clinical realities and financial opportunities. Nevertheless, Medicare Part B (provider reimbursement) specifically precluded nurse reimbursement.

One person's income or revenue stream is another's expense. Commercial insurance, as noted in the first chapter, exists to spread financial risk, and the well carry the sick financially, with costs of care spread through the group. Similarly, the cost of care for those in publicly funded insurance such as Medicare and Medicaid are spread in the society through taxes (see Figure 1.5 for an illustration of how insurance works). This means that even though individuals using the services may not feel the immediate financial impact of their use of services, in aggregate, the use of health care by individuals covered by Medicare and Medicaid uses tax dollars. In turn, less tax money remains for other goods and services; for example, public funding of higher education to keep college tuition affordable. Similarly, although employer-based insurance seems to be "paid for by my employer," it is actually a portion of the total compensation package the employee receives. Increased use of health services among those in the insurance pool will result in increased insurance costs. These costs are borne by employees as a reduction in possible wage increases, increased cost sharing when using health care, or a decrease in other fringe benefits.

Regardless of the source of the resources, taken as a whole, the availability of private insurance complemented by Medicare and Medicaid, all within a fee-for-service system, dramatically drove up the use of medical services. The use of the term "medical" services rather than "health" care here is intentional. Recall the orientation of the Flexner Report and its influence on medical education; Blue Shield was a physicians' organization, and the physicians were uniformly educated within the biological model of disease (see Table 2.1). The combination of forces created a health care system dependent on what physicians defined as illness. Physicians also determined treatment, including referral for additional treatment or testing, all unbundled from each other and charging for each piece of service without regard for costs, which were escalating impressively in the new regime.

TABLE 2.1 HOW DOES THE BIOMEDICAL MODEL OF HEALTH AND ILLNESS DIFFER FROM A HOLISTIC MODEL?

Biomedical Model Assumptions	Holistic Model Assumptions
Single underlying cause for a disease; removal of that cause will create health.[a]	Health and illness are multifactorial; not all abnormalities cause illness, and disease can occur without illness.
Health is the absence of disease.[a]	Health is a "state of complete physical, mental and social well-being and not merely the absence of disease or infirmity"[b]
Cure of disease is a goal; death is often viewed as a failure.	To cure and to heal are not the same. It is possible to have a healing death. Death is not an enemy.[c]
Emotional and mental disturbances are distinct from those of the body.[a]	There is a unifying interplay between mind and body; they cannot be separated.
The individual is independent of the environment and society.[a]	The human system is in dynamic, constant interaction with its social, spiritual, and physical environment.
People are victims with little responsibility for illness.[a]	People are full participants in their health and illness, and their actions and inactions matter. When ill, although not responsible for their condition, they are responsible to it.[c]
Patients are passive recipients of care.	Patients are active agents in their own recovery and always have choices in how they respond to their health and illness.

Sources: Adapted from [a]Wade, D., & Halligan, P. (2004). Do biomedical models of illness make for good healthcare systems? British Medical Journal, 329(7479), 1398–1401. https://doi.org/10.1136/bmj.329.7479.1398; [b]World Health Organization. (1946, June). Preamble to the constitution of the World Health Organization. Paper presented at the International Health Conference (Signed on 22 July 1946 by the representatives of 61 States [Official Records of the World Health Organization, No. 2, p. 100]); [c]Levine, S. (2010). Healing into life and death. Knopf Doubleday Publishing Group.

ATTEMPTS TO CHANGE FINANCIAL INCENTIVES TO CONTAIN COSTS

Health Maintenance Organizations

There were efforts to change the incentives that accelerate cost, emphasizing wellness and health promotion to contain costs. Notable among these attempts were HMOs. The HMO Act of 1973 was passed during the administration of Republican President Richard Nixon. This model, in its most undiluted sense, is the other side of the coin from fee-for-service. Instead of being reimbursed for each treatment, each service, each Q-tip used, there is a fixed sum per enrolee per month. This is called *capitation* or *capitation payments*, with the term capitation derived from *caput* and meaning "by head." All services used must be paid for within this fixed sum. Thus, unlike fee-for-service, which has an incentive for overtreatment and expensive, high-technology care, HMOs have a financial incentive for wellness, with the potential for undertreatment. As a result, early HMOs worked best when the insurance pool covered was largely healthy or had enough "well" members to carry or cover the costs for the sick ones. But physician income could be negatively impacted—remember, unlike fee-for-service setups in which providers treat, bill, and push those costs to third-party payers, HMO models have fixed pools of money to work with. In HMO models in which physicians share the risk for financial loss if there was more treatment than money gathered per enrolled patient, they stand to lose money. In this model, physicians bear the cost not only of their own decision-making but also that of other providers in their group. The impression of fewer services was also decried by many in the public at large who, largely unaware of the overtreatment potential fueled by fee-for-service, felt that this model of financing and reimbursement resulted in a lower quality of care. For these and other reasons, HMOs, which grew in the 1990s, faded in prominence thereafter (Bodenheimer & Grumbach, 2020).

PROSPECTIVE PAYMENT AND DIAGNOSTIC-RELATED GROUPS

Concerns about rising costs also caused Medicare to reconsider reimbursement strategies. In 1983, Medicare moved away from fee-for-service reimbursement to prospective payment via diagnosis-related groups, commonly known as DRGs. Instead of hospitals being paid "per diem"—reimbursed for each day that the patient was hospitalized—hospitals were now prospectively reimbursed a lump sum per episode of hospitalization. Ponder the difference in the incentives in these two models. In one, per diem, the hospital is paid for each day the patient is hospitalized. The author, for example, recalls being hospitalized for three full days for an uncomplicated wrist fracture in 1966, a procedure that required only simple casting and today would be managed in an hour or two in an outpatient setting. The treatment strategy has not changed, nor is the difference in hospitalization time due to new technology or novel healing strategies. Instead, in the per diem model, hospitals had a financial incentive for long hospitalizations and did not bear any financial risk for the efficiency with which the care was provided. Indeed, not only was there no incentive for efficient services, there was also a financial incentive for inefficient provision of care, a phenomenon called *perverse incentive*. Providers, both the hospital and the physician, were generously reimbursed in the pre-DRG years. The advent of Medicare DRGs shifted the financial risk for the length of stay to the hospital.

> *Nursing Student: 1976—pre-DRG*
> *Mary is excited to start her first clinical rotation at Big City Hospital. She is assigned just one patient, Mrs. Jensen, a 66-year-old having her gallbladder removed. Nurse faculty shares with Mary that faculty selected Mrs. Jensen because she is 2 days pre-op. Mary will have a chance to practice her interview skills with a lucid, well patient—a good start. Mrs. Jensen will have her pre-op lab test tomorrow, as well as a chest x-ray, as is standard for all patients undergoing surgery.*

The advent of DRGs dramatically changed this scenario because DRGs are based on a *prospective payment* in a set sum, rather than *retrospective payment* on a per diem rate. Therefore, before DRGs, the hospital would be reimbursed for each day Mrs. Jensen was in the hospital. The physician solely could decide how long she would stay in the hospital. The physician had no incentive for a timely discharge, and the hospital had an incentive to keep the patient as long as reasonably possible. Moreover, hospitals received additional compensation for complications, including ones caused by their care.

Financial Incentives in Diagnosis-Related Groups

Just as per diem reimbursement incentivized long hospital stays, the DRG payment scheme incentivizes early discharge. There are labor costs associated with a hospital stay—nurses and others—and the hospital now had the financial incentive to discharge the patient as quickly as possible because reimbursement would be the same, but the cost of care would be much less if the hospital stay were short. Conversely, in a very long stay, the hospital would actually lose money, as the cost of care would be greater than the reimbursement. If, instead, the patient could be moved through the hospital stay very quickly and the cost of providing care were less than the sum received from Medicare, the hospital would make money on that admission.

The speed with which a patient can be moved through a hospital or other setting—admission to discharge—is called *throughput*.

Impact of Diagnosis-Related Groups

Did this prospective, payment-by-diagnosis strategy impact the growth of health care expenditures, and how did it impact quality? Early reports suggested that this fundamental change slowed the growth of hospital inpatient costs without an impact on mortality rates and readmission (Davis & Rhodes, 1988). Later analyses found that although there was no impact on a long-standing trajectory toward better hospital care, there was an impact on patient stability at discharge (Kahn et al., 1991). The increase in readmission of patients—presumably due to being discharged too early—was clearly identified over time. In 2012 Rau noted:

> With nearly one in five Medicare patients returning to the hospital within a month of discharge, the government considers readmissions a prime symptom of an overly expensive and uncoordinated health system. Hospitals have had little financial incentive to ensure patients get the care they need once they leave, and in fact they benefit financially when patients don't recover and return for more treatment.
>
> Nearly 2 million Medicare beneficiaries are readmitted within 30 days of release each year, costing Medicare $17.5 billion in additional hospital bills. The national average readmission rate has remained steady at around 19% for several years, even as many hospitals have worked harder to lower theirs. (p. 1)

To address this perverse incentive, starting in 2009, hospitals were required to publicly report their readmission rate, which was then publicly available on the Hospital Compare website. There was no financial penalty for high readmission rates, and this new requirement had little, if any, impact on readmission rates (McIlvennan et al., 2015). Then, as part of the ACA and starting in October 2012, hospitals with a 30-day postdischarge readmission rate above a defined threshold are fined by Medicare. In the first year of the program, 2,217 hospitals forfeited more than $280 million in Medicare funds (Rau, 2012). This trend has remained relatively consistent, with 2,583 of 3,129 hospitals (83%) penalized in 2019, resulting in a loss of hospital revenue of $563 million (Rau, 2019). Over the period of a decade, 9 in 10 acute care general hospitals have been penalized at least once (Rau, 2021). Nevertheless, penalties actually dropped during the COVID-19 era (Advisory Board, 2023). This ACA policy action is called the Hospital Readmission Reduction Program and is just one payment reform strategy to address what was an unintended consequence of payment by diagnosis, specifically the possibility of premature discharge with a resulting rehospitalization. Other payment reform models also include penalties for readmission as well as other strategies to better link quality to payment. These are detailed in Chapter 4.

Clearly, patients can be harmed by a hospital discharge before they are ready. But recall also that there is harm related to keeping the patients in the hospital too long. This harm is in the form of excessive costs of care that are collectively borne by taxpayers (Medicare and Medicaid admissions) and employers and employees (commercial employer-based private insurance). Patients can also be harmed by longer exposure to medical error and hospital-acquired conditions. Nurses have an opportunity to play a key role in preventing readmission through patient education and discharge planning.

THE AFFORDABLE CARE ACT AND NEW (AND RENEWED) PAYMENT MODELS

The ACA will be detailed in Chapter 3, but key points are relevant to this discussion. The ACA, passed in 2010, attempts to address many of these issues and is a historic milestone. Along with Medicare and Medicaid in 1965, it is the first major piece of health reform legislation since the many failed attempts starting with Franklin D. Roosevelt (Morone, 2010). Designed to ensure that all Americans have financial access to health care, it also incentivizes new patterns of innovation and redesigned care models. Thus, it not only proposes to finance health care in new, more comprehensive ways ensuring coverage for all but also intends to change reimbursement. This latter aspect, changes in reimbursement strategies, is termed *payment reform*. Payment reform seeks to dramatically change provider behavior. Therefore, to effectively lead in a changing health care environment, nurses must understand the financial incentives and disincentives in a reformed care system. As just one example, nurses can play a leading role in preventing readmission of patients to the hospital and are in a prime position to redesign care models to ensure this end. Therefore, it is valuable to understand just how important this is in the hospital's bottom line when articulating a plan of care.

HOW DOES THE AFFORDABLE CARE ACT ATTEMPT TO ENSURE FINANCIAL ACCESS TO HEALTH CARE?

The ACA financing model builds on the existing employer-based health care system to ensure that all Americans have financial access to health care. In general, universal coverage may be financed in three ways. These are as follows:

1. Publicly funded through taxes, often called *single payer*

2. Funded through a requirement that all employers offer health insurance and requiring workers to sign up for this insurance (called an *employer mandate*)
3. Funded through a requirement that all individuals have health insurance (called an *individual mandate*)

The ACA, as originally enacted, used all three approaches. Different nations have used various combinations of these and other financing models. Switzerland, for example, uses an individual mandate as its financing vehicle to achieve universal financial access for all its citizens, while Canada uses a single-payer vehicle. It is important to note, however, that each nation's health care system reflects the values and historical evolution within that nation and its culture. Therefore, even when using similar financing mechanisms, the health care system may spawn very diverse provider behaviors because of different reimbursement (payment) strategies. As one example, Canada's single-payer system reimburses providers in a fee-for-service system, so—while publicly funded through taxes—it retains the potential for the opportunities and challenges inherent in fee-for-service systems. Currently in the United States, political views about a single-payer system are polarized. Nevertheless, the popular Medicare system is essentially a publicly funded single-payer system for those 65 and older, with the sources of revenue coming from a range of sources including payroll taxes and beneficiary cost sharing (see Figure 2.1) Medicaid is a publicly funded single-payer system for low-income individuals and some with disabilities. The U.S. employer-based system created challenges during COVID-19.

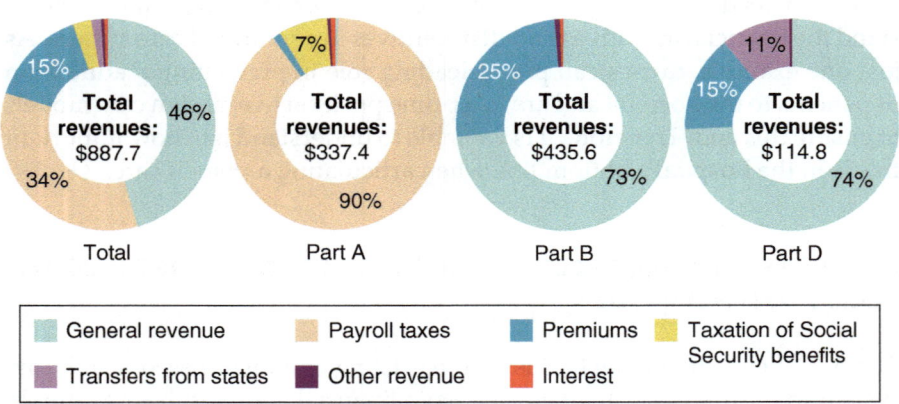

FIGURE 2.1: Revenue sources for Medicare Parts A, B, and D. Medicare revenues come from different sources, primarily general revenues, payroll taxes, and premiums paid by beneficiaries.

Source: Kaiser Family Foundation. Used with permission. https://www.kff.org/medicare/issue-brief/what-to-know-about-medicare-spending-and-financing.

COVID-19

The U.S. employer-based system created challenges during COVID-19 This global health emergency brought to light the enormous challenges stemming from the manner in which health care is financed and delivered in the United States, including hospitals' dependence on elective procedures for financial viability. The challenges, arguably foundational flaws, are multifold, as follows:

1. Americans who obtained their health insurance through their employers faced not only loss of income but also loss of health insurance when furloughed.
2. Hospitals curtailed their elective procedures to prepare for the potential surge of COVID-19 patients. Not only was care of this population expensive but the revenue from elective procedures also evaporated. High-revenue procedures include orthopedic procedures and certain diagnostic tests, for example, sleep studies. Even when hospitals promoted themselves as "safe to reopen," volumes were slow to re-emerge. Presumably, people were reluctant to put themselves in a potentially vulnerable position vis-à-vis the virus. Also, recall the magnitude of waste and unnecessary care in the United States. Perhaps some people merely concluded that they didn't need the offered service after all.

The pandemic accelerated calls for global budgets for rural hospitals (Fried et al., 2020), among others, as well value-based payments (Livingston, 2020). These and other forms of payment reform are detailed in Chapter 4. Other lessons from COVID-19 will be discussed in Chapter 13.

End-of-Chapter Resources

THOUGHT QUESTIONS

1. What might the U.S. health care system look like if the Flexner Report was never written?
2. Why do some Americans support Medicare yet oppose governmental involvement in health care?
3. What are the strategies that enable universal financial access to health care? Is one strategy better than others? Why or why not?
4. The pandemic clearly underscored deficiencies in the U.S. health care financing and delivery system. What strategies offer corrective steps? Who are the stakeholders? How do you get them engaged?
5. Define the following key terms:
    Capitation
    Health maintenance organizations

Payment reform
Per diem reimbursement
Perverse incentives
Retrospective reimbursement
Throughput
Unbundled services

EXERCISES

1. Prepare a short presentation on the evolution of the health care system in the United States from the early 1900s to the present day.
2. Develop a presentation on the pros and cons of the three financing approaches in the ACA.

QUIZ

True or False

1. One characteristic of the biomedical model is that the concept of *health* includes physical, mental/emotional, spiritual, and social aspects.
2. In the early 1900s, hospitals were the most highly preferred settings for medical treatment.
3. In response to the Flexner Report, nursing became a more highly compensated profession, with resulting increased social status for nurses.
4. The first U.S. employer-based health insurance was offered to Dallas schoolteachers for $6 a year.
5. The American Hospital Association established Blue Cross, which enabled insurees to have a choice of hospitals.
6. Blue Shield was established to ensure physician reimbursement for care provided.
7. National health insurance was considered for inclusion in the original Social Security Act during the administration of President Franklin D. Roosevelt.
8. Medicare and Medicaid were enacted in 1965 as a potential solution to the unintended consequences of employer-based health insurance.
9. Hospital nursing services have largely remained bundled into hospital room charges.
10. Capitated reimbursement within HMOs creates the same treatment incentives as fee-for-service reimbursement.

Multiple Choice

11. Holistic models of health
    A. Consider *health* to be the absence of disease
    B. Consider the human mind–body interplay and the interplay of the mind–body with physical, social, and spiritual environments
    C. Both A and B
    D. Neither A nor B
12. Which of the following is *not* true: As a result of the Flexner Report
    A. Medical education became longer and more expensive
    B. Medical education opportunities for women and people of color increased
    C. Most of the programs in homeopathy, naturopathy, and osteopathy were forced to close
    D. Physician specialization rather than primary care was emphasized
13. Employer-based health insurance
    A. Grew dramatically due to wage and price controls during World War II
    B. Is a pre-tax fringe benefit
    C. Excludes retired and unemployed individuals
    D. All of the above
14. The enactment of Medicare and Medicaid within fee-for-service reimbursement
    A. Fueled rapid growth in the health care industry
    B. Fueled unbundling of services, so that each piece of health care service would be charged individually
    C. Both A and B
    D. Neither A nor B
15. Medicare
    A. Began paying hospitals prospectively by diagnosis-related groups (DRGs) starting in 1983
    B. Is publicly funded through taxes and beneficiaries cost sharing
    C. Both A and B
    D. Neither A nor B
16. Hospital reimbursement via diagnosis-related groups (DRGs)
    A. Financially incentivizes long hospital stays
    B. Creates the potential for premature hospital discharge of patients
    C. Removes incentives to enhance hospital throughput
    D. All of the above

17. As originally enacted, the ACA financing model included
    A. Public funding through taxes
    B. Employer insurance mandates
    C. Individual insurance mandates
    D. All of the above

NOTE

1. The story of Papa John is a true story based on the author's father, who was actually born in 1914. Nick was his younger brother.

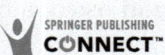 A robust set of instructor resources designed to supplement this text is located at http://connect.springerpub.com/content/book/978-0-8261-7236-5. Qualifying instructors may request access by emailing textbook@springerpub.com.

REFERENCES

Advisory Board. (2023). *The drop in hospital readmission penalties, charted*. Author. https://www.advisory.com/daily-briefing/2022/10/14/readmission-penalties

Barkin, S., Fuentes-Afflick, E., Brosco, J., & Tuchman, A. (2010). Unintended consequences of the Flexner Report: Women in pediatrics. *Pediatrics, 126*, 1055–1057. https://doi.org/10.1542/peds.2010-2050

Bodenheimer, T., & Grumbach, K. (2020). *Understanding health policy: A clinical approach* (8th ed.). Lange/McGraw Hill.

Davis, C., & Rhodes, D. (1988). The impact of DRGs on the cost and quality of health care in the United States. *Health Policy, 9*(2), 117–131. https://doi.org/10.1016/0168-8510(88)90029-2

DeLew, N. (2000). Medicare: 35 years of service. *Health Care Financing Review, 22*(1), 75–102.

Duffy, T. (2011). The Flexner Report—100 years later. *Yale Journal of Biology and Medicine, 84*, 269–276.

Ervin, S. (2021). History of nursing education in the United States. In S. S. DeBoor (Ed.), *Keating's curriculum development and evaluation in nursing education* (5th ed.). Springer Publishing. https://connect.springerpub.com/content/book/978-0-8261-7442-0/part/part01/chapter/ch01

Fried, J., Liebers, D., & Roberts, E. (2020). Sustaining rural hospitals after COVID-19: The case for global budgets. *Journal of the American Medical Association, 324*(2), 137–138. https://doi.org/10.1001/jama.2020.9744

Harley, E. (2006). The forgotten history of defunct Black medical schools in the 19th and 20th centuries and the impact of the Flexner Report. *Journal of the National Medical Association, 98*, 1425–1429.

Kahn, K., Draper, D., Keeler, E., Rogers, W., Rubenstein, L., Kosecoff, M., Sherwood, M. J., Harrison, E. R., Carney, M. F., & Brook, R. (1991). *The effects of the DRG-based prospective payment system of quality of care for hospitalized Medicare patients: Executive summary*. RAND Corporation.

Laws, T. (2021). How should we respond to racist legacies in health professions education originating in the Flexner Report? *AMA Journal of Ethics, 23*(3), E271–E275. https://doi.org/10.1001/amajethics.2021.271

Livingston, S. (2020, June 13). *COVID-19 may end up boosting value-based payment*. Modern Healthcare. https://www.modernhealthcare.com/insurance/covid-19-may-end-up-boosting-value-based-payment

McIlvennan, C., Eapen, Z., & Allen, L. (2015). Hospital readmissions reduction program. *Circulation, 131*(20), 1796–1803. https://doi.org/10.1161/CIRCULATIONAHA.114.010270

Morone, J. (2010). Presidents and health reform: From Franklin D. Roosevelt to Barack Obama. *Health Affairs, 29*(6), 1096–1100. https://doi.org/10.1377/hlthaff.2010.0420

Order of Saint Benedict. (n.d.). *The rule of Saint Benedict*. Retrieved July 30, 2014, from https://www.solesmes.com/sites/default/files/upload/pdf/rule_of_st_benedict.pdf

Prislin, M., Saultz, J., & Geyman, J. (2010). The generalist disciplines in American medicine one hundred years following the Flexner Report: A case study of unintended consequences and some proposals for post-Flexnerian reform. *Academic Medicine, 85*, 228–235. https://doi.org/10.1097/ACM.0b013e3181c877bf

Rau, J. (2012). *Medicare to penalize 2,217 hospitals for excess readmissions*. Kaiser Health News. Retrieved August 5, 2014, from http://www.kaiserhealthnews.org/Stories/2012/August/13/medicare-hospitals-readmissions-penalties.aspx

Rau, J. (2019, October 1). *New round of Medicare readmission penalties hits 2,582 hospitals*. Kaiser Health News. https://khn.org/news/hospital-readmission-penalties-medicare-2583-hospitals/

Rau, J. (2021). *10 Years of hospital readmission penalties*. Kaiser Family Foundation. https://www.kff.org/health-reform/slide/10-years-of-hospital-readmissions-penalties/

Shahriar, A., Puram, V., Miller, J., Sagi, V., Prasad, S., Castanon-Gonzalez, L., & Crichlow, R. (2022). Socioeconomic diversity of the matriculating US medical students by race, ethnicity and sex, 2017–2019. *JAMA Network Open, 5*(3), e222621. https://doi.org/10.1001/jamanetworkopen.2022.2621

Stahnisch, F., & Verhoef, M. (2012). The Flexner Report of 1910 and its impact on complementary and alternative medicine and psychiatry in North America in the 20th century. *Evidence-Based Complementary and Alternative Medicine, 2012*, 647896. https://doi.org/10.1155/2012/647896

Starr, P. (1982). *The social transformation of American medicine: The rise of a sovereign profession and the making of a vast industry*. Basic Books.

Sultz, H., & Young, K. (2011). Hospitals: Origin, organization, and performance. In J. G. Carroll (Ed.), *Health care USA: Understanding its organization and delivery* (7th ed.). Jones and Bartlett Learning.

Yakusheva, O., & Rambur, B. (2023). *How the hospital reimbursement model harms nursing quality—and what to do about it*. Health Affairs Forefront. https://www.healthaffairs.org/content/forefront/hospital-reimbursement-model-harms-nursing-quality-and-do

CHAPTER 3

Navigating the Health Care Landscape Shaped by the Patient Protection and Affordable Care Act of 2010, Subsequent Federal Legislation and Judicial Action

CHAPTER 3 details the Patient Protection and Affordable Care Act (ACA) of 2010 and subsequent key health care federal legislation. These include the 2015 Medicare Access and CHIP Reauthorization Act (MACRA); the 21st Century Cures Act of 2016; the Tax Cuts and Jobs Act (TCJA) of 2017; the Opioid Crisis Response Act of 2018; the Consolidated Appropriations Act (CAA) of 2023, and one major component of it, the Inflation Reduction Act of 2023. Relevant federal Supreme Court reviews and decisions are also described as well as historic laws that impact insurance reform, specifically, the Employer Retirement Income Security Act (ERISA) of 1974.

Following completion of this chapter, you will be able to:

- Detail insurance reform elements of the ACA.
- Discuss aspects of the ACA designed to increase Americans' access to health care insurance as well as transparency of the U.S. system.
- Discuss aspects of the ACA designed to address health care costs.
- Describe significant federal post-ACA legislation.
- Consider the impact of federal court decisions relevant to the ACA and other U.S. policies.

THE PATIENT PROTECTION AND AFFORDABLE CARE ACT OF 2010

The Patient Protection and ACA of 2010, colloquially known as "Obamacare," is the most sweeping piece of health care legislation passed since the initiation of Medicare and Medicaid in 1965. It is also poorly understood by many Americans and is often supported or decried without firm understanding by those voicing a verdict. At heart, the provisions within the ACA are not partisan issues, although they are often cast as such. Although both the 1965 and

2010 reforms passed while there was a Democrat in the White House, many presidents have taken up the issue of reform, including Republican President Richard Nixon. Indeed, Nixon supported a much more radical option than the ACA. It was, for example, inclusive of "a public option" whereby individuals could opt into a public payer, a feature initially in the ACA but removed following an outcry led by the insurance industry and conservatives, who perceived it as a first step toward a single-payer system (Halpin & Harbage, 2010). Although there was widespread momentum for the Nixon plan at the time, the Watergate scandal put an end to this effort. Stuart Altman, one of the architects of reform in both Democratic and Republican administrations, notes: "Had the Nixon plan passed, the level of opposition would have been much, much less than it is today. It would have become the law of the land, and it would've been every bit as accepted as Medicare is today" (Health Affairs, 2012, para 13). Yet the impetus for change did not start with Nixon. Instead, the need for change, rooted in a sense of crisis, has been ongoing for 50 years and is "still going strong" (Millenson, 2018).

What It Is Not

The ACA is not socialized medicine. In socialized medicine, the health care facilities are owned by the government and health care workers are governmental employees. Examples in the United States that fit this definition are the Veterans Affairs and Indian Health Services, whose services are limited to veterans and American Indians, respectively. An international example is Britain's National Health Service, a system currently ranked fourth among 11 wealthy nations, as the United States constantly ranks last (Schneider et al., 2021). Other nations achieve universal access to insurance coverage using private approaches rather than governmental approaches. Switzerland (ranked ninth) and the Netherlands (ranked second), for example, have an individual mandate, meaning people must have health insurance that they obtain from regulated, private insurance companies. Germany (ranked fifth) has an employer-based health care system in which both employers and employees each pay roughly 7.5% in a multipayer system that covers all citizens. Canada (ranked tenth) has a publicly funded single-payer system; however, unlike Great Britain, most hospitals are owned by charitable, religious organizations or nonprofit organizations, and most providers are not public employees. Thus, although publicly funded, Canadian health services are privately delivered and, like in the United States, are largely reimbursed through *fee-for-service*, a payment mechanism that will be discussed in detail in later chapters. In summary, there is not a single approach to ensuring access to health insurance (termed *universal coverage*), and access to health insurance does not necessarily ensure access to needed health care. Nevertheless, it is a key step, as most people cannot bear the financial burden of contemporary health care without some mechanism to mitigate the cost.

Although international rankings shift, the U.S. consistently ranks last among wealthy nations and, unlike other wealthy nations, does not guarantee access to insurance to all Americans. The ACA aimed to address this gap and builds on the U.S. model of *public and private financing* for a largely *privately delivered system* (see Box 3.1 for definitions of public and private).

If Not Socialized Medicine, What Is It Then?

The ACA is a hybrid model toward universal access to health insurance, built on the existing U.S. financing model that is a mix of public and private payers. It also has provisions for greater transparency in the U.S. health care system and authority to test new payment models. But first, why is it important that everyone is insured?

As the COVID-19 pandemic graphically illustrated, illness does not assess insurance status before striking, and health care workers, including nurses, legitimately want and deserve to be paid for the work they do. Moreover, the pandemic demonstrated the importance of ensuring that everyone has access to needed medical care, not only for their own well-being but also for the good of all. This is not just a humanitarian ideal; it is pragmatic. This pragmatism is not just health related but also economic. Recall that care for the uninsured does not provide any compensation to those hospitals and clinicians who serve them. These expenses don't disappear. Instead, they are transferred to those with commercial insurance for payment through the cost shift (recall Figure 1.4). So how does the ACA attempt to ensure that all Americans have a mechanism to defray the financial impact of seeking health care?

 BOX 3.1

UNDERSTANDING PUBLIC AND PRIVATE CONFIGURATIONS IN HEALTH CARE

Publicly Financed	Privately Financed
Revenue for health care services are derived from taxes	Revenues for health care services are derived from individuals/families and employers who pay premiums to insurance companies
Publicly Delivered	**Privately Delivered**
Health care services are delivered by health care workers, including nurses, who are employees of the government	Health care services are delivered by health care workers, including nurses, who are employed by the organization they work for

Note: Private organizations (right-hand column) such as insurance companies and health care organizations can be nonprofit or for-profit. In the case of the latter, the mission includes returning dividends to company stockholders.

The ACA can be conceptualized as three main components: insurance market reform to facilitate access to health care insurance, strategies for transparency (further detailed in Chapter 6) and testing of delivery innovation through payment reform (detailed in Chapter 4).

INSURANCE ACCESS—EMPLOYER MANDATES AND MEDICAID EXPANSION

The ACA, as initially passed, required that everyone have health insurance. As previously detailed, the U.S. health system has evolved as an *employer-based system*, meaning that most Americans who have commercial (nongovernmental) insurance obtain it through their employer. The ACA imposed an employer mandate; employers with more than 50 full-time employees (30 hours/week or more) must offer health insurance or face a financial penalty. Although it was predicted by some, including the Congressional Budget Office, that this element of the law would lead to a reduction in full-time employees as employers attempt to elude the mandate, some evidence to date does not support this prediction (Anots & Capretta, 2016; Van de Water, 2018). Conversely, Dillender et al. (2022) report that this provision of the ACA resulted in an increase of low-hours, involuntary part-time employment for 500,000 to 700,000 workers in selected industries that can circumvent the mandate, for example, food services and retail.

The ACA also retained the governmental payers started in the 1960s: Medicare and Medicaid. As passed, the ACA required all states to raise their Medicaid eligibility to 133% of the federal poverty level (FPL), set at $41,496.00 for a family of four in 2024. As a federal program largely under state control, this provision of the ACA did not withstand the Supreme Court decision in June 2012. Specifically, the ACA's federal requirement that states expand Medicaid to at least 133% of FPL to receive any matching federal funds was deemed to be unconstitutionally coercive of states. Thus, in contrast to the original intent of the law, Medicaid eligibility expansion is optional for states rather than mandatory (Kaiser Family Foundation [KFF], 2012). (A vote to strike down the entire ACA at that time was not supported in the June 2012 Supreme Court ruling, in a 4–5 vote.)

Medicaid expansion has been polarized largely along partisan lines, with the so-called "blue states" (Democratic and/or liberal) largely supportive and "red states" (Republican and/or conservative) offering more opposition. Over time, however, many states that initially did not expand Medicaid have chosen to do so, in some cases through a popular vote ballot initiative to circumvent reluctant legislators or governors. As this book goes to press, 40 states and the District of Columbia have expanded Medicaid and 10 have not (KFF, 2024). An updated interactive map can be found at https://www.kff.org/medicaid/issue-brief/status-of-state-medicaid-expansion-decisions-interactive-map.

COVID-19 created new incentives for states that had not expanded Medicaid to do so (Mann, 2020), and in July 2020 following a statewide vote, Oklahoma became the first state to expand Medicaid during the pandemic. Passing by less than one percentage point, the statewide vote created a new article in the Oklahoma state constitution that allowed adults with incomes up to 133% of FPL to be eligible. Nationwide, it was anticipated that more Americans will be eligible for and accept Medicaid due to COVID-induced job losses. Indeed, in the first months of the pandemic—February to May 2020—5.4 million laid-off workers became uninsured (Dorn, 2020). Congress passed the Family First Coronavirus Response Act (FFCRA) in 2020. This act required that the nation's Medicaid programs maintain coverage until the end of the COVID-19 public health emergency (PHE), ensuring continuous coverage for those on Medicaid at that time. This coverage provision ended with the enactment of the Consolidated Appropriation Act of 2023, a law that will be discussed in greater depth later in this chapter. An anticipated 8 to 24 million people were projected to lose their Medicaid coverage, and different states launched varying strategies to address those individuals who are now newly uninsured (Tolbert & Ammula, 2023). As such, the ultimate impact of the end of this provision is unclear as this book goes to press. Coleman (2023) reports that as of July 2023, 3.8 million people have lost their Medicaid coverage when the PHE ended. Prior to this massive disenrollment, however, the uninsured rate in the United States was at the lowest ever, reaching 7.7% among all U.S. residents in early 2023 (Assistant Secretary for Planning and Evaluation [ASPE], 2023).

AFFORDABLE CARE ACT STRATEGIES TO EXPAND ACCESS TO HEALTH CARE THROUGH INSURANCE ELIGIBILITY REFORMS

Of course, people prefer lower monthly premiums, so those insurance policies with lower cost premiums have a competitive advantage over those with higher premiums. One way a group's health care insurance premiums can be kept low is to exclude those with known health conditions from the insurance pool. Prior to the passage of the ACA, strategies to limit the cost of an insurance product through exclusion of some people were allowed. These were (a) *preexisting health condition exclusions*, meaning that if individuals have a health condition or have had a health condition when they apply for insurance and that condition is judged to make them liable to need extensive and/or expensive health care, they may be excluded from an insurance group, termed *denied coverage*, and (b) limits on how much insurance companies will pay over a lifetime, called *lifetime caps*. This can pose real problems if a person or family is suddenly faced with a catastrophe with ongoing health consequences or if they have chronic conditions and reach the cap. Although these strategies can keep a group's insurance premium lower, it denies health insurance to those in greatest need of care, which violates the very rationale for insurance in the first place.

The ACA has addressed these and other elements of the way health insurance has worked in the United States. The ACA requires insurance companies to remove the lifetime caps on the amount that can be paid for the care of an individual. It also ends the provisions that allowed insurance companies to deny insurance to an individual based on a preexisting health condition. This opens the opportunity for those previously uninsurable to be able to access health insurance. The ACA also allows adult children to stay on their parent's health insurance policy up to the age of 26, even when they are not dependents for income tax purposes, in college, or are married. Other provisions limit the difference between the least expensive and most expensive insurance premium, called *rating bands*, to one to three and removed gender as an insurance rating factor. Some states had already removed gender as a potential rating factor, but in those that had not, health insurance for young women could be much more expensive than that for a health- and age-matched male because of the women's potential "experience" of pregnancy. Overall, these ACA provisions increase access to health insurance, but they do not inherently decrease the overall cost of insurance. Nor does health insurance ensure access to care. Instead, these are strategies to enhance access to health insurance to mitigate financial disincentives to care.

WHAT ABOUT THOSE WHO ARE STILL NOT COVERED BY ONE OF THESE MECHANISMS?

The ACA represented a policy directed toward ensuring that all citizens are covered by one or a combination of the forms of insurance coverage listed in Figure 1.4. As such, it is a *hybrid financing model* with multiple payers. As initially passed, individuals who are not covered by Medicare or Medicaid were required to have commercial insurance. This requirement is termed a *mandate*. In addition to the *employer mandates* already described, there are *individual mandates*.

Individual Mandates

As originally passed, an individual who does not have employer-based insurance, Medicare, or Medicaid is required to have insurance or, similar to the employer mandate, pay a penalty. The individual mandate survived a 2012 Supreme Court challenge to its constitutionality and remains the law of the land as this text goes to press. However, the TCJA of 2017 dramatically modified the impact of this portion of the law. Although individual mandates remain in the ACA, the TCJA changed the penalty for not having insurance to zero dollars, thereby invalidating this portion of the ACA. Subsequently, a Texas federal trial court judge ruled that this in turn invalidates the entire ACA (KFF, 2019). At stake was the issue of *severability;* that is, can a portion of the ACA be severed and the remainder of the ACA stay intact? This consideration became the basis of a federal case filed by the attorneys general of 18 Republican states and the Trump administration, who argued that the entire ACA must be struck down now that the individual mandate was effectively nullified. If the ACA were ever to be fully struck down, key elements of the law, such as the provision that children can stay on their parents' health insurance until age 26 and the removal of gender as a rating factor would no longer be the law of the land, but instead subject to insurance regulation in each state. The U.S. Supreme Court agreed to hear this case and did so on November 10, 2020. In July 2021 the Supreme Court ruled that the challengers "lacked standing" (Center on Budget and Policy Priorities [CBPP], n.d., para 1). A full review of this decision can be found at https://www.cbpp.org/research/health/aca-survives-legal-challenge-protecting-coverage-for-tens-of-millions. Table 3.1 details the major elements of the ACA and any subsequent modifications. Again, note that if the ACA were ever to be struck down, insurance companies would not be subject to the ACA provisions, although a state may enact some or all of them. In the latter situation—state regulation of insurance companies—a different federal law, the ERISA, prevents state laws from governing employer-based health insurance, the most common form of nongovernmental insurance in the United States. This "dilutes states' ability to enact cost-control reforms" (McCuskey, 2023, para 1). Revision of ERISA is again emerging as a potential bipartisan area of consideration and support. See Box 3.2 for a summary of ERISA.

What About Individuals Who Cannot Afford to Comply With the Individual Mandate?

What about those who cannot afford to purchase health insurance? The ACA also has provisions for financial assistance to help those who cannot afford the cost of insurance. This form of financial assistance is called a *subsidy.* In addition, the law includes provisions that create the opportunity for individuals to better understand what they are buying when they purchase health insurance. To help individuals make the best choice for themselves in terms of both cost and coverage, the law also includes the *health insurance marketplace,* typically referred to as *health care exchanges.* The exchange is actually a menu of options designed to enable individuals and small businesses to see what insurance packages are available and compare cost and other trade-offs. Despite the rocky rollout of the exchanges due to the complexities of the technological interfaces and demands, the overall concept behind the exchanges is simple: comparison as a basis for choice.

TABLE 3.1 SUMMARY OF THE PATIENT PROTECTION AND AFFORDABLE CARE ACT OF 2010

ACA as Initially Passed	Rationale/Comments	Modifications, Updates, or Mechanism of Change, If Any
Enhanced Access to Health Insurance		
Employer mandate	Builds on existing employer-based system, but adds the requirement that all employers of 50 or more employees provide adequate and affordable health insurance coverage to their employees or pay a fine to the federal government.	
Medicaid expansion	Builds on a system in place since 1965; aimed to create more uniformity across states. Initially a requirement to access federal matching fund.	Eliminated following Supreme Court decision (2012).
Individual mandate	Builds on existing system to ensure that all have health insurance, given that uninsured (charity care) costs are shifted to those with commercial insurance and those without health insurance may have a financial barrier to access.	Survived a Supreme Court review of its constitutionality (2012), but the Tax Cuts and Jobs Act (2017) modified it so the penalty for not having health insurance is $0.[a]
Insurers cannot deny insurance coverage based on a preexisting condition	Although preexisting condition exclusions create a lower-cost insurance pool for others, they deny insurance to those who have been ill and are potentially in the most need. This was already law in many states; the ACA made it law for all states.	
Removal of lifetime caps on insurance coverage	Although lifetime caps create a lower-cost insurance pool for others, they deny insurance coverage to those who have been ill and are potentially in the most need	

Children can stay on their parent's health insurance policy until age 26, even if they are no longer dependents for insurance coverage or are married	A very popular provision that may reflect that young adults, including those with college degrees, may not be employed or are employed without benefits and thus cannot access employer-based insurance.
1:3 insurance band ratings based on age in the small business (fewer than 50 employees) and individual markets, meaning the difference between the lowest-cost and highest-cost premium component related to age, can only be three-fold	Creates less expensive insurance for those insurance groups who are older, for example, near Medicare eligibility and, in general, have more health conditions; creates higher-cost insurance for the young/healthy. Many states had already instituted rate bands to minimize the rate differences for older or higher-risk groups. The ACA made this a federal rule applying to all states.
Eliminates health status as a rating factor in the small group and individual markets	This provision prohibits insurers from charging those with poor health more than those with better health. The only exception noted is that insurers are allowed to increase rates for those who use tobacco.
Removes gender as a rating factor, meaning, as one example, a young woman's health insurance will not be more expensive than a man's because of the potential for pregnancy costs	Some states already eliminated gender as a rating factor. The ACA made it federal law.
Maximum out-of-pocket (MOOP) limits for health insurance products purchased on the exchange	Allows families to know the maximum costs they will incur in a given year.

(continued)

TABLE 3.1 SUMMARY OF THE PATIENT PROTECTION AND AFFORDABLE CARE ACT OF 2010 (continued)

ACA as Initially Passed	Rationale/Comments	Modifications, Updates, or Mechanism of Change, If Any
Premium tax credit creates a discounted monthly premium on a sliding scale based on income	Available to those purchasing on the health insurance exchange only.	
Subsidies for those who cannot afford out-of-pocket expenses for insurance products, termed CSRs	Lowers the cost of health care for eligible low-income individuals through reduced deductibles, copayments, and coinsurance.	Funding halted by the Trump administration on October 12, 2017, but insurance companies were still obligated to provide the financial support. Litigation ensued, and the Federal Circuit agreed with lower courts that Section 1402 provided "unambiguous obligation" on the part of the government to make CSR payments.
Establishment of health insurance marketplace (aka, "exchange"). Different iterations range from those in states that developed their own exchange, to state-based exchanges that used the federal IT platform, to the federally facilitated exchange, Healthcare.gov	The ACA requires that business and individuals have health insurance, yet making the best selection is challenging. The exchanges were to serve as an online "marketplace."	The various kinds of exchanges became a focus in the second Supreme Court review of the ACA, due to language in the original law directing tax subsidies to those in state exchanges, designed to help poor and middle-class people afford health insurance. In June 2015 the court ruled 6–3 that the intention of the law was also to include those in federally facilitated exchanges.
Transparency/Accountability		
Sunshine Act	Requires product manufacturers to report to CMS any payments or transfer of value to physicians and teaching hospitals in recognition that people have a right to know if their health care provider is financially connected to a recommendation they are making.	

Shared decision-making	Providers and patients work together to make health care decisions that are aligned with the patient's values and aims, with clear understanding of the pros and cons of treatment and other options, including watchful waiting.	
Community benefit	Formalizes the process by which nonprofit hospitals increase their relationship with the health needs of their community. A formal "community health needs assessment process" must be conducted for the hospital to be tax exempt. (See Rosenbaum et al., n.d., for details on the history and update.)	The tax-exempt status of hospitals has increasingly been questioned by policy makers, following data finding that a proportion of hospitals receive this favorable tax treatment without providing any community benefit. In 2023, leading Republican and Democratic senators asked the IRS to assess if hospitals are misusing their tax exempt status and not meeting their corollary responsibilities to their communities.
Metal levels and essential benefits	It can be difficult to understand what one is purchasing when selecting a health insurance plan. The ACA requires that all insurance products include "essential benefits." Products on the exchange must include these but do vary on the amount of cost sharing by the consumer: 40% cost sharing for bronze (actuarial value, i.e., AV of 60%); 30% cost sharing for silver (AV = 70%) 20% cost sharing for gold (AV-80%), and 10% cost sharing for platinum (90% AV).	Remains in the law, but an administrative rule now allows states to determine what constitutes "essential benefits" for insurance products sold within their borders. In 2024, dental care could also be considered an essential benefit at the discretion of the individual state.
Medical loss ratio	Lauded as a major consumer protection element of the ACA (Hall & McCue, 2019), insurance companies that cover individuals and small businesses are required to spend at least 80% of their premiums on health care claims and quality improvement. The remaining 20% may be used for marketing, administrative costs, and profits or contribution to reserves. In large group insurance markets, 85% is required to go the claims or quality improvement.	

(continued)

TABLE 3.1 SUMMARY OF THE PATIENT PROTECTION AND AFFORDABLE CARE ACT OF 2010 (continued)

ACA as Initially Passed	Rationale/Comments	Modifications, Updates, or Mechanism of Change, If Any
Stabilization of the individual and small group insurance market	The ACA required that insurance companies now cover all who apply. Although actuaries can predict costs with a high degree of accuracy when they have historical trend data (a measure of the amount and types of services used in the past), this was not possible when the law was newly enacted. Stabilizers were put in place for the first several years of the Affordable Care Act to ensure the insurance companies remained solvent (did not go bankrupt or be unable to reimburse claims for services used) and to encourage them to offer products on the exchange. These stabilizers are reinsurance, risk corridors and risk adjustment. See Table 3.2 for details.	
Quality-Focused Initiatives		
Medicare Shared Savings Program—Accountable Care organizations	Creates incentives for attention to outcomes of care as well as cost.	Ongoing, with increasing emphasis on the need for provider risk-bearing that is, accountability for outcomes *and* cost.
Hospital value-based purchasing	Goal is to better align payment with quality and avoid financially rewarding hospitals for cost consequences they created (for example, surgical site infection; also addressed the patient experience and cost). This program is detailed in Chapter 6.	
Hospital-Acquired Condition Reduction Program	Goal is to better align payment with quality and avoid financially rewarding hospitals for negative patient and cost consequences they created. The program is detailed in Chapter 6.	

Hospital-Readmission Reduction Program	Goal is to better align payment with quality and avoid financially rewarding hospitals for negative patient and cost consequences they created, specifically, too early discharge without adequate planning and postacute support. This program is detailed in Chapter 6.	
Quality improvement and cost reduction testing of new models of payment and delivery—Establishment of CMMI	Many of the strategies listed previously largely address insurance access and insurance market reform; only a few address the quality and overall cost of health care. Instead, this is addressed by testing new models of paying for services, which in turn spawns new models of care.	This area is in rapid evolution. What follows is a summary overview of some of the initiatives with a direct genesis in the ACA.
State innovation model	Creates an opportunity for states to develop and try out new models of payment and care delivery. They are multipayer or all payer in scope.	A total of 34 states, three territories, and the District of Columbia, impacting 61% of the U.S. population. Complex and diverse approaches, responding to the needs and opportunities for improved care and lowered costs in different states. See https://www.cms.gov/priorities/innovation/where-innovation-happening for details
Patient-centered medical homes	Goal is to transform and strengthen primary care. The Agency for Healthcare Research and Quality at CMS defines the PCMH as having five main features: • Comprehensive care • Patient-centered • Coordinated care • Improved access to services • Commitment to quality and safety	

(continued)

TABLE 3.1 SUMMARY OF THE PATIENT PROTECTION AND AFFORDABLE CARE ACT OF 2010 (continued)

ACA as Initially Passed	Rationale/Comments	Modifications, Updates, or Mechanism of Change, If Any
Comprehensive primary care	Goal is to transform and strengthen primary care through provider–payer partnerships; program offered participating physician practices enhanced payment, technical assistance, and performance feedback	
Bundled payments	Goal is to better coordinate an episode of care among diverse providers; to improve outcomes; and to reduce waste, redundancies, and cost.	
ACO Realizing Equity, Access, and Community Health (ACO REACH)	Launched in 2025, REACH aims to support health equity by bringing benefits of accountable care to Medicare beneficiaries in underserved areas.	
Guiding an Improved Dementia Experience Model (GUIDE)	Launched in 2024, GUIDE aims to reduce strain on unpaid care givers and improve quality of life for those with dementia and their caregivers.	
Other		
Tax on tanning beds		
An excise tax on high AV plans, also called "the Cadillac Tax"		A 40% tax on employer-sponsored care that exceeds a certain amount, designed to slow cost growth. The implementation date was repeatedly pushed back, and it was eventually repealed.

CLASS Plan	A publicly administered, voluntary, long-term care insurance program.	Never fully developed or administered. Repealed in 2013.
Establishment of the National Health Care Workforce Commission	Better align health workforce development with the nation's health needs.	Never funded and thus not implemented. The designated chair was to be nurse economist, Peter Buerhaus.
Community health benefit requirement for tax-exempt hospitals	Private tax-exempt hospitals are exempt from federal, state, and local taxes, yet their community value for this $24 billion expenditure has been questioned by policy makers. The ACA requires these hospitals to conduct community health needs assessments every 3 years; the intention is to direct more resources to community/population health needs.	Remains in the law. Data suggest that community benefit spending has changed little (Young et al., 2018) and that nonprofit health care organizations do not necessarily provide more charity care/community benefit than for-profit health care.

Notes: The author acknowledges the helpful suggestions of Elizabeth Howlett in the development of this table.

This table is not intended to be a full account of the ACA, and others may conceptualize the components in a different manner. It is designed to help the reader grasp the expanse of this law and further their understanding of the law and contemporary policy issues.

ACA, Affordable Care Act; AV, actuarial value; CLASS, Community Living Assistance Services and Supports; CMMI, Centers for Medicare and Medicaid Innovation; CMS, Centers for Medicare & Medicaid Services; CSRs, cost-sharing reductions; MOOP, maximum out of pocket; PCMH, patient-centered medical home.

Sources: Rosenbaum, S., Byrnes, M., & Hurt, N. (n.d.). *Community benefit and the ACA a brief history and update.* https://nchh.org/resource-library/HCF_CBACA%20overview.pdf; Young, G. J., Flaherty, S., Zepeda, D., Singh, S. R., & Cramer, G. R. (2018). *Community benefit spending By tax-exempt hospitals changed little after ACA* https://www.healthaffairs.org/doi/10.13//hlthaff.2017.1028.

BOX 3.2

WHAT IS ERISA?

ERISA stands for the Employer Income Security Act, which passed in 1974. The law was intended to protect the retirement assets of American workers but had unforeseen impacts on a state's capacity to contain health care costs. McCuskey (2023) notes that this law creates a situation in which state health reform "remains subject to one of the broadest federal preemptions in any area of the law . . . even when those laws do not directly conflict with federal requirements" (para 5). For example, a state may pass a law requiring that health care insurance claims be submitted to an all-payer claims database (APCD) to support state tracking of health cost trends. Employer-based health insurance plans do not need to follow this state law, as it is preempted under ERISA. This orientation was further codified in the 2016 *Gobeille v. Liberty Mutual Insurance Company*. In their 6–2 Supreme Court decision, the Court ruled that ERISA superseded existing state law that required submission to an APCD. This ruling had broad, largely negative consequences for health care cost control, transparency, and quality improvement (Fuse Brown & King, 2016). The exponentially growing concern about health care costs, however, has created political space for consideration of a range of potential ways to revise ERISA (see McCuskey, 2023 for details).

WHAT DOES THE HEALTH CARE EXCHANGE DO?

Comparing health insurance plans can be confusing. Therefore, to be sure there are apples-to-apples comparisons, each plan must cover the same set of basic benefits. These basic, core benefits are termed *essential health benefits* (see Box 3.3). The essential health benefits also include some elements of prevention and screening that must be provided at no charge to the patient, meaning the financial disincentives to use these services have been removed. The definition of what services must be included is an important one; prior to this requirement, an individual may have purchased less expensive health insurance, only to find it was less expensive because it did not cover many services and left the person unexpectedly responsible for services they received. During the Obama era, the law was initially interpreted to mean that each state must have the same essential benefits for insurance plans sold within their borders. The Trump administration promulgated an administrative rule that allows states to determine their own essential health benefits, arguing that this allows more tailored plans. Conversely, opponents of this change raised concerns about insufficient coverage as well as variability among states. Indeed, states who opted to determine what constitutes essential benefits for insurance products sold in their states did so in remarkably different ways, as illustrated in the first two states to pursue this option: Alabama and Illinois. Alabama proposed reducing the prescription drugs that plans must cover, with the stated intention of decreasing costs and mitigating the opioid epidemic. Illinois proposed the coverage of alternative chronic pain treatment

BOX 3.3

ESSENTIAL HEALTH BENEFITS REQUIRED BY THE AFFORDABLE CARE ACT

Ambulatory patient services

Chronic disease management

Emergency services

Hospitalizations

Laboratory tests

Maternity and newborn care

Mental health and substance use disorder services, including behavioral health treatment (this includes counseling and psychotherapy)

Pediatric services

Prescription drugs

Preventive services

Rehabilitative services and devices

Source: HealthCare.gov. (n.d.). *What marketplace health insurance plans cover.* https://www.healthcare.gov/what-does-marketplace-health-insurance-cover.

---

and expanded access to mental health services via telehealth (Livingston, 2018). Since passage of the ACA, the health care landscape has been dramatically altered by COVID-19, a greater use of digital care, an increase in the use of providers who are not physicians, including nurse practitioners (NPs), and a greater recognition of the impact of social determinants of health. An update of what constitutes "essential" health benefits is under consideration (Jost, 2023) and in April 2024 CMS announced expanded essential benefit policies that allow states the option of adding adult routine dental services, among other updates (U.S. Department of Health and Human Services [USDHHS], 2024). Notably, because determination of essential benefits is now held by the states, states would need to act to allow or require adult dental services to be an essential benefit in that state (Burroughs et al., 2024).

The ACA also requires that insurance companies cover a range of preventative services without patient cost sharing in the form of copayments, deductibles, or co-insurance. These have been modified over time, following recommendations of the U.S. Preventive Services Task Force, an independent panel of scientists and physicians, and the Advisory Committee on Immunization Practices, a federal committee of immunization experts. Covered services fall within four broad categories: evidence-based screenings and counseling, routine immunizations, preventative services for women, and preventative services for youth and children (see https://www.kff.org/womens-health-policy/fact-sheet/preventive-services-covered-by-private-health-plans for a detailed summary of services).

When Health Insurance Plans Have the Same Essential Benefits, What Is Different Among Them?

Although the ACA required that minimum health benefits be the same, what does differ among the options is the balance between monthly premiums and associated *cost sharing*, that is, the amount that a person enrolled in that plan would pay out of pocket. Lower monthly premium plans will have higher patient *out-of-pocket cost sharing* (copayments at the time the patient uses health care services, deductibles that must be reached before insurance coverage starts, and co-insurance, a percentage of cost paid when using health services). Because of their name—*bronze, silver, gold,* and *platinum*—the different categories of essential health benefit plans within the exchange are sometimes termed *metals* or *metal levels*.

To underscore, these metals differ not in the minimum services that are covered, but rather in how individuals choose to balance the cost of care they use. Platinum, for example, has the highest monthly premium but the lowest out-of-pocket expense when using services. Bronze has the lowest monthly premium of the metals but the highest out-of-pocket expenses when using health services. There is even a term for the average proportion of health care that is paid for by the individual out of pocket. This term, *actuarial value*, is set at roughly 60%, 70%, 80%, and 90% for bronze, silver, gold, and platinum, respectively. So, for example, a bronze plan pays for 60% of services used; platinum pays for 90%. As a result, in a bronze plan, the person using health services would pay roughly 40% out-of-pocket but only 10% in a platinum plan. Recall, however, that the platinum plan will have a higher monthly premium that is paid regardless of health services used.

So, why would anyone choose a bronze plan? The trade-off is in the ongoing cost of the monthly premium, which is lowest in the bronze plan. Young persons who are betting that they will not need health services may choose a bronze plan with the lowest monthly premiums, seeing that as a better value than paying higher monthly insurance premiums for care they do not expect to use. Conversely, persons with any chronic conditions may choose to pay more each month, the platinum plan, for example, because they know that they use a lot of health care services and want the reassurance that 90% will be covered, especially if that is 90% of a very large health care bill. *Premium subsidies* and *cost-sharing subsidies*, the latter termed *cost-sharing reductions* (*CSRs*), were a provision of the ACA designed to help financially needy people pay the difference between their expected contribution to insurance and what they actually pay. Premium subsidies are provided to income-eligible people in the exchange, and CSRs are for the lowest-income people who are above the Medicaid eligibility threshold. By law, the subsidies are *benchmarked to silver*, meaning you must choose a silver plan to obtain subsidies.

There has been dramatic polarization around the CSR program, with many conservatives decrying this portion of the law, considering the payment illegal because it was appropriated by the executive branch of the government and not Congress (Bryan, 2017). For this and other reasons, there was largely conservative support for President Trump's action to cut CSRs. Conversely, CSRs are supported by many Democrats and at least some moderate Republicans. Both sides of the aisle can agree that health care is too expensive. Thus, it is likely that CSRs will reclaim a place in the national health care debate at some point in time. Rules are complex, with special provisions for American Indians and Alaskan Natives (Fernandez, 2024). A summary is available at https://crsreports.congress.gov/product/pdf/R/R44425.

Are There Other Low-Cost Plans in the Exchange?

There is one more category of health insurance plans in the exchanges required by the ACA. These are termed *catastrophic plans*. These plans also cover the essential health benefits to some degree and emergency care after the deductible is met, but differ from the bronze plans in that catastrophic plans do not cover 60% of the health care costs. Federally funded tax credits and subsidies are not available for individuals covered by catastrophic plans, and participation is limited to those under 30. Individuals over the age of 30 must meet one of two conditions to be eligible for a catastrophe plan: They cannot find coverage for less than 8% of their income (the affordability criterion) or they have experienced a financial hardship such as homelessness, eviction, domestic violence, or a natural disaster; etc. (the hardship criterion) (Healthcare.gov, n.d.-a.).

THE AFFORDABLE CARE ACT AND OUT-OF-POCKET MAXIMUMS

For individuals choosing the bronze, silver, or catastrophic coverage, the decision to keep money in their pocket each month may also be reinforced by another provision of the ACA that sets limits on the total amount of health care costs an individual or family will pay each year. This is termed *maximum out-of-pocket* (MOOP) or *out-of-pocket limits*, set at no more than $9,450 for individuals and $18,900 for a family in 2024. These are reviewed annually by the Internal Revenue Service and typically increased on an annual basis. Note that although a commercial insurance company may have included a MOOP, there was no required limit prior to the ACA. Although the defined MOOP still represents a sizable amount of money, a single hospitalization can far exceed this amount. This, then, would have fallen to the underinsured or uninsured family to pay or would have been a financial loss to the hospital as *charity care* or *bad debt*, the cost of which is shifted to those with commercial insurance (again, review Box 1.4).

OTHER NOTEWORTHY ASPECTS OF THE AFFORDABLE CARE ACT

The ACA includes several other noteworthy provisions. Efforts to stabilize the insurance market were undertaken. Why? Insurance companies were required to take all who applied, and it was impossible for them to predict what that insurance pool would look like (how well or ill new enrollees would be) and, thus, how the insurance products should be priced. Recall that if an insurance company underprices their product, there may be more claims than they can pay. This would result in a drop in reimbursement to health care providers, including those facilities that employ and pay nurses, or the insolvency of the insurance company. The "three Rs"—reinsurance, risk corridors, and risk adjustment—were designed to prevent an insurance company from becoming insolvent. These are described in Table 3.2.

TABLE 3.2 *THE THREE Rs:* REINSURANCE, RISK CORRIDORS, AND RISK ADJUSTMENT

Stabilization Strategy	Rationale and Strategy	Years in Effect
Reinsurance	Designed to protect plans that enroll high-cost individuals; plans are reimbursed for enrollees whose costs exceed a predetermined threshold (termed *attachment point*) up to a predetermined reinsurance cap	2014–2016 (temporary)
Risk corridors	Designed to limit insurance companies' losses and gains beyond an acceptable limit in the early years of the ACA; plans with lower-than-expected claims were required to redistributed funds to companies with higher-than-expected claims	2014–2016 (temporary)
Risk adjustment	Designed to prevent *adverse selection* (aka *cherry picking*) in which insurance plans disproportionately enroll well, low-cost populations; funds are redistributed from plans with lower-risk enrollees to those with higher-risk, and therefore more expensive, enrollees	2014 onward (permanent)

Note: The ACA, as originally passed, required everyone to have health insurance. The provisions of *the three Rs* were put in place to ensure that companies remained financially viable, termed *solvent*, in the early years when they did not have an accurate way to gauge who would purchase their insurance products and how much it would cost to insure their beneficiaries.

ACA, Affordable Care Act.

Source: Adapted from Cox, C., Semanskee, A., Claxton, G., & Levitt, L. (2016, August 17). *Explaining health care reform: Risk adjustment, reinsurance, and risk corridors*. Kaiser Family Foundation. https://www.kff.org/health-reform/issue-brief/explaining-health-care-reform-risk-adjustment-reinsurance-and-risk-corridors.

Notably, risk corridors were the subject of a 2020 Supreme Court decision. This time-limited strategy was deemed essential to stabilize the insurance market by redistributing funds from those insurance plans that earned excessively large profits to those who incurred excessively large losses (Jost, 2016). The goal was to remove disincentives insurers may have about offering products on the exchange, given that they could not know the health status, and thus the cost of coverage, of newly insured individuals. The strategy was modeled on a similar approach that was successful in Medicare Part D, prescription drug coverage, passed during the presidency of George W. Bush. The ACA limited risk corridors to the first 3 years of ACA implementation, yet some Republicans decried the program as an insurance company "bailout" and prohibited the use of tax dollars for funding, which in turn destabilized the program. In April 2020, the Supreme Court, in an 8–1 vote, ruled that Congress ruled that the nation must keep the repayment promise, stating: "These holdings reflect a principle as old as the Nation itself: The Government should honor its obligations" (*Maine Community Health Options v. United States*, 2019).

Two other major provisions of the ACA conceptually align with other major topics in this text: emerging reimbursement models (Chapter 4) and strategies to enhance transparency in the U.S system, specifically the Shared Decision Making and the Sunshine Act, both detailed in Chapter 6. Before we leave Chapter 3, however, please take a moment to again review the basic elements of the ACA detailed in Table 3.1. How many of these aspects were you aware of?

WHERE CAN A NURSE DIRECT A PATIENT WHO ASKS QUESTIONS ABOUT HOW TO NAVIGATE THE COMPLEX TERRAIN OF HEALTH INSURANCE?

Nurses are well-trusted health professionals, and patient education across a range of issues is a core competency of nurses. That said, the decision of which health plan to choose can have enormous consequences for a family; nurses who are asked for advice on health insurance should be prepared with the general knowledge heretofore described, but may—understandably and appropriately—still feel at a loss to provide specific direction. Fortunately, *navigators* have been trained to help people find their way through the health insurance exchange. Nurses can feel confident about referring patients who ask questions about the exchange to these trained navigators. Take a moment to determine where navigators can be found in your region. Some states have also attempted to create user-friendly exchange websites in which individuals can include personal information like income to readily determine which plan would offer them the greatest financial or other advantage, including subsidies and tax credits. Take a moment to review the health insurance exchange website in your state. Similarly, every state has a

State Health Insurance Assistant Program (SHIP). SHIP counselors offer free counseling and assistance to help people chose the best Medicare option for themseles. Information and contacts for individual states may be found at https://www.shiphelp.org/.

INSURANCE LESSONS FROM COVID-19

The many lessons of COVID-19 will be discussed in later sections of this text, but insurance cost implications offer worthy illustration at this point. Recall that people received care whether they were insured or not; costs of the uninsured are shifted to those with commercial insurance. Moreover, Congress banned cost sharing for COVID-19 testing for some plans, and many other plans not required to eliminate cost sharing nevertheless followed this action as a public health priority. Yet these costs don't vanish. Instead, insurers must cover the full costs and shift excessive costs to next year's price hike request. In late spring 2020, insurers in New York, for example, requested an average rate increase of 11.7% for 2021 (Spector, 2020). Conversely, some insurance companies prospered financially during COVID-19, as fewer people sought and used elective health care services during the pandemic (Maddipatla & Humer, 2020). KFF (2023) reports that the average annual cost of employer-sponsored, single-plan health insurance premiums rose from $7,911 in 2022 to $8,435 in 2023 and family plans during that time rose from $22,463 to $23,968. Conversely, median family income dropped during that same time, from $76,330 to $74,580 (Guzman & Kollar, 2023), further illustrating the affordability gap. As Americans "catch up" on care missed during the pandemic, premiums are expected to continue to rise (Roy & Satija, 2024), placing more financial pressure on American families.

OTHER SIGNIFICANT HEALTH CARE LAWS POST ACA

The ACA was the most significant major health care legislation since the passage of Medicare and Medicaid in 1965. It is, however, not the only significant health care legislation.

THE MEDICARE ACCESS AND CHIPS REAUTHORIZATION ACT OF 2015

The Medicare Access and CHIPS Reauthorization Act of 2015 (MACRA) passed with broad bipartisan support. The law replaced a wildly unpopular formula for reimbursement for physicians and others in Medicare Part B, including NPs, with a new model that requires reimbursement via one of two paths: a qualified advanced alternative payment model (Q-APM) or subject to the Merit-Incentive Payment System (MIPS). Both pathways require that providers accept financial risk for the cost of care; qualified advanced alternative payment models are, by definition, risk-bearing. Providers who are in a Q-APM are exempt from MIPS and have received a 5% additional participation bonus (as this text goes to press, the bonus payment is scheduled to sunset at the end of 2024. An act of Congress would be needed to change this). Providers in the MIPS track are not subject to an automatic reimbursement increase. Instead, reimbursement for providers in the MIPS lane is determined by a composite score that, over time, increasingly included financial risk bearing; reimbursement based on MIPS increased over time and could range from −9% to −9%.

The 2024 MIPS weights in the composite score determining payment vary by practice size (Table 3.3).

Physician groups have been vocally negative about the reporting requirement in MIPS and, starting in 2024, a new, more streamlined reporting model, the MIPS Value Pathway, was introduced. Details are available at https://qpp.cms.gov/mips/mips-value-pathways. Note, however, that in all of these models RNs can directly impact payment if they understand the metrics, and NPs are subject to MACRA unless their practice falls below the prescribed threshold of patients.

THE 21ST CENTURY CURES ACT

The U.S. Food and Drug Administration (USFDA) states that the 21st Century Cures Act of 2016 is "designed to help accelerate medical product development and bring new innovations and advances to patients who need them faster and more efficiently" (USFDA, 2020, para 1). In addition to the development of coordinating intercenter institutes, expedited options for eligible biologic products (the Regenerative Medicine Advanced Therapy initiative) and innovative medical devices (the Breakthrough Devices Program) are a key focus, at a cost of $500 million over 9 years (USFDA, 2020).

TABLE 3.3 MIPS WEIGHTS

Standard MIPS Weights	Standard MIPS Weights for Small Practices
Quality—30%	Quality—40%
Cost—30%	Cost—30%
Improvement activities—15%	Improvement activities—30%
Promoting intraoperatively—25%	Improving interoperability—0%

MIPS, Merit-Incentive Payment System.

THE OPIOID CRISIS RESPONSE ACT OF 2018

The bill emerged from clear congressional consensus on the need for legislation to address the U.S. opioid epidemic. It included legislation that (a) requires the U.S Postal Service to prevent the flow illegal drugs to the United States: the Synthetics Trafficking and Overdose Prevention Act or STOP Act; (b) requires the FDA to package opioids in limited amounts, for example, 3 to 7 days; (c) provides financial support for comprehensive recovery centers; and (d) develops an interagency task force on trauma-informed care, including recommendations for best practices for children and youth as well as babies born in opioid withdrawal. The law builds on the previous Comprehensive Addiction and Recovery Act (CARA) that allowed qualified NPs and PAs to receive waivers to prescribe buprenorphine in office-based settings through October 2021. Such regulatory language was needed because the original waivers for prescribing medication-assisted treatment was for physicians with limited panels of people being treated by these physicians. The temporary CARA provision was made permanent in 2018 in the Substance Use Disorder Prevention that Promotes Opioid Recovery and Treatment (SUPPORT) Act. Section 3201 of the SUPPORT Act made the authority permanent for nurse practitioners (NPs) and physician assistants (PAs) and then granted certified nurse midwives, clinical nurse specialists, and certified registered nurse anesthestists the 5-year temporary authority that NPs and PAs received in CARA. Section 1262 of the CAA of 2023 (to be discussed shortly) removed many of the barriers that impeded providers, including NPs, from providing medication-assisted treament (MAT) for people with opiod use disorder (see Box 3.4). See Leveille and Rambur (2024) for a history of nurses and MAT.

BOX 3.4

PRESCRIBING OF BUPRENORPHINE FOR TREATMENT OF OPIOID USE DISORDER

"Section 1262 of the 'Consolidated Appropriations Act of 2023 (PDF | 3.8 MB)' removes the federal requirement for practitioners to apply for a special waiver prior to prescribing buprenorphine for the treatment of opioid use disorder. It also removes other federal requirements associated with the waiver such as discipline restrictions, patient limits, and certification related to provision of counseling. Separately, section 1263 of the 'Consolidated Appropriations Act of 2023 (PDF | 3.8 MB)' requires new or renewing Drug Enforcement Administration (DEA) registrants,

(continued)

BOX 3.4

PRESCRIBING OF BUPRENORPHINE FOR TREATMENT OF OPIOID USE DISORDER (*CONTINUED*)

starting June 27, 2023, upon submission of their application, to have at least one of the following:

- A total of eight hours of training from certain organizations on opioid or other substance use disorders for practitioners renewing or newly applying for a registration from the DEA to prescribe any Schedule II-V controlled medications;
- Board certification in addiction medicine or addiction psychiatry from the American Board of Medical Specialties, American Board of Addiction Medicine, or the American Osteopathic Association; or
- Graduation within five years and status in good standing from medical, advanced practice nursing, or physician assistant (PA) school in the United States that included successful completion of an opioid or other substance use disorder curriculum of at least eight hours."

Source: Substance Abuse and Mental Health Services Administration (2023, June 7). *Waiver elimination (MAT Act)* (para 5). https://www.samhsa.gov/medications-substance-use-disorders/waiver-elimination-mat-act.

THE CONSOLIDATED APPROPRIATIONS ACT OF 2023 (CAA)

This sweeping legislation represents an effort to address various challenges. This $1.7 trillion omnibus legislation tackles a wide array of issues both within and outside of health and health care. An example of the former as this book goes to print is U.S. aid to Ukraine in its war with Russia. Full description of this over 1,600-page law is beyond the scope of this text. What follows, therefore, is a summary of issues of greatest immediate relevance to nurses, both as professionals and as taxpayers and users of health care (Box 3.5).

The No Surprises Act. The law protects patients from medical bills that are unexpected because the person unwittingly used out-of-network services inclusive of emergency services and air ambulances. These unexpected expenses are often referred to as "surprise billing." The law also requires that people are only responsible for cost sharing that is equivalent to the amount they would be liable for if the service was provided in-network. The background to this issue and its significance will be discussed in Section II of this text.

BOX 3.5

WHAT IS OMNIBUS SPENDING LEGISLATION?

The term omnibus spending refers to legislation that funds diverse, often unrelated issues.

Prescription drug price reporting. Another element of the CAA designed to address transparency relates to prescription drug prices. Called RxDR, for prescription drug (Rx) data reporting (DR), insurance companies and employer-based health insurance plans must submit information on prescription drugs health care spending. Although termed *Rx*DR, the required DR expands beyond drugs to include reports on health care services spending and premiums paid by members and employers. These data are collected by CMS for the Department of Health and Human Services, the Department of Labor, the Department of Treasury, and the Office of Personnel Management. The aim is to understand what drugs are used most frequently and drive overall costs up. It also aims to provide more clarity on the impact of prices on the cost sharing paid by the insured. These data will be publicly reported on the U.S. Department of Labor website as well as that of the U.S. Department of Treasury.

The Mental Health Parity and Addiction Equity Act (MHPAEA). This massive regulation requires that health plans and insurance companies collect and analyze data and provider reimbursement rates to ensure that the provider network (see Box 3.6) for mental health is not more restrictive than other networks, for example, medical-surgical networks. The overall goal is to ensure that access to substance abuse treatment or mental health services is on par with access to other forms of health care. Execution of these provisions are much more complicated than they appear. As this text goes to press, there are nearly 400 pages of proposed regulations for this element of the CAA alone.

Telehealth and digital care. The CAA extended the flexibility to telehealth rules that were instituted during the COVID-19 pandemic. These flexibilities were originally linked to the formal PHE, and the CAA decoupled many flexibilities from the formal PHE, which ended in May 2023. Telehealth and digital regulations are under rapid evolution. Readers are advised to view current policies at https://telehealth.hhs.gov/providers.

Health care workforce shortages. The CAA provided authorization for 200 new graduate medical education slots, with at least 100 directed to the area of psychiatry at an expense of $1.8 billion over 10 years. The nation currently spends roughly $18 billion on graduate medical education and roughly $0.5 billion on nursing education. Workforce issues will be further detailed in

BOX 3.6

WHAT IS A PROVIDER NETWORK?

The term *provider network* refers to a group of health care providers such as physicians, NPs, PAs, or hospitals who negotiate with payers such as insurance companies and are then contracted to provide services at an agreed-upon discounted rate. These providers agree to not bill above the discounted contracted amount. Providers who are out-of-network do not have this agreement in place and may bill at a higher rate.

Chapter 14. The law also provided $39.2 billion to health-related programs within the Department of Defense, including S582.5 million for cancer (House Committee on Appropriations, n.d.). The full legislation can be found at https://www.congress.gov/117/bills/hr2617/BILLS-117hr2617enr.pdf.

Inflation Reduction Act, This expansive legislation attempts to address inflation and other issues and includes a substantial focus on green energy, particularly through the tax code. The law's impact on health care is largely, although not exclusively, through Medicare. It includes removal of the long-standing prohibition on Medicare's negotiation with pharmaceutical companies on drug prices and caps the price of insulin at $35/month. The full text of the law is available at https://www.congress.gov/117/bills/hr5376/BILLS-117hr5376enr.pdf.

Arguably, the governmental action with the most sweeping impact on health care is not within these congressional directed actions. On June 24, 2022, the Supreme Court voted to overturn *Roe v. Wade*, the landmark legislation that created legal access to abortion in all states. The role of the Supreme Court will be discussed in detail in Chapter 12.

SUMMARY

In Chapter 3, we reviewed the ACA and selected subsequent legislation. Elements of the ACA directed toward enhancing Americans' access to health insurance were highlighted. Notably, although these may increase access, they do not address the overall underlying cost challenges facing the nation. In fact, including those with preexisting conditions, those who have reached what would have been lifetime caps, and allowing young, healthy adults to stay on their parent's insurance—although popular provisions—can increase the cost for others in the insurance pool (fewer well enrollees to carry the sick). Instead, changing what we pay for and how—termed payment reform—more directly addresses the excessive cost in the U.S. system. Payment reform is the focus of Chapter 4.

End-of-Chapter Resources

THOUGHT QUESTIONS

1. What might the U.S. health care system look like if Richard Nixon's proposal had become law?
2. Why do some Americans support the Patient Protection and Affordable Care Act and others so strongly oppose it?

3. What are the pros and cons of allowing easy access to telehealth?
4. Define the following key terms:
   Cost sharing
   Cost-sharing reduction
   Employer mandate
   Essential benefits
   Individual mandate
   Metal levels
   Rating bands
   Rating factors
   Reinsurance
   Risk adjustment
   Risk corridors
   Transparency in health care

EXERCISES

1. Interview peers, coworkers, or family on what they know about the Patient Protection and Affordable Care Act (ACA). What do they know about Obamacare? How many elements of the ACA listed in Box 3.1 could they name? Is their support or opposition based on an understanding of the facts? Why or why not?
2. Develop a presentation detailing the insurance-related elements of the Patient Protection and Affordable Care Act.

QUIZ

True and False

1. The Patient Protection and Affordable Care Act of 2010 is a form of socialized medicine.
2. The Patient Protection and Affordable Care Act of 2010 requires that a person select a bronze plan on the exchange to receive a subsidy.
3. The Patient Protection and Affordable Care Act of 2010 required Medicaid expansion, which was deemed unconstitutional by the U.S. Supreme Court in 2012.
4. The Patient Protection and Affordable Care Act of 2010 remains intact exactly as passed.
5. The Patient Protection and Affordable Care Act of 2010 replaced Obamacare.

Multiple Choice

6. Which of the following statements about the Patient Protection and Affordable Care Act of 2010 is NOT true?
   A. It represents the most sweeping health reform law since the introduction of Medicare and Medicaid in 1965.
   B. It includes a tax on tanning beds.
   C. It includes payment reform that attempts to remove perverse incentives for higher-cost, lower-quality care.
   D. It includes a public option whereby people can opt in to Medicare, regardless of age.
7. Which of the following statements about the Patient Protection and Affordable Care Act of 2010 is TRUE?
   A. As passed, it included an individual mandate, which was deemed unconstitutional in 2012.
   B. As passed, it included an employer mandate, which was deemed unconstitutional in 2012.
   C. As passed, it included provisions to merge Medicare and Medicaid.
   D. As passed, it included strategies to stabilize the health insurance market.
8. The Patient Protection and Affordable Care Act had as a goal enhanced access to health insurance. Which of the following mechanisms were used? **Select all that apply**.
   A. Insurance companies can no longer deny health insurance to people with preexisting health conditions.
   B. Young adults can remain on their parent's health insurance plan as long as they are unmarried and dependent on their parent's income tax.
   C. Insurance companies cannot enforce lifetime caps on reimbursement.
   D. Gender cannot be used as a rating factor.
9. In which of the following health insurance plans would you pay the most out of pocket when using health services?
   A. Bronze
   B. Silver
   C. Gold
   D. Platinum
   E. In each of these, you would pay the same amount out of pocket when using health services

10. In which of the following health insurance plans would you pay the least out of pocket when using health services?
    A. Bronze
    B. Silver
    C. Gold
    D. Platinum
    E. In each of these, you would pay the same amount out of pocket when using health services

ACKNOWLEDGMENT

The author acknowledges the helpful critique of Elizabeth Howlett on an earlier version of this chapter.

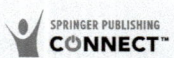

A robust set of instructor resources designed to supplement this text is located at http://connect.springerpub.com/content/book/978-0-8261-7236-5. Qualifying instructors may request access by emailing textbook@springerpub.com.

REFERENCES

Anots, J., & Capretta, J. (2016). *The ACA and its employment effects*. Health Affairs Forefront. https://www.healthaffairs.org/content/forefront/aca-and-its-employment-effects

Assistant Secretary for Planning and Evaluation. (2023, August 3). *National uninsured rate reaches an all-time low in early 2023 after the close of the ACA open enrollment period*. https://aspe.hhs.gov/sites/default/files/documents/e06a66dfc6f62afc8bb809038dfaebe4/Uninsured-Record-Low-Q12023.pdf

Bryan, B. (2017, October 12). *Trump just made a huge move that could blow up Obamacare*. Business Insider. https://www.businessinsider.com/trump-ends-cost-sharing-reduction-csr-payments-2017-10

Burroughs, M., Wilson, K., & Matsonm, M. (2024, May 8). *New ACA policy expands access to dental care. Now, states need to act*. Health Affairs Forefront. https://www.healthaffairs.org/content/forefront/new-aca-policy-expands-access-dental-care-now-states-need-act

Center on Budget and Policy Priorities. (n.d.). *ACA survives legal challenge, protecting coverage for tens of millions*. Author. https://www.cbpp.org/research/health/aca-survives-legal-challenge-protecting-coverage-for-tens-of-millions

Coleman, A. (2023, August 9). *Almost 3.8 million people have lost their Medicaid coverage since the end of the COVID-19 public health emergency*. Commonwealth Foundation. https://www.commonwealthfund.org/blog/2023/almost-38-million-people-have-lost-their-medicaid-coverage-end-covid-19-public-health

Dillender, M., Henirich, C., & Housemen. (2022). Effects of the Affordable Care Act on part-time employment: Early evidence. *Journal of Human Resources*, 0718-9623R2. https://doi.org/10.3368/jhr.57.4.0718-9623R2

Dorn, S. (2020, July 13). *The COVID-19 pandemic and resulting economic crash have caused the greatest health insurance losses in American history*. Families USA. https://www.familiesusa.org/resources/the-covid-19-pandemic-and-resulting-economic-crash-have-caused-the-greatest-health-insurance-losses-in-american-history/

Fernandez, B. (2024, February 14). *Health insurance premium tax credit and cost-sharing reductions*. Congressional Research Service. https://crsreports.congress.gov/product/pdf/R/R44425

Fuse Brown, E., & King, J. (2016). *The consequences of Gobeille v. Liberty Mutual for health care cost control*. Health Affairs Forefront. https://www.healthaffairs.org/content/forefront/consequences-em-gobeille-em-span-class-lowercase-v-span-em-liberty-mutual-em-health

Guzman, G., & Kollar, M. (2023, September 12). *Income in the United States: 2022*. United States Census Bureau. https://www.census.gov/library/publications/2023/demo/p60-279.html

Halpin, H., & Harbage, P. (2010). The origins and demise of the public option. *Health Affairs, 29*(6), 1117–1124. https://doi.org/10.1377/hlthaff.2010.0363

Hall, M., & McCue, M. (2019, July 2). *How the ACA's medical loss ratio rule protects consumers and insurers against ongoing uncertainty*. Commonwealth Foundation. https://www.commonwealthfund.org/publications/issue-briefs/2019/jul/how-aca-medical-loss-ratio-rule-protects-consumers-insurers

Health Affairs. (2012). *A giant of health policy reflects on past reforms*. Health Affairs. https://www.healthaffairs.org/doi/full/10.1377/hlthaff.2012.0841

HealthCare.gov. (n.d.-a). *Health coverage exemptions, forms & how to apply*. Author. https://www.healthcare.gov/health-coverage-exemptions/forms-how-to-apply/

House Committee on Appropriations. (n.d.). *Consolidated appropriations act 2023: Summary of appropriations provisions by subcommittee*. https://democrats-appropriations.house.gov/sites/evo-subsites/democrats-appropriations.house.gov/files/FY23%20Summary%20of%20Appropriations%20Provisions.pdf

Jost, T. S. (2016, October/November). *Stabling forces*. The Actuary. https://www.theactuarymagazine.org/stabilizing-forces/

Jost, T. S. (2023, January 11). *HHS considers updating the essential health benefits*. The Commonwealth Foundation. https://www.commonwealthfund.org/blog/2023/hhs-considers-updating-essential-health-benefits

Kaiser Family Foundation. (2012). *A guide to the Supreme Court's decision on the ACA's Medicaid expansion*. https://www.kff.org/wp-content/uploads/2013/01/8347.pdf

Kaiser Family Foundation. (2019, November 27). *Potential impact of California v. Decisions on key provisions of the Affordable Care Act*. https://www.kff.org/health-reform/fact-sheet/potential-impact-of-texas-v-u-s-decision-on-key-provisions-of-the-affordable-care-act/

Kaiser Family Foundation. (2023, July 27). *Status of state Medicaid expansion decisions: Interactive map*. https://www.kff.org/medicaid/issue-brief/status-of-state-medicaid-expansion-decisions-interactive-map/

Kaiser Family Foundation. (2024, February 28). *Preventive services covered by private health plans under the Affordable Care Act*. Author. https://www.kff.org/womens-health-policy/fact-sheet/preventive-services-covered-by-private-health-plans

Kaiser Family Foundation. (2023, October 18). *Premiums and worker contributions among workers covered by employer-sponsored coverage, 1999-2023*.

Author. https://www.kff.org/interactive/premiums-and-worker
-contributions-among-workers-covered-by-employer-sponsored
-coverage/

Leveille, M., & Rambur, B. (2024). Nurse-led opioid disorder treatment. *Policy, Politics, & Nursing Practice, 25*(1), 4–5. https://doi.org/10.1177/15271544231210700

Livingston, S. (2018, July 24). *How states are defining essential health benefits.* Modern Healthcare. https://www.modernhealthcare.com/article/20180724/NEWS/180729957/how-states-are-defining-essential-health-benefits

Maddipatla, M., & Humer, C. (2020, April 27). *U.S. health insurers benefit as elective care cuts offset coronavirus costs.* Reuters. https://www.reuters.com/article/us-health-coronavirus-usa-healthinsurance-idUSKCN2291DY

Maine Community Health Options vs. United States. (2019). *No. 18–1023. Argued December 10, 2019—Decided April 2, 2020.* https://www.supremecourt.gov/opinions/19pdf/18-1023_m64o.pdf

Mann, C. (2020, April 15). *The COVID-19 crisis is giving states that haven't expanded Medicaid new reasons to reconsider.* The Commonwealth Fund. https://www.commonwealthfund.org/blog/2020/covid-19-crisis-giving-states-havent-expanded-medicaid-new-reconsideration

Millenson, M. (2018, September 12). Half a century of the health care crisis (and still going strong), *Health Affairs Forefront.* https://www.healthaffairs.org/content/forefront/half-century-health-care-crisis-and-still-going-strong

McCuskey, E. (2023). *Reforming ERISA to help states control health care costs.* The Commonwealth Foundation. https://www.commonwealthfund.org/publications/issue-briefs/2023/feb/reforming-erisa-help-states-control-health-care-costs

Rosenbaum, S., Byrnes, M., & Hurt, N. (n.d.). *Community benefit and the ACA a brief history and update.* https://nchh.org/resource-library/HCF_CBACA%20overview.pdf

Roy, S., & Satija, B. (2024, February 13). *US hospitals see post pandemic catch-up behind insurer healthcare costs.* Reuters. https://www.reuters.com/world/us/us-hospitals-see-post-pandemic-catch-up-behind-insurer-healthcare-costs-2024-02-13/

Schneider, E., Shah, A., Doty, M., Tikkanen, R., Fields, K., & Williams, R. (2021). *Mirror, mirror 2021: Reflecting poorly: Health care in the U.S. compared to other high-income countries.* Commonwealth Fund. https://www.commonwealthfund.org/publications/fund-reports/2021/aug/mirror-mirror-2021-reflecting-poorly

Spector, J. (2020, June 8). *NY insurers, citing COVID-19 costs, seek double digit rate hikes in 2021. Check your plan.* https://www.democratandchronicle.com/story/news/politics/albany/2020/06/08/new-york-insurance-rates-citing-coronavirus-costs-seek-big-hikes-2021/3172713001/

Tolbert, J., & Ammula, M. (2023, June 9). *10 things to know about the unwinding of the Medicaid continuous enrollment provision.* Kaiser Family Foundation. https://www.kff.org/medicaid/issue-brief/10-things-to-know-about-the-unwinding-of-the-medicaid-continuous-enrollment-provision/#:~:text=At%20the%20start%20of%20the,exchange%20for%20enhanced%20federal%20funding

U.S. Department of Health and Human Services. (2024, April 2). *HHS finalized policies to make marketplace coverage more accessible and expand essential benefits.* Author. https://www.hhs.gov/about/news/2024/04/02/hhs-finalizes-policies-make-marketplace-coverage-more-accessible-expand-essential-health-benefits.html

U.S. Food and Drug Administration. (2020, January 31). *The 21st century cures act*. https://www.fda.gov/regulatory-information/selected-amendments-fdc-act/21st-century-cures-act

Van de Water, P. (2018). Raising threshold for health reform's employer mandate would put more workers at risk. Center on Budget amnd Policy Priorities. https://www.cbpp.org/research/health-reform-not-causing-significant-shift-to-part-time-work

Young, G. J., Flaherty, S., Zepeda, D., Singh, S. R., & Cramer, G. R. (2018). *Community benefit spending By tax-exempt hospitals changed little after ACA*. https://www.healthaffairs.org/doi/10.1377/hlthaff.2017.1028

CHAPTER 4

Payment Reform: Improving Care Delivery by Changing Who Is Reimbursed, How, and for What

CHAPTER 4 details payment reform models and describes the impact on the roles, responsibilities, and knowledge needs of entry-level RNs, seasoned professionals, advanced practice clinicians, and nurse leaders. Following completion of this chapter, you will be able to:

- Describe the limitation of fee-for-service reimbursement for health care services.
- Illustrate essential dimensions of emerging payment models along a range from fee-for-service at one end to the other end of the continuum: fixed revenue global capitation.
- Discuss essential nursing knowledge in the reformed health system.
- Detail parameters of value-informed nursing practice for nurses at all levels of education and practice.

> *Cissy has enjoyed her 12 years as an RN in the surgical ICU of a community hospital. She is aware that changes seem to be happening, and there are rumblings of financial strain at the hospital, particularly since COVID-19. Cissy is glad that all of that has nothing to do with her. Her indifference was shattered when the chief nursing officer (CNO) invited Cissy and two other ICU nurses together for a meeting. The CNO opens by sharing that Cissy and her colleagues have been exemplary nurses, but that they will "soon be dinosaurs." "The inpatient book of business is shrinking," the CNO states, "and we need to downsize that portion of our workforce or lay people off." Cissy is stunned—and defensive! The CNO details the hospital situation with terms Cissy is not familiar with: "shared savings programs," "bundled payments," "value-based care," and "per member per month global budgets." The CNO concludes with the following statement: "I don't want to lose you three... how about retooling for virtual transitional care?" Flash-forward 1 year later: Cissy loves her new role managing transitions for the chronically ill population in the hospital service area.*[1]

The previous chapters detailed the rise of the medical establishment within the fee-for-service milieu. Incentives in fee-for-service systems push toward higher volumes and thus reward or incentivize *more* care rather than *better* care. Fee-for-service models incentivize behavior that fragments care and creates disincentives for coordination and integration. Fee-for-service also contributes to the nation's difficulty containing health care costs. Thus, payment reform, a key element of health care reform, is creating new and different incentives and disincentives than we have seen previously in health care. Understanding emerging payment models helps nurses make sense of the clinical arena and their own work, as it did for Cissy. Understanding incentives and disincentives is also necessary to provide leadership in the redesign of health care. To aid understanding, the models for payment reform described in this chapter are presented along a continuum from most like fee-for-service to progressively less like fee-for-service and ending with global budgets. Payment models that are not fee-for-service are sometimes termed alternative payment models because they are alternative to traditional fee-for-service. Another common term is value-based payments (VBPs), with value being the quotient of quality outcomes divided by cost. Another catch-all term is pay for performance (P4P) because the payment is shaped by or totally dependent on processes or outcomes determined by performance measures. Many of these models are under development and testing, and still others are in flux. Moreover, the exact elements may vary from setting to setting or state to state.

Nevertheless, the substantial hospital financial downturn during COVID-19 illustrated the serious problems stemming from a hospital system dependent on the volume of elective procedures done, in which April 2020 was the worst month ever for hospital operating margins (net revenue after expenses). Margins dropped a staggering 282% relative to the same period just 1 year earlier (Kacik, 2020), with prognostications that COVID-19 will accelerate the move to VBP (Livingston, 2020). Roiland et al. note that the capacity of organizations to respond to pandemic-induced challenges depended on large part on their reimbursement models, with participation in VBP associated with "more financial flexibility and stability" (Roiland et al., 2020, para 2). In particular, they detail the manner in which VBPs enabled organizations to (a) leverage and expand virtual care; (b) reorient staff and workflows; (c) address social needs, including home delivery of essential goods, meals, and medications; and (d) shift sites of service to settings with a lower risk of disease transmission. Finally, Noël (2022) concludes that COVID-19 made the case for value more "vital and urgent" (para 7) and lowered barriers to change, for example, the enhanced adoption of telehealth and digital innovation. In 2021 the Centers for Medicare and Medicaid Innovation (CMMI) set a goal of having 100% of beneficiaries in traditional Medicare and most people in Medicaid in a VBP model by 2030 (Fowler et al., 2022). But what exactly are these VBPs? And what do they have to do with you?

FROM VOLUME TO VALUE: PAYMENT MODELS THAT MOVE AWAY FROM FEE-FOR-SERVICE REIMBURSEMENT

First, four general models will be detailed. These are *advanced primary care*, iterations of which are also known by the term *patient-centered medical home* (PCMH); *accountable care organizations (ACOs)*; *bundled payments*, sometimes called *payment by episode or episode payment models*; and *global budgets*. A key differentiation among models is the magnitude of financial risk bearing. So, first, let's review that key concept.

In traditional fee-for-service reimbursement, providers do not bear any financial risk for the cost of care. Effective or ineffective, providers are reimbursed. Moreover, prior to relatively recent penalties or nonreimbursement for low-quality care or harmful care, providers were often reimbursed more for poor-quality care than excellent care. An example is when hospitals were reimbursed for complications they caused in the first place, a dynamic that changed with the introduction of Hospital Value-Based Purchasing, a specific initiative that will be discussed fully in Chapter 6. For now, let's review overall payment reform models and the concept of risk.

Emerging payment models shift the dynamic of paying more for poor care than excellent care by adding two elements. The first, present in all of them, is heightened accountability for the outcomes of care, with some reimbursement linked to patient outcomes. The second, present in some, is heightened accountability for not only outcomes but also cost. This is termed financial risk. It can be *shared risk* or *full risk*; *upside only* or *two sided* inclusive of *downside risk*.

In shared risk, providers who deliver care for less than projected share those savings with the payer, which can be Medicare, Medicaid, and/or commercial insurance. They also share financial loss if care is more costly than projected. In full risk bearing, providers fully receive the financial gain of delivering less costly care but bear all the lost revenue when care is more costly than projected. This latter model is also called two sided, in that providers can benefit by receiving more revenue but also lose revenue. In upside only—also known as *one-sided* risk—providers financially benefit from care delivered that is less costly than projected, but do not bear any potentially negative financial consequences for costly care. Forty different alternative payment models are in play at the time of this writing, a circumstance on which Chernew et al. (2020) reflect: "The dizzying array of options and rules may distract from the hard work of transforming care" (p. 415). Recall that these are alternatives to fee-for-service. Although fee-for-service is simple to understand and manipulate, it easily and often slides into unnecessary, low-value care and is widely recognized as a driver of the United States' vexing cost and quality conundrum.

Pay for Performance—An Overview

P4P builds on fee-for-service by providing additional financial incentives to providers who achieve quality metrics (see Box 4.1). It is an attempt to better align the business case with the case for quality within the clinical setting. It is not an alternative to fee-for-service, but typically instead provides complementary, additional reimbursement when selected metrics are met. This additional reimbursement can occur at the individual (typically physician) level, a group-of-providers (again usually physician) level, or the institutional level. The logic for additional reimbursement for achievement of certain quality and outcome metrics is that under fee-for-service, poor-quality care receives the same compensation as high-quality care. In some cases, poor-quality care receives more reimbursement than high-quality care, and errors, inefficiencies, and unnecessary care are all reimbursed, indicating a mismatch between the provider's financial incentives and patient needs. P4P injects the new variable of objective measures of quality that theoretically promote better alignment between provider behavior and better outcomes for patients. At the same time, many P4Ps do not require that providers take on financial or other risks for their clinical judgments and behaviors. Instead, it relies on measures that are intended to be an objective reflection of their performance. As such, this small step in payment reform is more palatable to some providers. Moreover, although a small step, it is a radical move away from the relative lack of accountability inherent in the fee-for-service system.

A challenge in P4P—indeed, in any payment system linked to outcomes—is the choice of metrics. There is the potential for metric-driven behavior (Mannion & Braithwaite, 2012) that results in metric-driven patient harm (Rambur et al., 2013). Examples of behavior that can lead to metric-driven

BOX 4.1

WHAT ARE QUALITY METRICS?

Concepts such as *health* or *good care* can be difficult to define and measure. Quality metrics use something that can be measured to serve as a proxy for health, health improvement, efficiency, or effectiveness. Some metrics focus on process; others on outcomes. Measurement may include the patient experience, including patient satisfaction and cost. By using metrics, individuals, organizations, health systems, or nations may compare their performance relative to peers as well as those they aspire to be like. In some settings, individual providers such as nurse practitioners and physicians in PCMHs or ACOs can compare their performance and cost with that of their peer providers. On the other end of the spectrum, the United States can compare the performance of U.S. health care with that delivered in other nations. Comparison can be a powerful incentive toward improvement; no one—whether an individual, organization, or nation—wants to be the highest-cost entity delivering lower-quality care. This form of comparison is termed *benchmarking*.

harm include gaming and measure fixation (see Box 4.2 for a full list). In addition, to date, the outcomes of P4P are mixed, with some early studies finding quality improvement (Calikoglu et al., 2012) and others in the same era finding no improvement in quality when compared to hospitals not under a P4P system (Ryan et al., 2012). Similarly, studies in other settings such as nursing homes did not find consistent improvement using P4P models (Werner et al., 2013). A 2017 systematic review of 69 studies noted that many of the studies reporting positive outcomes were conducted in the United Kingdom, a nation where the incentives are greater than in the United States. Based on the review, these authors concluded that "consistently positive associations with improved health outcomes have not been demonstrated in any setting" (Mendelson et al., 2017, p. 341). Chernew et al. reported a lack of evidence of cost savings but also noted that many such initiatives have not been evaluated. Finally, Kim et al.'s (2020) systematic review found that surgical care P4P inclusive of penalties for poor performance had positive outcomes in 5 of 10 studies. They suggest that inducing providers to improve surgical care is more likely to succeed in

BOX 4.2

METRIC-DRIVEN UNINTENDED CONSEQUENCES

Tunnel vision refers to the prioritization of financially incentivized care over other valuable care or a prioritization of measured elements of care over unmeasured elements of care of equal or greater value.

Measure fixation is a focus on particular measurement without reflection on how maximization of the particular outcome can miss or even be in opposition to the underlying objective of care. It also refers to focus on a particular measurement without attention to the distress caused to a patient by maximization of the metric.

Acontextual actions or cherry picking refers to the potential to choose patients who can maximize positive measurement while deferring or refusing to treat more vulnerable, more seriously ill patients.

Misrepresentation refers to the deliberate *manipulation of data* so that the reported behavior differs from the actual behavior.

Gaming refers to *manipulation of behavior* to meet targets. It differs from misrepresentation in that it is a contortion of *actual* behavior, not merely *reported* data.

Myopia refers to a focus on short-term, measurable performance at the expense of legitimate long-term consequences and goals.

Suboptimization is the pursuit of narrow local objectives by managers at the expense of the objectives of the organization as a whole.

Ossification is the inhibition of innovation. It may include organizational paralysis brought about by an excessively rigid system of performance measures.

Source: Adapted from Smith, P. (1995). On the unintended consequences of publishing performance data in the public sector. *International Journal of Public Administration*, 18(2–3), 277–310. https://doi.org/10.1080/01900699508525011

penalty-based models or those with rewards and penalties rather than reward-only payment models. An example of a reward-only model would be an "upside only" track.

Finally, it could be argued that physicians and other providers should inherently strive for quality, as many do, rather than needing additional financial incentives to do so. From this perspective, a system like P4P may be an inherently ethically flawed approach. To illustrate the ethical knot, ponder the following: An analogy to P4P would be paying for college with tuition funds, but if it could be demonstrated that a student actually learned not only what was expected but also beyond that, then the faculty member or the faculty group teaching in that discipline would receive additional compensation. A system in which providers need to be incentivized to embrace quality outcomes seems antithetical to fundamental ethical principles like *beneficence* and professional responsibility. We return to this issue of ethics and, specifically, *ethinomics,* the intersection of ethics and economics, in Chapter 8. For now, let's explore some specific P4P models in evolution in the United States. (Provider- and hospital-based value-based reimbursement models codified into law are detailed in Chapter 6.)

Patient-Centered Medical Homes

PCMHs represent a team-based P4P model of care delivery. Unlike episodic, physician-centric care, the idea behind PCMHs is that comprehensive personalized care can best be delivered by a team (see Figure 4.1). This team may include different combinations of skill sets for different patients and includes the use of registries and electronic health record data for individual- and population-based care. The use of these data can, in turn, help the medical home determine which patients are in need of some aspect of care. PCMHs also rely on *community health teams* and *health coaches* for an array of supportive services. Community health teams were defined in the Affordable Care Act (ACA) to potentially include "medical specialists, nurses, pharmacists, nutritionists, dietitians, social workers, behavioral and mental health providers (including substance use disorder prevention and treatment providers), doctors of chiropractic, licensed complementary and alternative medicine practitioners, and physician assistants" (American College of Physicians, 2013, p. 1), whereas health coaches are individuals who work with patients to change behavior and improve health. The overall premise is that such an approach will create higher-quality care at a lower cost. Many states have used the PCMH model for their Medicaid population (Kaiser Family Foundation, 2023).

Despite logical elegance, studies do not fully support the founding hypothesis of higher-quality, lower-cost care as a result of this model. A 3-year pilot study with 32 primary care practices, six health plans, and roughly 120,000 patients did not find a reduction in patients' use of hospitals or EDs

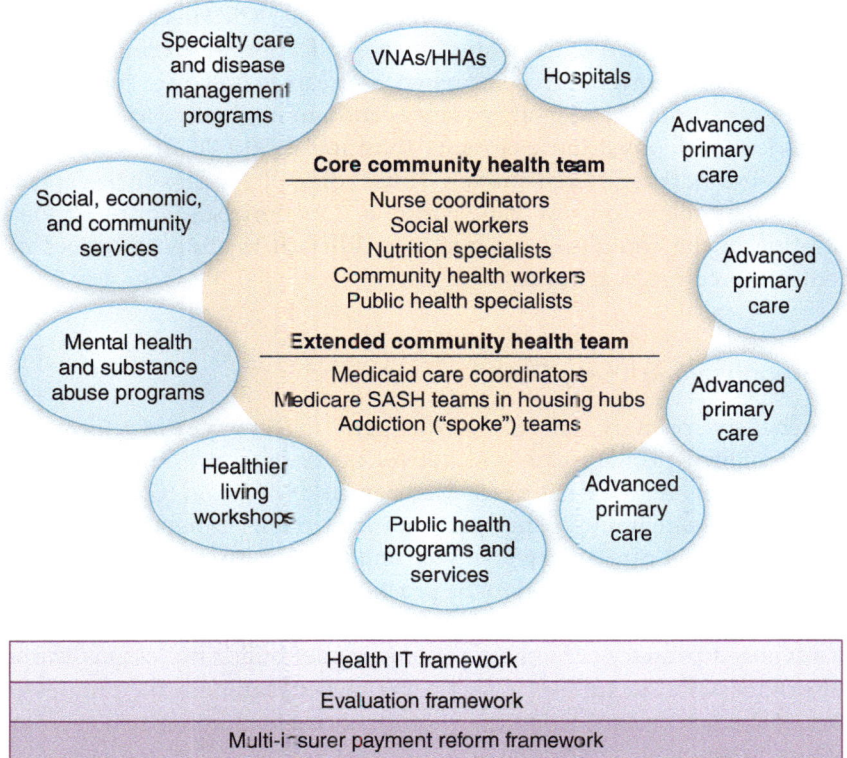

FIGURE 4.1: Patient-centered medical home.
Source: Adapted from Department of Vermont Health Access. (2014). *Vermont blueprint for health: 2013 annual report*. Retrieved February 20, 2015, from http://hcr.vermont.gov/sites/hcr/files/pdfs/VTBlueprintforHealthAnnualReport2013.pdf.

or a reduction in total cost of care in this model and found only limited improvement in quality. At the same time, the primary care physicians in the participating practices received accumulated average bonuses of $92,000 per physician during the 3-year trial (Friedberg et al., 2014). A more recent systematic review by Veet et al. (2020) found decreased ED utilization and increased use of primary care, while Nielson et al. (2015) report improvement in many metrics, including cost, across 20 studies. Finally, Fortuna et al. (2021) found improvement in patient care metrics, for example, diabetes and hypertension control and breast and colorectal cancer screening, but PCMH adoption was not associated with improved provider and nurse measures of satisfaction, work–life balance, teamwork, or professional experience.

It is quite possible that the fundamental approach is sound, but the settings with poor results are either not constituted optimally or there has not been sufficient time to achieve high-quality, lower cost care. As illustrated in Figure 4.1, *teamness* is a central construct in a PCMH, yet the optimal nature and composition of the teams await explication. A documented challenge in implementing truly comprehensive team-based care includes the physician-centric nature of many practices and unimaginative roles for nurse practitioners and physician assistants (Nutting et al., 2012) to which the author would add registered nurses. Thus, some of the less-than-expected outcomes may relate to team composition or function. See Figure 4.2 for an illustration of the continuum of care for addiction treatment services in a patient-centered medical home.

Comprehensive Primary Care

Comprehensive primary care (CPC) is designed to test payment reform models to strengthen primary care and deliver better care at a lower cost. In a collaboration among the Centers for Medicare and Medicaid (CMS) and commercial and state insurance plans, participating primary care practices receive a monthly nonvisit care management fee and the opportunity to share in any net savings in the care delivered to the practice's Medicare patients. CPC is the foundation for Comprehensive Primary Care Plus (CPC+) that started in 2017. This advanced primary care medical home model builds on lessons learned in the original CPC, including "insights on practice readiness, the progression of care delivery redesign, actionable performance-based initiatives, necessary health information technology and claims data sharing" (CMS, n.d.-a, para. 2).

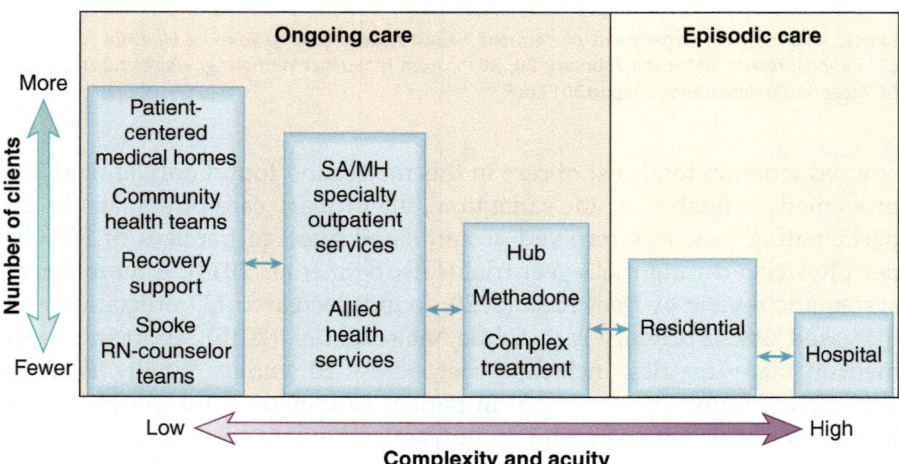

FIGURE 4.2: Continuum of health services for addiction treatment.

Source: Adapted from Department of Vermont Health Access. (2014). *Vermont blueprint for health: 2013 annual report*. Retrieved February 20, 2015, from http://hcr.vermont.gov/sites/hcr/files/pdfs/VTBlueprintforHealthAnnualReport2013.pdf.

In 2023, a new iteration of this model was announced. Called *Making Care Primary*, this 10.5-year model intends to improve care management and care coordination and support primary care connections with specialists and Medicaid as well as community connections for health-related social needs such as nutrition and housing (cms.gov, n.d.-a). It is not yet clear if this new model will improve the mixed outcomes to date. Compared to matched practices, CPC sites slowed ED use by 2%, but overall spending was not sufficient to cover the cost of care management. Moreover, physician and patient experiences were not improved, nor was practice improved as measured by a limited set of quality measures (Peikes et al., 2018). Nevertheless, these models in which care is reconfigured and outcomes measured may be a useful strategy, and perhaps even a necessary step, toward accountability for outcomes and cost. Payment models that include explicit and, in some cases, substantial financial risk will now be described.

Accountable Care Organizations

The ACA provided the impetus for the formation of ACOs. ACOs are an attempt to shift the locus of care to a population, with a focus on *value of service* rather than *volume of service*. In this way, ACOs—at least theoretically—are a dramatic departure from fee-for-service, which incentivizes volume of care over the actual value of that care. This challenges nurses and others to embrace a new manner of thinking; just because services are being provided (volume) does not mean that this treatment has value, or as ethicist Virginia Sharpe noted, dissecting the difference between what *can* be done and what *should* be done.

An ACO may be further defined as a group of providers who *agree* to be accountable for the cost and quality of care for a defined population. Although these terms do not seem revolutionary in and of themselves, this is indeed a radical departure from the traditional fee-for-service approach in which accountability for cost was largely absent and aggregated accountability for outcomes was loose, at best, and frequently nonexistent. Moreover, ACOs typically depend on complex data management, aiding the analysis of both cost and quality (see Figure 4.3), and the sophistication required to create and maintain the necessary supporting software and hardware is a relatively new capacity in the health care arena and is still underdeveloped in many places, making ACOs difficult without that support. Note: At this time, ACOs are a voluntary coalition of providers across different types of services and organizations.

Importantly, ACOs are not health maintenance organizations (HMOs). In fact, elements of ACOs emerge from what had been viewed as failures or limitations in HMOs. An ACO, for example, does not typically limit beneficiaries' access or choice of providers, and there is no gatekeeper. The term *gatekeeper* refers to an element of HMOs in which patients cannot directly

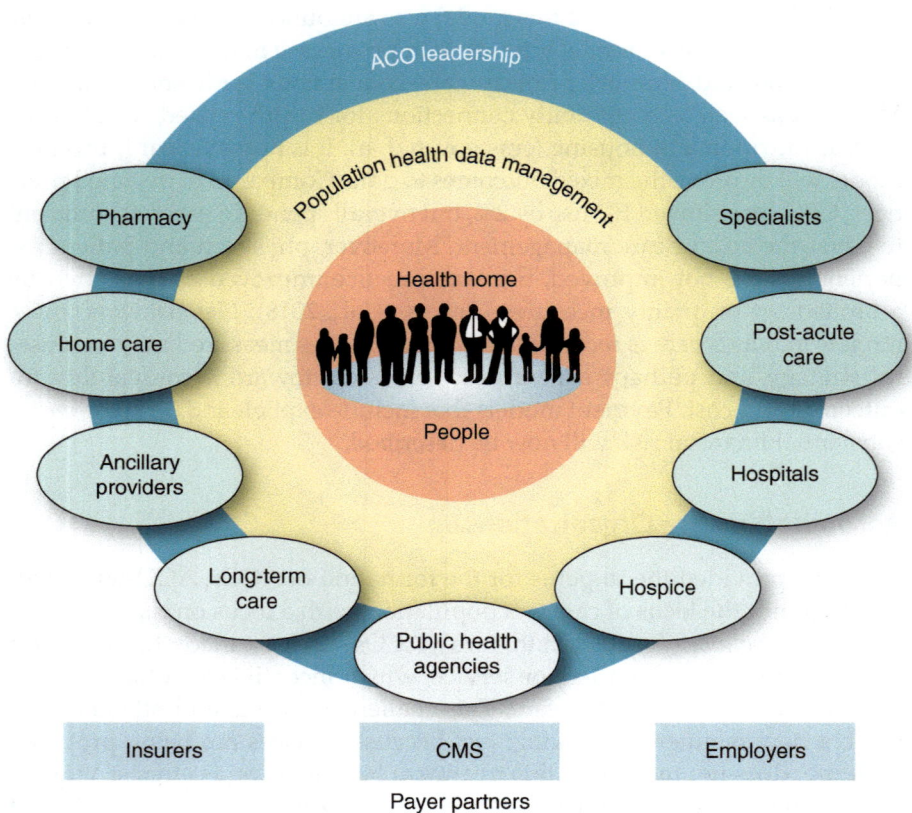

FIGURE 4.3: Accountable care organization structure.
Source: Used with permission from Xcenda, an AmerisourceBergen company.

access specialists or any provider other than their primary care provider, who needs to refer the patient if the services are to be covered financially by the third-party payer.

Accountable Care Iterations

There have been various iterations of ACOs, but the concept is most easily understood by examining the one that is codified into the ACA law: the Medicare Shared Savings Program (MSSP). Others on the federal level are being tested through the authority of the CMMI, and there are state-level Medicaid ACOs as well as commercial insurance ACOs.

SSP ACOs allow savings from innovation and care redesign to be shared between the providers and the payer. Such funding provides a financial bridge between treatment cultures rooted in volume of treatment as the marker of financial success—the "more is better" model—and new ones referencing a more complex mix of quality and cost outcomes. Specifically, SSPs differ from a traditional fee-for-service arrangement in a number of important ways. First, it is a *performance-based contract* between a *payer* (such as private insurance or Medicare) and a *provider organization*; savings from delivery of more cost-effective care are shared between the payer and the provider as long as performance metrics are met. The assumption is that the potential for financial return will drive innovation, coordination, and redesign of care processes and infrastructure. Care coordination and redesign is an area where there is substantial opportunity for nurses to influence the value of care.

> Laticia is an RN in a clinic that is part of a physician–hospital organization that employs 1,500 physicians. The clinic is affiliated with an academic medical center, and most of the physicians have admitting privileges. Laticia is concerned about inefficiencies in the patient scheduling process. She completes a literature review and identifies two models that could be more efficient. She shares these with her supervisor, who then asks Laticia to present her findings and recommendations to the senior leadership team. They adopt Laticia's redesigned model for flow and patient throughput. The subsequent performance data suggest that Laticia's model results in far shorter waiting periods for patients with emergent conditions and higher patient satisfaction, with an overall reduction in unexpected hospital admissions for acute exacerbations in patients with chronic conditions. Because overall expenditures were less than projected, the clinic group receives a portion of these savings. Laticia knows it took someone "on the ground" and close to the working surface to see both the problem and the potential for such an innovative solution. As a result of her excellent work, Laticia is promoted to a new role, director of innovation. A key responsibility is to interact with staff nurses and employed physicians to identify and implement workflow redesign as well as clinical service delivery innovations that decrease unnecessary utilization of services, reduce overall costs, and meet key quality metrics.

SHARING SAVINGS

So how is the amount that could be shared determined? The payer and the ACO, guided by quality targets that must be met, determine the projected expenditures—expenditures expected in a traditional fee-for-service delivery model—for a population of patients. These projections are *risk adjusted*, meaning the expenditure projections take into consideration the health and illness status of the population. Thus, the model recognizes that a group with more severe illnesses typically uses more services and thus incurs higher costs. Then, over time, the actual expenditures are compared with the projected expenditures, and any savings are then shared by predefined formulas (see Figure 4.4). This is called *upside risk*. Note that quality targets must be met. The cost savings cannot be at the expense of quality.

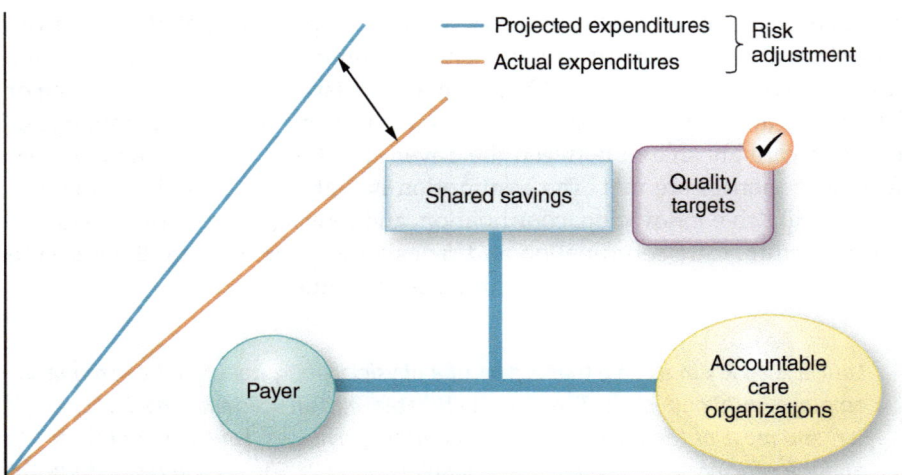

FIGURE 4.4: Calculating shared savings.
Source: Courtesy of Kara Suter, MS. Used with permission.

What if the new models actually fail to yield savings or the actual expenditures are higher than expected? This latter is termed *downside risk*. The acceptance of downside risk would mean that the provider groups in a shared savings model would be held financially accountable for some portion of expenditures above the projection (see Figure 4.5). In the traditional fee-for-service models of health care, that extra cost is instead reflected in higher insurance premiums the next year. Acceptance of downside risk places provider groups in the situation of being financially accountable not only for what goes right financially, receiving some portion of the savings, but also for

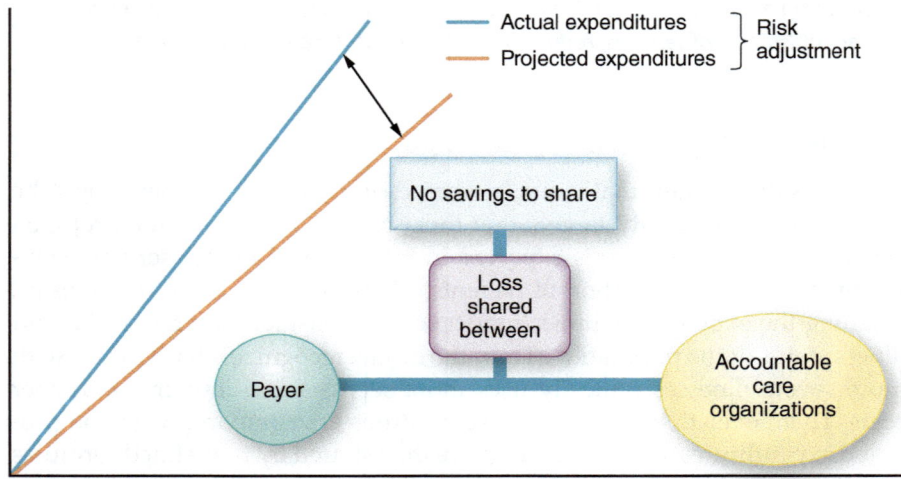

FIGURE 4.5: Shared savings illustrating downside risk.

some of the excessive cost if things do not go well financially. Although Medicare pilot trials designed to test shared savings ACOs give providers who accept downside risk a larger portion of the savings, many providers had been reluctant to accept downside risk, particularly those in small practices. In 2012, for example, roughly 28% of the Medicare ACOs accepted downside risk to create a *two-sided risk* model, that is, both upside and downside; by 2018, the rate of two-sided risk was up modestly, to 33% (Rosenberg, 2019). Peck et al. (2019) note that although ACOs with downside risk are increasing, they remain in the minority, with the greatest obstacle to adoption being provider reluctance (Healthcare Financial Management Association, 2023).

It is important to understand that this downside risk does not simply evaporate. In the traditional fee-for-service Medicare program, for example, excessive costs are borne by taxpayers and Medicare beneficiaries. In the private insurance market fee-for-sevice model, these costs will be borne by the insurance company in the short term but passed on to those insured in the form of higher premiums.

Empirical evidence supports greater cost savings in two-sided risk models (Gonzalez-Smith et al., 2019). Similarly, Haverkamp et al. (2018) have found that ACOs with risk-bearing experience are more likely to take steps to reduce low-value care. This is logical, because they are accountable for cost and outcomes of care; low-value care creates cost without improved outcomes. The contribution nurses can make toward positive redesign, and the value of such redesign, is substantial. Specific skills are detailed in Table 4.1.

In general, ACOs are primary care grounded, even if the ACO is hospital led. This is because primary care providers are typically the *attributed provider*, that is, the provider accountable for the cost and outcomes of care. Notably, nurse practitioners (NPs) and physician assistants/associates (PAs) are playing increasing roles in ACOs, with NP prevalence increasing from 17.6% to 25% and PAs increasing from less than 1% to over 13%, with a concomitant decrease in physicians (Nyweide et al., 2020; analysis of 2013 to 2018). Perloff et al. (2023) found that allowing NPs to be Medicare attribution–eligible results in more patients being attributed to ACOs without increasing patient complexity. They conclude that such attribution is a worthy approach for those organizations interested in growing Medicare ACOs.

Clearly, understanding ACOs and financial risk is essential nursing knowledge. Nurse practitioners may be attributed providers, and entry-level nurses can play key roles in high-quality, cost-effective care when they understand the underlying payment and performance dynamics.

Bundled Payments

ACO accountability is for all care received, while bundled payments replace fee-for-service payment and its incentives with a fixed amount by episode or condition. This bundled payment is across the care continuum, inclusive of

TABLE 4.1 KEY NURSING SKILLS IN THE VALUE-BASED VIRTUAL WORLD

Baccalaureate	Advanced Practice Nurses (*in Addition to the Baccalaureate Skills*)
Cultural proficiency	Design, lead, and evaluate population-level care
Appreciation of social determinants of health, coupled with the capacity to sensitively intervene at personal/family care levels as well as politically (see Berwick et al., 2020 for explication of ways to address moral determinants of health)	Build, develop, maintain, and modify teams to maximize positive outcomes/minimize cost
Commitment to shared decision-making, including the ability to effectively communicate with physicians when care trajectory does not align with the known wishes of the person and family	Mentor BS-prepared nurses to maximize their role in primary care
Ability to participate in, maintain, and support effective interprofessional teams	Cultivate cultural fluency within practice/work setting and throughout the community served
Recognize wasteful and unnecessary care and effectively communicate to ensure resolution (e.g., proactively taking steps to address standing orders that create waste)	Lead shared decision-making initiatives
Redesign inefficient delivery that is within the RN's span of control, for example, address rigid standing orders	Troubleshoot and problem-solve to create solutions for barriers to practice change
Use findings of predictive and prescriptive analytics derived from multiple data sets (big data) to modify care at individual and population cohort levels (e.g., a cohort with congestive heart failure or diabetes)	Propose and test reconfigured models of care; disseminate promising practices
Propose strategies to use artificial intelligence to improve outcomes and decrease costs	Implement promising artificial intelligence strategies; test outcomes and disseminate findings broadly; support the scaling of effective approaches
Clear understanding of the cost of outcomes of their own care (see Yakusheva et al., 2020, for one strategy toward this end)	Direct initiative to decrease waste and unnecessary care
Direct environmental modification to maximize health (e.g., home visits to address allergens and mold abatement in a child with asthma)	Lead policy initiatives to support healthy environmental policies at the local, regional, national, and international levels

(continued)

TABLE 4.1 KEY NURSING SKILLS IN THE VALUE-BASED VIRTUAL WORLD (*continued*)

Baccalaureate	Advanced Practice Nurses (*in Addition to the Baccalaureate Skills*)
Provide telehealth, virtual, and digitally supported care to individuals and families in their homes or other environment; use broad data sets inclusive of self-monitoring data to modify plans of care; technical competencies to troubleshoot and resolve evolving technical challenges	Analyze outcomes of telehealth, virtual, and digitally supported care, with particular attention to outcomes in disadvantaged or underrepresented groups; propose new apps or innovations to improve access outcomes and decrease cost
Capacity to triage and make appropriate referrals and also delegate	Analyze systems of care and nurse skill mix; promote role differentiation
Support person/family self-management of acute and chronic illness	Lead teams providing care populations with complex health needs; measure outcomes and disseminate findings
Appreciate the process and outcomes measures that direct payment in their setting (for example, Hospital Value-Based Purchasing) and the rationale for these policies (align the economic case for care decisions with the quality case)	Be a resource for others struggling to understand the intersection of measurement and payment; support and, in some cases, direct learning agendas for others

postacute care and readmissions. Bundled payments typically target types of care that have been expensive or populations that are frequent users of a health service; for example, those diagnosed and frequently admitted with congestive heart failure (CHF). In a fee-for-service system, there is little financial incentive to, for example, keep a patient out of the ED, use palliative care when appropriate, or provide nurse and social worker support to the individual and the family. Indeed, the types of services not provided by someone who can bill, for example, an RN rather than an MD, are uncompensated in fee-for-service.

In bundled payment models, integrated care delivery is financially incentivized, and there is a strong incentive to prevent avoidable complications. Under the Obama administration, regions of the country were randomly assigned to test bundled payments for joint replacement surgery, with plans to add more conditions. The first Trump administration originally only supported voluntary provider participation with bundled payments, but in 2018 reversed course to support adoption of mandatory bundles. Mandatory bundles represent payment obligations. In other words, providers who treat Medicare patients for a condition that is a mandatory bundle will be required to participate within the quality and financial parameters assigned to that episode of care if they expect to be reimbursed by Medicare. Conceptually, it is like diagnosis-related groups for hospital care, but it extends beyond the hospital walls to be a single lump sum for all care associated with a particular diagnosis or episode of care such as joint replacement or radiation oncology. Bundles are also being tested in Medicaid and commercial insurance populations.

Using a bundled care payment model for a person with CHF as an example, types of care may include the hospital, acute care hospital at home, home health care, skilled nursing faculty, and specialty physicians as necessary. The care provided by the hospital, however, would—or certainly should—look very different than in a fee-for-service system. The hospital may hire nurses to specifically develop individualized plans of care with ongoing support to keep these patients out of the hospital.

Other studies have found that bundled payments for the management of cancer resulted in a 34% decrease in the expected cost but a paradoxical increase in the cost of chemotherapeutic agents. Nonetheless, it still netted dramatic overall cost savings with no alteration in quality (Newcomer et al., 2014). This study also tested the sharing of physician performance information as a means to enhance quality, raising the potential that physician behavior changed because outcomes were being measured. Nevertheless, this payment strategy offers refreshing promise. An eight-country study of 23 bundled payment initiatives for procedures (e.g., total joint replacement and cardiac surgery) and management of chronic conditions (e.g., diabetes and breast cancer) found predominantly positive cost and quality of care impacts (Struijs et al., 2020); analysis in the United States, however, has found improved quality while lowering costs in lower extremity joint replacement, but not other conditions (Agarwal et al., 2020). Still other analyses found that bundled payments resulted in decreased costs for hospitals for both medical and surgical admissions, but surgical only for physician groups (Liao et al., 2022).

The bundled payment program remains in evolution, as do empirical findings, but a shift from voluntary to obligatory is underway. In 2024 CMS payment rules for fiscal year 2025 proposed a new mandatory bundle payment initiative, the *Transforming Episode Accountability Model* (TEAM) that would replace traditional fee-for-service in selected hospitals, which have not yet been named as this text goes to print. Five conditions are included, with the bundled payment for all acute and postacute care (up to 30 days). The conditions selected were chosen because they have "sufficient volume to warrant standard care pathways during the acute and post-acute portions of the episode" (Hut, 2024, para 7). These conditions are (a) coronary artery bypass graft, (b) lower-extremity joint replacement, (c) major bowel procedures, (d) spinal fusion, and (e) surgical hip or femur fracture treatment.

Another disease-specific model that may be of great interest to nurses is the Guiding an Improved Dementia Experience (GUIDE) model. Announced on July 3, 2023, with an implementation date of January 1, 2024, this eight-year model is unique in that it focuses not only on the person living with dementia but also their unpaid caregiver, with an overall aim of enabling people to live in their homes and communities. A broad range of nurse-relevant and nurse-led services is envisioned, including care coordination and management, caregiver support, and respite services (CMS, n.d.-b). Nurses, with broad education across different populations and settings, coupled with their understanding of human behavior, therapeutic human environments, family dynamics, and analytics, are in a powerful position to maximize the potential of these and other bundled payment models.

Finally, bundled payments for end-stage renal disease (ESRD) are being tested in the United States and elsewhere around the globe. Recall that people with ESRD are Medicare eligible and they represent a growing, comparatively costly population. Emrani et al.'s (2023) scoping review of 59 studies (64% from the United States) on payment systems for dialysis and payment effects found a trend: a shift from retrospective fee-for-service payments to prospective and P4P models. The former was associated with undertreatment of unpaid and inexpensive services and overtreatment of payable services, and the latter was associated with cost savings, shifting services outside the bundle, and variable impacts on quality of care. A continued U.S. focus on ESRD payment models is likely to continue or accelerate given its dramatic increase (doubling from 2000 to 2019, driven by hypertension and diabetes) and the substantial racial and ethnic disparities, including an increase of 149.5% among people of Asian descent (Kuehn, 2022).

Global Budgets

Global budgets take many of the incentive forces in bundled payments to the next level by bundling all services in a particular setting, such as hospitals. Global budgets for hospitals means all-payer (Medicare, Medicaid, and commercial insurance) payments to hospitals—who in turn pay their staff, including nurses—and their employed physicians. This may be based on the *historical revenue* for a defined period of time, usually a year. You can think of the concept of historical revenue as analogous to your income from the previous year. Although the hospitals will be guaranteed their revenue for the upcoming year, they will have significant incentives to reduce avoidable utilization, coordinate care better, and manage their costs in order to enhance the quality of care and improve their margins, or the amount that remains after they have paid their expenses. Over time, of course, the hospital budget may need to increase to reflect legitimate increases in expenses (e.g., raises for the nurses) within an overall orientation of cost control. Thus, as a means to control the growth in health care spending, increases in a hospital's global budget from year to year may be based on economic indicators that reflect the overall growth in the economy, such as the consumer price index, market basket index, or gross state product. Another approach to global budgets would be to reimburse hospitals on a risk-adjusted *per member per month (PMPM)* method.

Overall, the incentives in global budgets are very different from the volume-based incentives under fee-for-service reimbursement. Quality performance measures and efficiency standards can be incorporated into the global budget formula to modify overall payments over time, offering additional incentives for enhancement of the quality of care.

Why would a setting such as a hospital consider a global budget? R. Slusky et al. (personal communication, December 19, 2013) offer the following perspectives.

Unlike fee-for-service payments, global budgets provide the participating hospitals predictable revenues, while at the same time incentivizing the hospital to focus more on cost management rather than revenue enhancement. Global budgets are also a way to link the payment system to the goals of population-based health care. Over time, a global budget can reflect the total amount a community ought to spend, based on the demographics and health care needs of the population being served by the hospital and other community providers. A hospital reimbursed in a global budget model in a region with many families of childbearing age, for example, would likely offer dramatically different combinations of services than a hospital serving a large community of elders. Providers also have greater flexibility to determine how to spend human and capital resources to meet community needs. And, like a household budget, the hospital has strong incentives to reduce unnecessary care and care of little value, particularly if it is expensive, invasive care.

Maryland has experimented with a hospital (rather than all setting) global budget through its all-payer rate setting model. In place for decades through a Medicare waiver, the state of Maryland negotiated a new Medicare waiver in 2014. It required the state to implement hospital global budgets within a 5-year period; in 2017 the CMS and Maryland partnership was expanded with the Care Redesign Program. The overall intent of these approaches in Maryland is to control the growth of health care expenditures over time based on a predetermined trend factor and provide incentives for the hospitals to increase their margins by better management of their costs relative to their budgets. Maryland has been ahead of schedule and in the first 3 years achieved $554 million in hospital Medicare savings without shifting costs to other parts of the system outside the global budget (Haber et al., 2019); Medicare spending fell 2.8% relative to a comparison group, with a 4.1% reduction in hospital expenditures, but only a modest impact on quality was found (Japinga & McClellan, 2020). At the same time, the number of Maryland ambulatory surgical centers (ASCs) per capita is the highest in the nation at 56.7 ASCs/100,000 people (Durda, 2021); ASCs are not within the hospital rate setting budget, likely reflecting the finding noted in ESRD bundled payments—care shifts outside the bundle and the associated financial limits.

Pennsylvania has adopted a global budget model for rural hospitals, with an anticipated performance period end date of December 31, 2024 (CMS, n.d.-c). Other states (Massachusetts and Rhode Island) have set expenditure targets, and still others have set price caps as a multiplier of Medicare rates (Montana, Oregon, and Washington) (Pany et al., 2022).

These authors note that "competition and market-based policies have not succeeded in meaningfully constraining healthcare prices" (para 8); thus stakeholders are exploring price regulation through caps on prices, growth targets, and global budgets. Although targets are not caps or full global budgets, evidence to date suggests even the comparatively modest step of expenditure targets has slowed health care spending in Massachusetts (Waugh & McCarthy, 2020). In the wake of COVID-19, Fried et al. (2020) have called for global budgets as a strategy to sustain rural hospitals. Building on these models, the Community Transformation Track of the Community Health Access and Rural Transformation (CHART) model expands on the Maryland and Pennsylvania experience to include participating hospitals in Alabama, South Dakota, Texas, and Washington (Kalata et al., 2023).

Kalata et al. (2023) suggest that global budgets in rural areas are particularly appealing because they may stabilize revenue and allow otherwise financially distressed institutions to avoid closure.

NURSING ROLES WITHIN EMERGING PAYMENT MODELS

Emerging payment models offer tremendous opportunities for nurses to bring their knowledge, skills, and abilities into play in new ways. Educated across provider settings—hospitals, nursing homes, and home health practice specialties, and at individual, family, and population levels—the generalist scope of practice of a baccalaureate or higher-degree RN is an excellent fit with the societal need to address health care costs. Indeed, nurses have the potential to be the glue in the new health system. Some skills are new domains for nurses, whereas others are not new, but rather renewed skills, preparation, and education that are dormant. Notably, in the fee-for-service system, a nurse is viewed as a *labor cost* rather than a *knowledge worker*. The emerging models recognize that all care is a cost, and unlike in fee-for-service, in which physicians and hospitals are perceived as *revenue drivers* creating cash flow, these models better recognize the parallel societal costs. Worthy value-based nursing skills for entry-level and advanced practice skills are detailed in Table 4.1.

Are nurses ready to lead care redesign within new payment models? Fraher et al. (2013) argue that too little attention has been paid to the learning needs of those who are not physicians, which remains relevant today. These authors suggest:

> [B]ecause of sheer numbers—the U.S. healthcare system employs 2 7 million registered nurses—it is nurses who are arguably in the most pivotal position to drive system change. Nurses are providing patient education and care coordination, improving care transitions between community and acute care settings, conducting home visits for patients with complex chronic conditions, enhancing patient and family engagement, improving population health management, and increasing

community outreach. These efforts have reduced unnecessary hospitalizations and readmissions, improved patients' experiences, increased the quality of care provided, and lowered costs (p. 1813).

As of 2024, there are 5.2 million nurses, 4.6 million of whom are working. The sheer numbers are even more manifold than a decade ago, underscoring nurses' pivotal role in care models reshaped by payment reform.

OTHER LEADERSHIP OPPORTUNITIES FOR NURSES

Superutilizers have been a successful target of nursing-led coordinated care. Superutilizers are people with recurring, preventable health care needs that result in the use of high-cost care such as the ED. Notably, the documented financial cost to individuals and the system fails to consider the additional emotional and physical cost borne by these individuals and their family. Superutilizers represent just 1% of the U.S. population, yet they are responsible for 22% of the cost. In Medicaid, this imbalance is even more dramatic: 5% of the population represents 55% of the cost (Mann, 2013). Lantz notes that these individuals have complex medical and social needs, and interventions need to address this complexity inclusive of "nonmedical problems such as poverty, food insecurity, housing instability, transportation challenges, and social isolation" (Lantz, 2020, p. 31). Nurses' broad background suggests they are in an ideal position to lead such interventions. One successful model employs teams of nurses and social workers for individual *and* population management. Such care depends on the use of robust data, and strong analytic skills are needed by the field-based care managers and care coordinators. Using this approach, the Vermont Chronic Care Collaborative, for example, has demonstrated promising early results in cost savings after expenses, reduction in inpatient and ED utilization, and decreased 30-day readmission rate (Vermont Chronic Care Initiative, 2019). Mann (2013) notes common characteristics across successful care collaboration programs, such as:

1. **Web-based provider portals with easy access to patient data:** These data can then be used to discern patterns of health care utilization, such as when there is a visit to the ED versus a primary care visit. Understanding individual patterns of utilization provides the foundation for development of tailored interventions for each patient.
2. **Real-time data:** This is useful to develop effective, tailored, strategies for care management. Any lags in data must be minimal. ED utilization reports from 6 months to a year ago would not help a care coordinator develop timely interventions to address the root cause of the ED visits.
3. **Decision-support tools:** These can help the care manager use the data in meaningful ways, supporting the transition from information, to

knowledge, to a plan for action by offering prompts, to action under defined conditions of data patterns.

Still other studies have found nurse-led primary care of a patient population with common chronic complications of hypertension (coronary heart disease, heart attack, and stroke) had better outcomes than traditional physician-led primary care, with a resulting $3.7 million in cost savings (Wagner & Zabler, 2024).

In the post–fee-for-service world, outcomes matter, demanding fresh attention to the skills needed in today's health care system. Skills such as "prevention, care coordination, care process reengineering, dissemination of best practices, team-based care, continuous quality improvement, and the use of data to support a transformed system" (CMMI, cited in Fraher et al., 2013, p. 1813) are well suited to nurses' skill sets and interests, yet demand a broad and deep understanding of health economics. Thus, Section II (Chapters 5–7) expands on the foundation developed in Chapters 1 to 4 to further explicate the nuances of health economics as foundational nursing knowledge in the emerging era. To aid understanding and application, health economics is illustrated in contrast to examples of classic economics that are common in nurses' everyday lives.

End-of-Chapter Resources

THOUGHT QUESTIONS

1. In which payment model would you prefer to be? Provide a rationale for your response.
   A. A 28-year-old with poorly controlled type 1 diabetes
   B. An older person with multiple chronic conditions
   C. A pediatric neurosurgeon
   D. An RN
   E. A taxpayer
   F. A Medicare beneficiary
2. What are the potential unintended consequences of each of the payment reform models?
3. Define the following key terms:
   Accountable care organization
   Benchmarking
   Global budget
   Patient-centered medical home

Pay for performance
Risk adjusted
Shared savings program

EXERCISE

1. Develop a presentation to explain payment reform models to your peers, including a description of how each model works, its value to society, and its strengths and weaknesses.
2. Consider your most recent clinical experience. How might care be redesigned to improve outcomes and decrease cost? Which payment model would be the best strategy toward that end? Defend your answer.

QUIZ

True or False

1. All forms of reimbursement create the same treatment incentives and disincentives.
2. The acronym P4P refers to a form of health care reimbursement termed *preferred for payment*.
3. Another term for PCMHs is advanced primary care.
4. The ACA defined potential members of the community health team.
5. The optimal configuration of team members in a PCMH has been defined and is firmly supported by empirical evidence.
6. An ACO may be defined as a group of providers who agree to be accountable for the cost and quality of the care provided.
7. The term *superutilizer* refers to individuals who use a disproportionally high amount of health care.
8. Hospital global budgets provide hospitals with a predictable revenue outlook.
9. Under fee-for-service reimbursement, hospital-employed nurses are often viewed by management as a labor cost.
10. Bundled payments create a financial incentive to coordinate care across the entire episode of illness or condition management.

Multiple Choice

11. Fee-for-service reimbursement
    A. Creates strong incentives for care coordination
    B. Contributes to the nation's difficulty containing health care costs
    C. Both A and B
    D. Neither A nor B

12. Linking reimbursement to achievement of quality metrics
    A. May result in better health care outcomes
    B. May create metric-driven behavior that creates metric-driven patient harm
    C. Both A and B
    D. Neither A nor B
13. In addition to employing physicians and nurses, PCMHs rely on
    A. Community health teams
    B. Health coaches
    C. Both A and B
    D. Neither A nor B
14. ACO shared savings programs
    A. Create opportunities for nurses to influence the value of care provided through care coordination and care redesign
    B. Require that quality thresholds be met before savings from expected expenditures are shared among the payer and the ACO
    C. Both A and B
    D. Neither A nor B
15. Global budgets in health care
    A. Create financial incentives to reduce avoidable health care utilization
    B. Create financial incentives to coordinate care
    C. Both A and B
    D. Neither A nor B
16. Fee-for-service reimbursement
    A. Creates financial incentives to reduce avoidable health care utilization
    B. Creates financial incentives to coordinate care
    C. Both A and B
    D. Neither A nor B
17. Nursing skills valued in a reformed health care system include
    A. Care process reengineering
    B. Care coordination
    C. Systematic use of data
    D. All of the above

NOTE

1. True story, shared with the author in May 2014. The nurse described was successful in her role and subsequently started a company to help organizations deploy this model.

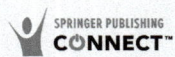

A robust set of instructor resources designed to supplement this text is located at http://connect.springerpub.com/content/book/978-0-8261-7236-5. Qualifying instructors may request access by emailing textbook@springerpub.com.

REFERENCES

Agarwal, R., Liao, J., Gupta, A., & Navathe, A. (2020). The impact of bundled payments health care spending, utilization, and quality: A systematic review. *Health Affairs, 39*(1) 50–57. https://doi.org/10.1377/hlthaff.2019.00784

American College of Physicians. (2013). *Community health teams to support the patient centered medical home.* Retrieved August 18, 2014, from https://www.acponline.org/sites/default/files/documents/advocacy/where_we_stand/assets/ii12-community-health-teams.pdf

Berwick, D. (2020). Moral determinants of health. *Journal of American Medical Association, 324,* 225–226. https://doi.org/10.1001/jama.2020.11129

Calikoglu, S., Murray, R., & Feeney, D. (2012). Hospital pay-for-performance programs in Maryland produced strong results, including reduced hospital-acquired conditions. *Health Affairs, 31*(12), 2649–2658. https://doi.org/10.1377/hlthaff.2012.0357

Centers for Medicare and Medicaid Services. (n.d.-a). *Comprehensive primary care initiative.* Author. https://www.cms.gov/priorities/innovation/innovation-models/comprehensive-primary-care-initiative

Centers for Medicare and Medicaid Services. (n.d.-b). *Guiding and improved dementia experience (GUIDE) model.* Author. https://www.cms.gov/priorities/innovation/innovation-models/guide

Centers for Medicare and Medicaid Services (n.d.-c). *Pennsylvania Rural Health Model.* https://www.cms.gov/priorities/innovation/innovation-models/pa-rural-health-model

Chernew, M., Conway, P., & Frakt, A. (2020). Transforming Medicare's payment systems: Progress shaped by the ACA. *Health Affairs, 39*(3), 413–420. https://doi.org/10.1377/hlthaff.2019.01410

Durda, L. (2021, June 8). *10 States with the highest number of ASCs per capita.* Becker's Hospital News. https://www.beckersasc.com/benchmarking/10-states-with-the-highest-number-of-ascs-per-capita.html

Emrani, Z., Amiresmaili, M., Daroudi, R., Najafi, M. T., & Akbari Sari, A. (2023). Payment systems for dialysis and their effects: A scoping review. *BMC Health Services Research, 23*(1), 45. https://doi.org/10.1186/s12913-022-08974-4

Fortuna, R. J., Johnson, W., Clark, J. S., Messing, S., Flynn, S., & Judge, S. R. (2021). Impact of Patient-Centered Medical Home transformation on providers, staff, and quality. *Population Health Management, 24*(2), 207–213. https://doi.org/10.1089/pop.2020.0007

Fowler, L., Rowal, P., Fogler, S., Waldersen, B., O'Connell, M., & Quinton, J. (2022). *The CMS innovation center's strategy to support person-centered, value-based specialty care.* https://www.cms.gov/blog/cms-innovation-centers-strategy-support-person-centered-value-based-specialty-care

Fraher, E., Ricketts, T., Lefebvre, A., & Newton, W. (2013). The role of academic health centers and their partners in reconfiguring and retooling the existing workforce to practice in a transformed health system. *Academic Medicine, 88*(12), 1812–1816. https://doi.org/10.1097/ACM.0000000000000024

Fried, J., Liebers, D., & Roberts, E. (2020, June 10). Sustaining rural hospitals after COVID-10: The case for global budgets. *Journal of American Medical Association, 324*(2), 137–138. https://doi.org/10.1001/jama.2020.9744

Friedberg, M., Schneider, E., Rosenthal, M., Volpp, K., & Werner, R. (2014). Association between participation in a multipayer medical home intervention and changes in quality, utilization, and costs of care. *Journal of the American Medical Association, 311*(8), 815–825. https://doi.org/10.1001/jama.2014.353

Gonzalez-Smith, J., Bleser, W., Muhlestein, D., Richards, R., McClellan, M., & Saunders, R. (2019, October 25). *Medicare ACO results for 2018: More downside risk adoption, more savings, and all ACO types now averaging savings*. Health Affairs Blog. https://www.healthaffairs.org/do/10.1377/hblog20191024.65681/full/

Haber, S., Beil, H., Morrison, M., Greenwald, L., Perry, R., Jiang, L., Masters, S., Rutledge, R., Berzin, O., Cole-Beebe, M., Feinberg, R., Zichittella, L., Kluckman, M., Parish, W., Keyes, V., Kendrick, D., Schneider, J., Hooper, E., Mittman, L., . . . Amico, P. (2019). *Evaluation of the Maryland all-payer model, Volume 1: Final report*. RTI International. https://downloads.cms.gov/files/md-allpayer-finalevalrpt.pdf

Haverkamp, M. H., Peiris, D., Mainor, A. J., Westert, G. P., Rosenthal, M. B., Sequist, T. D., & Colla, C. H. (2018). ACOs with risk-bearing experience are likely taking steps to reduce low-value medical services. *The American Journal of Managed Care, 24*(7), e216–e221.

Healthcare Financial Management Association. (2023). *2023 Perspectives on value-based care*. Terry Group. https://terrygroup.com/app/uploads/2023/09/Terry-Health-2023-VBC-Survey-Report.pdf

Hut, N. (2024, April 16). *CMS calls for hospitals to be subject to a new bundled payment model and data-reporting requirement*. Healthcare Finance Management Association. https://www.hfma.org/payment-reimbursement-and-managed-care/medicare-payment-and-reimbursement/cms-calls-for-hospitals-to-be-subject-to-a-new-bundled-payment-model-and-data-reporting-requirements/

Japinga, M., & McClellan, M. (2020, June 15). *Uniquely similar: New results from Maryland's all-payer model and paths forward for value-based care*. Milbank Memorial Fund. https://www.milbank.org/publications/uniquely-similar-new-results-from-marylands-all-payer-model-and-paths-forward-for-value-based-care

Kacik, A. (2020, May 21). *April was the worst month ever for hospital operating margins*. Modern Healthcare. https://www.modernhealthcare.com/finance/april-was-worst-month-ever-hospital-operating-margins

Kaiser Family Foundation. (2023). *States that reported patient centered medical homes in place*. https://www.kff.org/medicaid/state-indicator/states-that-reported-patient-centered-medical-homes-in-place/?currentTimeframe=0&sortModel=%7B%22colId%22:%22Location%22,%22sort%22:%22asc%22%7D

Kalata, S., Nathan, H., & Ibrahim, A. M. (2023). Understanding community health access and rural transformation reform—implications for rural surgical care. *JAMA Surgery, 158*(5):437–438. https://doi.org/10.1001/jamasurg.2022.6834

Kim, K. M., Max, W., White, J. S., Chapman, S. A., & Muench, U. (2020). Do penalty-based pay-for-performance programs improve surgical care more effectively than other payment strategies? A systematic review. *Annals of Medicine and Surgery, 60*, 623–630. https://doi.org/10.1016/j.amsu.2020.11.060

Kuehn, B. M. (2022). End-stage kidney disease doubles. *Journal of the American Medical Association*, 327(16), 1540. https://doi.org/10.1001/jama.2022.5342

Lantz, P. M. (2020). "Super-utilizer" interventions: What they reveal about evaluation research, wishful thinking, and health equity. *The Milbank Quarterly*, 98(1), 31–34. https://doi.org/10.1111/1468-0009.12449

Liao, J. M., Huang, Q., Wang, E., Linn, K., Shirk, T., Zhu, J., Cousins, D., & Navathe, A. S. (2022). Performance of physician groups and hospitals participating in bundled payments among Medicare beneficiaries. *JAMA Health Forum*, 3(12), e224889. https://doi.org/10.1001/jamahealthforum.2022.4889

Livingston, S. (2020). Covid-19 may end up boosting value-based payment. *Modern Healthcare*. https://www.modernhealthcare.com/insurance/covid-19-may-end-up-boosting-value-based-payment

Mann, C. (2013, July 24). *Targeting Medicaid super-utilizers to decrease cost and improve quality*. Centers for Medicare and Medicaid Services (CMS Informational Bulletin).

Mannion, R., & Braithwaite, J. (2012). Unintended consequences of performance measurement in healthcare. *Internal Medicine Journal*, 42(5), 569–574.

Mendelson, A., Kondo, K., Damberg, C., Low, A., Motuapuaka, M., Freeman, M., O'Neil, M., Relevo, R., & Kansagara, D. (2017). The effects of pay-for-performance programs on health, health care use, and processes of care: A systematic review. *Annals of Internal Medicine*, 166(5), 341–353. https://doi.org/10.7326/M16-1881

Newcomer, L., Gould, B., Page, R., Donelan, S., & Perkins, M. (2014). Changing physician incentives for affordable, quality cancer care: Results of an episode payment model. *Journal of Oncology Practice*, 10(5), 322–326. https://doi.org/10.1200/JOP.2014.001488

Nielson, M., Gibson, J., Buelt, L., Grundy, P., & Grumbach, K. (2015). *The patient-centered medical home's impact on cost and quality: An annual update of the evidence 2013–2014*. Milbank Memorial Fund.

Noël, F. (2022). Accelerating the pace of value-based transformation for more resilient and sustainable healthcare. *Future Healthcare Journal*, 9(3), 226–229. https://doi.org/10.7861/fhj.2022-0118

Nutting, P., Crabtree, B., & McDaniel, R. (2012). Small primary care practices face four hurdles—including a physician-centric mind-set—in becoming medical homes. *Health Affairs*, 31(11), 2417–2422. https://doi.org/10.1377/hlthaff.2011.0974

Nyweid, D., Lee, W., & Colla, C. (2020). Accountable Care Organizations' increase in nonphysician practitioners may signal shift for health care workforce. *Health Affairs*, 39(6), 1080–1086. https://doi.org/10.1377/hlthaff.2019.01144

Pany, M., Biniek Fuglesten, J., & Newman, T. (2022, May 31). *Price regulation, global budgets and spending targets: A road map to reduce health care spending, and improve affordability*. Kaiser Family Foundation. https://www.kff.org/health-costs/report/price-regulation-global-budgets-and-spending-targets-a-road-map-to-reduce-health-care-spending-and-improve-affordability/

Peck, K. A., Usadi, B., Mainor, A. J., Fisher, E. S., & Colla, C. H. (2019). ACO contracts with downside financial risk growing, but still in the minority. *Health Affairs (Project Hope)*, 38(7), 1201–1206. https://doi.org/10.1377/hlthaff.2018.05386

Peikes, D., Dale, S., Ghosh, A., Taylor, E., Swankoski, K., O'Malley, A., Day, T., Duda, N., Singh, P., Anglin, G., Sessums, L., & Brown, R. (2018). The comprehensive primary care initiative: Effects on spending, quality, patients and physicians. *Health Affairs, 37*(6), 890–899. https://doi.org/10.1377/hlthaff.2017.1678

Perloff, J., & O'Reilly-Jacob, M., Perlman, A., & Sobul, S. (2023). The impact of nurse practitioner attribution in Medicare Shared Savings ACOs. *American Journal of Managed Care, 11*(4), 20–29. https://doi.org/10.37765/ajac.2023.89475

Rambur, B., Vallett, C., Cohen, J., & Tarule, J. (2013). Metric-driven harm: An exploration of unintended consequences of performance measurement. *Applied Nursing Research, 26*(4), 269–275. https://doi.org/10.1016/j.apnr.2013.09.001

Roiland, R., Japinga, M., Singletary, E., Sharma, I., Gonzalez-Smith, J., Wang, G., Jacobs, J., Bleser, W., Saunders, R., & McClellen, M. (2020). *Value-based care in the COVID-19 era: Enabling health care response and resilience.* https://healthpolicy.duke.edu/sites/default/files/2020-07/best_practices_brief_final.pdf

Rosenberg, J. (2019, July 9) Despite growth, uptake of downside risk in ACO contracts remains low. *American Journal of Managed Care.* https://www.ajmc.com/focus-of-the-week/despite-growth-uptake-of-downside-risk-in-aco-contracts-remains-low

Ryan, A., Blustein, J., & Casalino, L. (2012). Medicare's flagship test of pay-for-performance did not spur more rapid quality improvement among low-performing hospitals. *Health Affairs, 31*(4), 2417–2422. https://doi.org/10.1377/hlthaff.2011.0626

Struijs, J., DeVries, E., Baan, C., van Gils, P., & Rosenthal, M. (2020, April 6). *Bundled payment models around the world: How they work, their impact.* The Commonwealth Fund. https://www.commonwealthfund.org/publications/2020/apr/bundled-payment-models-around-world-how-they-work-their-impact

Veet, C. A., Radomski, T. R., D'Avella, C., Hernandez. I., Wessel, C., Swart, E. C. S., Shrank, W. H., & Parekh, N. (2020). Impact of healthcare delivery system type on clinical, utilization, and cost outcomes of patient-centered medical homes: A systematic review. *Journal of General Internal Medicine, 35*(4), 1276–1284. https://doi.org/10.1007/s11606-019-05594-3

Vermont Chronic Care Initiative. (2019, December 6). *Vermont chronic care initiative: Health together.* https://dvha.vermont.gov/for-providers/vermont-chronic-care-initiatie-vcci1

Wagner, P., & Zabler, P. (2024). Costs saved by visiting a nurse-led primary care facility comparison of primary care models *Policy, Politics, & Nursing Practice, 0*(0). https://doi.org/10.1177/15271544241247767

Waugh, L., & MCarthy, D. (2020, March 5). *How the Massachusetts Health Policy Commission is fostering a statewide commitment to contain health care spending growth.* The Commonwealth Foundation. https://www.commonwealthfund.org/sites/default/files/2020-03/Waugh_Massachusetts_hlt_policy_comm_cs.pdf

Werner, R., Konetzka, R. T., & Polsky, D. (2013). The effect of pay-for-performance in nursing homes: Evidence from state Medicaid programs. *Health Services Research, 48*(4), 1393–1414. https://doi.org/10.1111/1475-6773.12035

Yakusheva, O., Needleman, J., Bettencourt, A. P., & Buerhaus, P. I. (2020). Is it time to peek under the hood of system-level approaches to quality and safety? *Nursing Outlook, 68*(2), 141–144. https://doi.org/10.1016/j.outlook.2019.11.004

SECTION II

Health Care Economics: A Pragmatic Overview

Health care markets differ from classic free markets in dramatic ways. Why is knowing this important to you? Many elements of health care and health reform are shaped by policy or payment attempts either to add elements of classic free markets to health care markets or to correct or control consequences of the manner in which health care markets work. Simply put, it is difficult to understand much of what happens in health care without understanding these principles. Fortunately, these principles and their consequences are easy to understand when they are contrasted with principles of classic free market theory that you are familiar with in your everyday life.

Chapter 5 describes a principle you are very familiar with: When you purchase something, you notice the price because you are paying for it, and the purchase is felt in your pocketbook. Health care differs in important ways, and these are detailed.

Chapter 6 describes the central role of information in classic markets, how health care markets differ from these, and the emerging trends that are increasing the role of information in health care policy and nursing practice. Although the Internet of Everything and artificial intelligence are broader than information, they—and other digital innovations—are included in this chapter for ease of understanding. Payments that stem from metrics, a form of information, are also described in this chapter.

Chapter 7 reviews two more principles that manifest along a range of things familiar to you—such as the licensing law that enables you to practice as an RN—to less familiar but important things like certificates of need and antitrust laws. Antitrust laws exist to ensure market competition and a decrease in market competition through mergers and acquisitions (termed market concentration) directly impacts the quality of care and nurses' salaries and opportunities. Thus, although these regulations may seem obscure, they directly impact your life and job.

Together, learning about health economics will enable you to better understand events and activities in your workplace and clinical setting as well as clarify overall principles of health reform. Importantly, it also provides an essential framework by which to understand health care and policy changes long into the future.

CHAPTER 5

How Health Care Markets Differ From Other Markets . . . and Why It Matters

CHAPTER 5 builds on the foundation in Chapters 1 to 4 to explicate the nuances of health economics more fully. To do so, health care markets are described in contrast to classic free markets. Following completion of this chapter, you will be able to:

- Contrast the implications of "the buyers bear the consequences of their decisions" between classic free markets and health care markets and decision-making.
- Explain key-related strategies such as cost sharing and price transparency legislation.
- Discuss the concept of demand in health care, including supplier-induced demand, small area variation, and moral hazard.

WHAT DOES IT MEAN TO BEAR THE FINANCIAL CONSEQUENCES OF DECISION-MAKING?

These two scenarios illustrate the first item.

> Cecily Jones, RN, is exhausted after a 12-hour shift and decides a bit of "retail therapy" is in order. She stops at the local upscale department store on her way home from work. There she is captivated by a pricey smartwatch she sorely desires. Recalling that the rent is due as well as the payment on her son's orthodontics, she decides to forgo the new watch. Determinedly, she also marches past the clothing sale rack, carried by the realization that right now she cannot afford anything new. What she has will simply have to do.

> Ms. Williams enters the ED with vague symptoms following a fall while skiing. Although she was wearing a helmet, she recalls a famous actress who died after a ski injury. Ms. Williams is worried. The ED triage finds nothing unusual, but Ms. Williams is very vocal in her concern, her anxiety accelerating.

> The busy attending physician, Joan Garcia, MD, plans watchful waiting with clear instructions on warning signs, but at Ms. Williams's insistence reconsiders. As Ms. Williams blathers, Dr. Garcia's attention shifts to the recent department meeting in which the fiscal status of the hospital was reviewed: Patient revenues are down, her department chair shared, and targets for higher inpatient volumes have been set. Thumbing the chart, Dr. Garcia notes that Ms. Williams has low-deductible, fee-for-service insurance. The waiting room is filled with patients needing immediate attention, and Dr. Garcia is eager to move on to the next patient. As she tries to move on, Ms. Williams attaches herself, barnacle-like, adamant that she wants a complete checkup. She slyly suggests that she "just may sue if not treated right." Although Dr. Garcia is convinced it probably is not necessary, she orders a CT scan. Ms. Williams now seems very happy with her care, calling to tell her son she likely will be admitted.

These scenarios illustrate one of the significant ways in which health care markets differ from classic free markets. In a classic free market, *buyers bear the financial consequences of their decisions to purchase* a product or service. The value of each potential purchase is weighed against other appealing options as well as other financial responsibilities. As a result, buyers *self-ration* purchases all the time. Few Americans, for example, drive a Rolls-Royce. It is simply too expensive a car for most people, and perhaps not even practical. Instead, cars are purchased with an appreciation of the impact of the cost of the purchase in relationship to other purchase opportunities, as well as the value of the potential purchase in relationship to other goods and services. Nurse Jones, for example, weighed the impact of the cost and value of a new watch and wardrobe against other responsibilities and desires. She chose not to make a purchase. Nurse Jones self-rationed. Similarly, an individual considering a new car will weigh the pros and cons of different options—different makes and models, new or used, current vehicle or public transportation—based on the cost and perceived value of the contribution the new purchase brings.

Less Immediate Cost Consequences in Health Care

Conversely, Ms. Williams had little incentive to moderate her desire for care. Ms. Williams does not bear the immediate financial impact of her decision to seek services. It is a bit like asking someone looking for a car if they want a Rolls-Royce and handing them the keys, or like a parent or other authority deciding that a Rolls is for you and handing you the keys. In each case, the cost of this interaction is largely hidden from view.

Ms. Williams may perceive that the services are "paid for anyway" by the insurance company. This arrangement masks the cost of seeking services, and thus there is little self-rationing among those with health insurance, in part because the immediate cost of the decision to purchase is not borne by the consumer. In economics, overuse of services because you "don't have skin in the game" is termed *moral hazard*. Moreover, the cost may even be difficult to ascertain, given that health care markets are characterized by a lack of *price transparency*. Federal legislation has emphasized price transparency as an important strategy toward better outcomes at a lower cost by passing legislation, for example, hospital price transparency rules effective January 1, 2021 (CMS.gov, 2023), with a substantial increase in penalty for noncompliance used to spur participation (Kacik, 2024). Price transparency legislation is a rare issue with bipartisan support, for example, the Lower Costs, More Transparency Act of 2023 that passed in the House with bipartisan support (Tong, 2023) and the Health Care PRICE Transparency Act 2.0 introduced in the Senate in 2024 with bipartisan sponsors.

Value transparency is a more complex issue than price transparency. The actual value of the service is very difficult to determine, and one of the things the patient is "purchasing" is information itself, assuming the provider is assessing the value. As Arrow (1963) notes, "When there is uncertainty, information or knowledge becomes a commodity" (p. 946). The role of information in markets is a critical issue, and these issues will be discussed in depth in Chapter 6.

Third-Party Payers

Simply put, Ms. Williams did not weigh the cost of treatment against her other financial demands. She showed up at the ED expecting treatment. Unlike a classic free market where the interaction is limited to two entities, a buyer and a seller, health care includes a *third party*. This third party is an insurance company; indeed, insurance companies are called *third-party payers* for exactly this reason.

Third-party payers exist to spread risk in the ways described in Chapter 1. At the same time, the cost of treatment is not apparent or visible to the individual because they do not bear that cost immediately and directly, nor can they read it on a price tag. Instead, that cost is spread to the group. Indeed, spreading the cost of care from one individual to many is the functional purpose of insurance groups to begin with. Insurance companies spread the risk, a strategy that can keep down individual financial risk and—if the individual is in a low-utilization group—the cost of insurance. Yet if there is a great deal of high-cost utilization within the group, insurance rates will increase the following year. Nevertheless, this event is chronologically disconnected from the individual's decision to seek treatment at a certain time, and the cost is an aggregate based on the sum of all care provided within a group that year.

The Promise of Providers Assuming Financial Risk

The providers in a fee-for-service system also have no incentive for nontreatment, assessing value, or limiting the cost of treatment. Recall that the *cost* borne by the insurance company or governmental payer—which is actually borne by the members in the group through their premiums or through taxes—is actually *revenue* to the provider. Thus, there is a misalignment between incentives, highlighting the importance of risk sharing and risk-bearing payment reform (see Table 5.1).

Health Care as a Vulnerable Purchase

There are other key ways health care markets differ from classic free markets, and many of these make it difficult to control costs. Unlike other goods

TABLE 5.1 FINANCIAL RISK TERMS

Financial risk comes in various types. Recall that "bearing" financial risk means that providers' care decisions are linked to cost accountability. These range from opportunities for additional payments or, on the other end of the spectrum, a loss of revenue. The main categories are as follows: one-sided risk, two-sided risk inclusive of downside risk, risk-sharing, and risk-bearing.

One-Sided Risk	Two-Sided Risk
One-sided risk is also called upside only. In one-sided risk arrangements, the cost of care for a population of patients is projected and, if providers deliver care for less cost than projected, they are financially rewarded with those savings. If they are in a **one-sided risk-sharing arrangement**, they share those financial rewards with the payer covering the individuals who received care; for example, Medicare, Medicaid, or commercial insurance. The parameters guiding the arrangement are detailed in advance, including quality measures that must be met before additional payment is received. This is to prevent lower costs being obtained at the expense of quality or patient access to care.	The term **two-sided risk** includes, as the name implies, both **upside and downside risk. Downside risk** refers to providers also being accountable for cost that is greater than projected. In a risk-sharing arrangement inclusive of downside risk (**a two-sided risk arrangement**), the providers would share with the payer the positive financial outcomes described herein as well as negative financial outcomes if cost of care is higher than projected. In **full risk bearing**, providers not only reap all the financial benefits of delivering care that is less than projected but also bear the full negative financial impact of delivering care that is more expensive than projected. Notably, these projections of cost of care for a given population include **risk adjustment**, meaning the cost of care for an ill population would be projected to be more than that for a well population. This is designed to prevent adverse selection, also called **cherry picking**, whereby providers would only be willing to accept risk for populations likely to be well and therefore generate little cost. Again, in **two-sided risk models** the parameters, including the quality metrics that must be met, are detailed in advance of the agreement to proceed with this form of payment reform

and services, health care is a vulnerable purchase. In a classic market, purchasing power is in the hands of the consumer. A consumer may buy what and when they want and walk away from a purchase without consequences. Nurse Jones, for example, although desirous of a smartwatch, does not bear dramatic consequences for not making the purchase, desire and disappointment notwithstanding. For Ms. Williams, however, things are more muddled. Although it is quite possible that Ms. Williams is best left untreated, it is also possible that she has anything from a concussion to a basilar skull fracture. Health care "purchases" are marked by *uncertainty*. This notion was first promulgated by Kenneth Arrow, the Nobel Prize–winning economist whose seminal ideas birthed the area of health care economics referenced in Chapter 1.

What Is Payment Reform?

Payment reform is the umbrella term used to define health care reimbursement strategies that move away from fee-for-service, as described in Chapter 4. These include an array of pay-for-performance models such as accountable care programs, bundled payments, and global budgets. Inherent in these strategies is *provider accountability* for selected outcomes and—in the case of the latter three—accountability for cost of clinical decision-making. This contrasts with fee-for-service, in which providers are not held financially accountable for the cost, or value, of their treatment decisions. In general, U.S. providers have been reluctant to accept downside risk, noting that many of the antecedents to health outcomes lie in social determinants. Nevertheless, it is unclear if the resistance is related to not appreciating the role of social determinants or being unclear on how to address them. Glenn et al. (2024), for example, found that 68.4% of physicians agreed or strongly agreed that social determinants impact their patient health outcomes. Only 24.1% felt their health care setting was set up to address social determinants; female physicians were more likely to prioritize social determinants, as were some specialties such as psychiatrists. Nurses have the potential to fill that gap in both understanding and application.

UNCERTAINTY AS AN ECONOMIC CONCEPT

Unlike Nurse Jones who could easily ascertain the rewards and costs of the new smartwatch, Ms. Williams cannot be certain about what she needs. She cannot assess what is unnecessary, what the potentially harmful consequences of actions and options are, and what the potentially harmful consequences of inaction are. Indeed, some of what Ms. Williams is seeking in health care is exactly this information. Dr. Garcia, although possessing more information than Ms. Williams, also cannot be fully certain of the consequences of either course. Arguably, the instinct of most Americans—both providers and patients—is toward treatment even if the result is overtreatment-induced harm. Without financial risk, providers also have few incentives and face organizational disincentives for watchful waiting, provided the patient—like Ms. Williams—has insurance that will cover the cost of care. Treatment momentum accelerates when patient satisfaction is an outcome metric and the patient clearly desires treatment. Unlike a classic free market in which assumption of the financial risk of the purchase moderates consumption, neither the provider nor the patient has an incentive to limit, or even question, treatment.

The scenario illustrated in the preceding text details an employer-based insurance scenario. Nevertheless, similar treatment incentives hold in all fee-for-service systems, including tax-funded ones like Medicare. Little has changed since Cassidy's (2013) observation that the current fee-for-service reimbursement scheme in Medicare "gives beneficiaries little incentive to see the highest value care or avoid unneeded care" (p. 4). Still other evidence finds that low-value testing in primary care during routine annual health exams of low-risk patients triggers subsequent costly specialist visits, procedures, and diagnostic tests (Bouck et al., 2020) and that general health checks did not reduce morbidity or mortality (Krogsbøll et al., 2012, a finding again more recently supported in a Cochrane systematic review (Krogsbøll et al., 2019). Similarly, Liss et al. (2021) found that ". . . general health checks were not associated with reduced mortality or cardiovascular events, but were associated with increased chronic disease recognition and treatment, risk factor control, preventive service uptake, and improved patient-reported outcomes." They suggest that "Primary care teams may reasonably offer general health checks, especially for groups at high risk of overdue preventive services, uncontrolled risk factors, low self-rated health, or poor connection or inadequate access to primary care" (2021, p. 2214). Yet the pervasiveness of the yearly screening as an unquestioned good is deeply rooted in American culture. Kherad et al. note: "In high-income countries, regular general health check-ups are part of the fabric of the healthcare systems. The hidden concept of general health check-ups, promoted for more than a century, is to identify diseases at a stage at which early intervention can be effective. However, there has been little evidence to support the benefits of such checkups." They further describe the need to shift patients and providers away from this "nonevidence based yet firmly entrenched practice of the general health check-up" (Kherad et al., 2023, p. 1). Clearly, professional nursing's promotion of evidence-based practice should include careful scrutiny of low value and wasteful care and implementation of strategies to reduce both.

Strategies Connect Patients to Financial Consequences of Treatment

Strategies to encourage consumers of health care to be cognizant of the cost of their actions exist and are well known to nurses. These include deductibles, copayments, and coinsurance (see Box 5.1). Together, these are termed *cost sharing*. Notably, the Affordable Care Act (ACA) has attempted to incentivize certain care by eliminating or subsidizing cost sharing for certain interventions or individuals. A child visiting a provider for immunizations, for example, would not have a copayment, while a sick child visit may, depending on the specifics of the plan, the heretofore mentioned benefits package. The overall policy objective for selective application of cost sharing is to remove disincentives for needed care, but not unneeded care. Similarly, during the 2020 coronavirus pandemic, states, commercial insurers, and a presidential executive order quickly eliminated cost sharing for COVID-19 testing. The goal was to remove all financial disincentives to seek a screening test that was deemed to have great utility not only to the individuals being tested but also to society at large.

The 2020 presidential election heralded calls for "first dollar coverage" for all care from some more liberal candidates. First dollar coverage means elimination of all cost sharing. Notably, many nations with universal coverage do not have first dollar coverage and instead incorporate cost sharing. They may also only cover a narrow set of health benefits rather than offering comprehensive coverage (Glied et al., 2019). Thus, when examining health plans as well as public policy, it is important to not only consider the magnitude of cost sharing but also the range of services that are eligible for reimbursement, that is, the benefit package. This important distinction is often overlooked in conversations about health reform, yet it is an extremely important consideration. The more comprehensive the benefit package, the more expensive the monthly premium. The greater the cost sharing, the lower the premium. Although the "Medicare for All" campaign plan of 2020 called for first dollar coverage (no cost sharing), beneficiaries

 BOX 5.1

TYPES OF COST SHARING

Deductible: The amount an individual needs to pay out of pocket before the insurance company begins its coverage for services.

Copayment: A payment owed by the individual at the time a covered service is received.

Coinsurance: A form of ongoing cost sharing between an individual and an insurance company in which the individual pays a percentage of covered services.

in traditional Medicare, in contrast to Medicare Advantage (MA), pay roughly 20% out of pocket in the form of cost sharing. In 2024 the deductible for Part A was $1,632 for each *benefit period,* and the monthly premium was $0. For Part B, the 2024 monthly premium was $174.40/month (or higher depending on income) and with a $240 deductible. The Part B deductible benefit period is 1 year, so that deductible amount is applicable to an entire year. Conversely, in Part A, there are no limits to the number of benefit periods in a year, meaning the deductible may need to be paid more than once a year (Medicare.gov, 2024), which, in the author's view, potentially creates confusion for many beneficiaries. A description of 2024 Medicare categories and eligibility can be found in Appendix A.

Deductibles, the amount an individual needs to pay out of pocket before the insurance company begins its coverage for services, are arrayed along a continuum from low to high, each with different utilization disincentives. There are plans with comparatively low deductibles—for example, a family employer-based insurance at $250/year/family. For individuals and families in which this is the only form of cost sharing, there is no disincentive to health care use once this relatively low-cost bar has been reached. High deductibles of up to $5,000 to $10,000 per family per year offer a substantial disincentive, even for needed care. The ACA has addressed this for insurance plans sold on the exchange by mandated *maximum out-of-pocket (MOOP)* limits. These are set annually by the federal government; for example, the 2024 MOOP for a single person was $9,450 and $18,900 for a family plan (Healthcare.gov, n.d.). MA plans also must set a MOOP, which in 2024 was $8,850 for in-network care. A preferred provider organization (PPO) MA will typically set two limits: one for in-network care and a higher one for out-of-network care (Medicare Interactive, 2024). Recall that an MA health maintenance organization (HMO) plan does not cover out-of-network care, so there is no MOOP for those individuals (MA will be further described later in this chapter). Also, recall that Medicare is always an individual plan, not a family plan, so there are no corollary family plan MOOPs in Medicare. Some states have additional out-of-pocket limits by category; for example, for prescription drugs. In the ACA, limits are aggregated into the overall MOOP.

Cost sharing pros and cons. Cost sharing decreases the use of services. Brot-Goldberg et al. (2017), for example, found that a switch from a noncost sharing plan to a high-deductible plan led to an overall spending reduction between 11.8% and 13.8%. The decrease stemmed from a reduction in the volume of services used, with no evidence of a reduction in cost related to price shopping. More recently, a systematic review found cost sharing impacted adherence to a medication, but less clear evidence on impact on overall clinical outcomes and cost (Fusco et al., 2023). Unlike Nurse Jones in our opening scenario, such data suggest that users of health care do not "shop around" for the best price and make decisions based on price and the perceived value, for reasons we will explore more deeply in upcoming chapters. To underscore, overuse of health services related to having coverage is termed *moral hazard*. So, all evidence suggests that cost sharing impacts the use of health services. How does it impact health? Well, it depends.

Cost Sharing: A Barrier to Needed Care or Opportunity to Decrease Unnecessary Utilization?

> Sarah Rossi has a stomachache. The persistent nagging pain in her side is now nearly constant and aggravated with movement. She feels "off"—tired, slightly nauseated, and lightheaded. She ponders calling her primary care provider, Ai Le, a nurse practitioner (NP), but suspects that the receptionist will just encourage her to see NP Le in the clinic or via telehealth. Sarah likes her provider, but the effort of going to the clinic seems exhausting, as does ramping up for an electronic visit. She also recalls that her employer-based insurance has just been switched to a high-deductible plan with a copayment due at the time of the visit. Sarah decides to "gut it out" and see how she feels in the morning.

Many individuals make the same decision as Sarah. Indeed, a seminal, classic RAND study found that when comparing those with no cost sharing to those in high-deductible plans, those in the former used 40% more health services (Newhouse, 1993). Does this impact their health? As health providers, it surely seems that what we do should matter and does matter! Surely, those individuals who do not seek treatment suffer health consequences? Although it would seem logical, the data do not consistently support negative health outcomes as the result of lower usage. Moreover, growing evidence also suggests that there is substantial overdiagnosis, overtreatment, and screening-induced harm (Commonwealth Foundation, 2023; Segal et al., 2023; Welch et al., 2011) in the U.S. system. Sarah's decision to forego treatment may evolve without further incidents or negative effects.

SELF-LIMITING HEALTH EVENTS

> Sarah goes to bed early and is awakened with severe stomach cramps and diarrhea. She recalls the party she was at the night before and wonders if this bout is the result of bad Brie. "Why do I eat things that taste bad?" she laments. She leaves the bathroom feeling better, quickly falls asleep, and awakens refreshed in the morning.

In this scenario in which Sarah had an acute, self-managed episode, the avoidance of medical intervention is positive.

WHAT ABOUT THOSE WITH CHRONIC ILLNESS?

High-deductible plans have had a different trajectory for those with chronic diseases. Specifically, high-deductible plans have been associated with a significant cost burden for those who, unlike Sarah's acute episode likely of food-borne origin, have chronic conditions and must seek and remain in regular treatment and make visits to their provider (Chandra et al., 2024; Galbraith et al., 2011).

How Do Deductibles Differ From Copayments?

Copayments, payments due at each visit, have also been associated with decreased use. Numerous studies have found, for example, that even relatively small copayments due at the time of an ED visit have reduced nonemergency utilization of the ED, although this was not found in a study of Medicaid enrollees (Mortensen, 2010). Other studies have found high deductibles to be associated with increased ED use, with the inference being that people did not seek community-based care that would have avoided an emergency room visit. Artiga and colleagues detail the reduction in health care use with even small, required copayments, stating:

> **Even relatively small levels of cost sharing in the range of $1 to $5 are associated with reduced use of care, including necessary services.** Research also finds that cost sharing can result in unintended consequences, such as increased use of the emergency room, and that cost sharing negatively affects access to care and health outcomes. For example, studies find that increases in cost sharing are associated with increased rates of uncontrolled hypertension and hypercholesterolemia and reduced treatment for children with asthma. Additionally, research finds that cost sharing increases financial burdens for families, causing some to cut back on necessities or borrow money to pay for care. (2017, para 3, bold in the original)

Other studies have found that when comparing no-copayment groups with both low- and high-copayment groups, the two copayment groups were less likely to seek care for minor symptoms, but the high-copayment groups were also less likely to seek care for serious symptoms. Given these findings, it is logical to assume that this copayment consequence would negatively impact health outcomes. Yet in this study, the health status, both physical and mental, was similar among all the copayment groups (Wong et al., 2001), suggesting that there were no long-term adverse effects of copayment cost sharing. Conversely, Loehrer et al. (2021) explored selected conditions and found that individuals with higher cost sharing were more likely to present with more complex surgical acute appendicitis and diverticulitis than those with lower cost sharing. This alternative scenario haunts every clinician.

> Sarah goes to bed early and is awakened by sharp pains in her shoulder. Almost too weak to stumble to the bathroom, she realizes she is now very, very sick. She calls her friend, who takes her to the ED. Sarah is diagnosed with a ruptured ectopic pregnancy, in which the bleeding is irritating the diaphragm. Nurse Jones tells Dr. Garcia, "This one looks shocky," and Dr. Garcia ponders if Sarah should be admitted to the regular unit or ICU. "How does someone let something like this go?" wonders Nurse Jones.

So, which scenario was Sarah headed for? Was the deductible and copayment a reasonable, important, and appropriate disincentive for seeking care, or did it prevent Sarah from receiving needed care in a timely manner? To date, the ability to systematically tease out when avoidance of care is positive and when it leads to adverse health outcomes remains elusive. Genuine need for health services, a seemingly straightforward phenomenon, is—like many things in health economics—a complicated issue with entwined components. Fortunately, there are new research strategies and tools, some of which are discussed in the following sections as well as in Chapter 6. Nurse leadership to support discernment of the value of care is sorely needed, particularly given the eroding trust in the U.S. health system (Keckley, 2023; Saad, 2023), the public's consistent trust in nurses' ethics and honesty (Brenan, 2023), and the perception of nurses' capacity to positively reform the health system (Commonwealth Fund/New York Times/Harvard School of Public Health, 2019).

WHAT IS MEDICARE ADVANTAGE?

The lack of provider incentives for careful attention to waste and low value care described earlier reflects traditional Medicare as well as fee-for-service commercial insurance plans. A growing proportion of Medicare beneficiaries, however, are covered by MA, reaching 54% in 2024 (Freed et al, 2024). MA, originally termed Medicare Part C, is Medicare administered by a private insurance company. In this payment arrangement, providers, again, do not assume financial risk. Instead, financial risk is borne primarily by the insurance company that in turn has a substantial financial incentive to decrease utilization across the board, both needed and wasteful. MA plans have been a highly successful line of business for many insurance companies, yet those savings, to date, have not been returned to taxpayers or Medicare beneficiaries (see Emanual, 2022 for more explication of this issue).

Why do people choose MA? First, many plans offer additional services such as some routine dental, vision, and hearing benefits, and some offer annual physical exams in addition to the wellness visit, although the amount of potential services covered—also termed *benefit package*—may not be clear to subscribers. Most recently, many of the MA plans have included significant over-the-counter benefit allowances, and some of the special needs plans (see Box 5.2) have "cash cards" for purchasing or paying for almost anything, Yet Jacobson et al. (2024) found that nearly one third of individuals enrolled in MA plans did not access any extra benefits for various reasons and nearly a quarter said they did not know what benefits are available to them. There are efforts to ensure MA enrollees are more aware of these benefits, an effort nurses can support (see https://www.medicare.gov/basics/get-started-with-medicare/get-more-coverage/your-coverage-options/compare-original-medicare-medicare-advantage for a side-by-side comparison of traditional Medicare and MA).

Rather than functioning like traditional insurance, including traditional Medicare, MA plans offer defined benefits that may be generous or, conversely, can be more costly and more challenging to access than traditional fee-for-service Medicare A and B benefits. It depends on (a) how much care is needed, (b) what care is needed, and (c) what providers are used. The third point, "providers used," is particularly important in MA because, unlike traditional Medicare, not all providers are in network or accept MA. Providers who do not accept MA do so for a variety of reasons. Emerson states "Hospitals are dropping Medicare Advantage plans left and right" (article title) and notes that the most commonly cited reasons are perceived prior authorization denials and slow payments" (2023). The clinical burden of preauthorization can be substantial. Recall that MA plans directly lose revenue when services are used and thus have a great incentive for utilization control. Other reasons for providers to no longer accept MA include lower payments than traditional Medicare.

MA plans may also require cost sharing (again, review Box 5.1) and thus can be considered a "pay as you go" model. This is also true of traditional Medicare if the individual doesn't have secondary coverage. Colloquially termed Medigap, this secondary coverage is obtained from a commercial insurance company for an additional premium.

 BOX 5.2

WHAT ARE MA SPECIAL NEED PLANS?

MA special need plans (SNP, often pronounced like the word snip) are MA plans targeting particular groups of high-need people, such as institutionalized beneficiaries, those with selected chronic conditions, and "dual eligibles," those eligible for both Medicare and Medicaid. ATI Advisory reports that dual beneficiaries "comprise a medically, functionally and socially complex population often forced to navigate two uncoordinated systems. As a result, these individuals tend to experience poor health outcomes and barriers to access, resulting in high spending across both the Medicaid and Medicare programs" (ATI Advisory, 2022, p. 3).

There are many tradeoffs and considerations for older adults pondering if traditional Medicare or MA is the best option for them. Approximately 11% of those in traditional Medicare have no secondary coverage. This can leave individuals with significant out-of-pocket exposure (consider the 20% cost sharing for Medicare Part B). There also is no annual MOOP in traditional Medicare, which can lead to medical debt and even bankruptcy. A study by Himmelstein et al. (2022) found that among Medicare beneficiaries, the percentage with medical debt was the lowest in those with traditional Medicare plus a supplement (7.52%) followed by those with MA (9.95%), and highest in those with traditional Medicare without a supplement (12.60%). Rakshit et al. (2024) note that people in the United States carry at least $220 billion in medical debt, with the highest proportion of such debt in the states of South Dakota, Mississippi, North Carolina, and West Virginia. Medical debt can impact those of any age and life situation, not just older adults. New mothers aged 18 to 35, for example, are twice as likely to have medical debt as women who did not recently give birth (Cox & Claxton, 2024).

Returning to the Medicare eligible, medical debt informs another reason people who are not eligible for employer-sponsored retiree insurance coverage or Medicaid and who cannot afford a Medicare "Medigap" supplement might choose MA plans. MA plans have defined MOOPs for in-network care and a higher out-of-network MOOP if a preferred provider organization (PPO) (recall that MA HMO plans do not reimburse for most services provided out of network). MA plans are required to cover the standard "medically necessary" benefits defined in traditional Medicare A and B, yet there are trade-offs. There may be obstacles to navigate, for example, the heretofore mentioned prior authorization. MA typically uses a more narrow network of providers, whereas traditional Medicare allows beneficiaries to have open access to providers. And, as previously noted, not all providers accept MA plans, leaving the individual to pay the entire bill.

In addition to concerns about network adequacy, people may not understand what extra benefits—those not provided in traditional Medicare—are covered. People may be surprised by large expenses related to, for example, major dental work that they assumed was covered by the dental insurance benefit. Defined benefit packages are standard course in U.S. dental "insurance." Gym membership and other perks are included in many MA plans, as are low or no copayments or deductibles or services to address social determinants, for example, health care–related transportation.

The trade-off? Again, MA plans limit the network of providers they cover, meaning a beneficiary may not have reimbursement coverage for services outside of the network unless truly emergent or urgent care. As such, they may have limited access to their choice of provider unless they have substantial financial reserves, that is, the financial freedom to seek second opinions from providers outside the designated network and pay for it out of pocket.

In the view of the author, the responsibility of the nurse is to understand these trade-offs and, when possible, help people understand the options so they can make an informed decision for themselves. When making coverage decisions for the coming year, individuals don't often think about many potential needs for sources of care they don't currently receive—for example, rehabilitation in a skilled nursing facility or home health—and their choice of these providers may be limited with MA plans. Unfortunately, plans, their coverage, and their cost can change every year, as can their network of providers. Provider directories are not always current, making it difficult to assess if your provider is in network and accepting MA. Also, once someone is enrolled in an MA plan, in many states, if they choose to leave and go to traditional Medicare, they may not be able purchase an affordable supplemental/Medigap coverage—or they can be denied a policy altogether. This is because private insurance companies are largely state regulated, and only four states—Connecticut, Maine, Massachusetts, and New York—prohibit medical underwriting for Medicare supplemental insurance plans. In the others, people can be denied coverage based on preexisting conditions (Kaiser Family Foundation, 2018).

Finally, it is critical to understand how networks operate and how that impacts access to care. For example, in a PPO MA plan, out-of-network providers would typically be covered, but with a much higher out-of-pocket expense by way of patient cost sharing. So, a person who has the financial means to cover large out-of-pocket costs for out-of-network services is relatively healthy, doesn't think they will need much medical care in the coming year, and has no plans to travel out of state (and potentially out of network) may choose this sort of plan because of the (a) lower monthly premium costs compared to traditional Medicare and a supplement/Medigap and (b) to access the additional benefits. Conversely, most MA HMO plans do not cover any out-of-network care other than truly urgent and emergent care. For most people, this would be an immutable impediment to access care out of network. The Commonwealth Foundation provides additional background on MA, including PPO versus HMO MA plans (Commonwealth Foundation, 2024). Discerning options can nevertheless be very challenging because of the magnitude of the choices—the average beneficiary has the option of 41 different plans (MedPAC, 2023)—and the opacity of the options.

Gina Upchurch with Senior PharmAssist, which provides Medicare counseling in Durham, North Carolina, among other things states: "Choice architecture to help Medicare beneficiaries make informed choices about their prescription and medical coverage is becoming more complex every year. Not only is it challenging to help people decide between receiving benefits via Traditional Medicare or MA, but also, to navigate the plethora of extra benefits with MA plans. The details of those benefits and what providers—doctors, hospitals, rehab facilities, and so forth—contract with these MA plans is almost impossible to keep up with, plus they change every year. This leads to decision-making paralysis or individuals being swayed by the loudest marketing or brokers and agents who benefit more from the sales of MA plans" (G. Upchurch, personal communication, April, 2024).

Linking back to the organizing concept of this section, health care markets are unlike classic free markets because people do not bear the financial impact of their decision-making. In MA plans, the insurance companies bear that risk and organize their offerings to minimize their expenses. This may mean better care coordination and addressing upstream social determinants or, on the other end of the spectrum, limited access to desired providers or needed care.

WHAT IDEAS HELP US UNDERSTAND OVERTREATMENT? THE EXAMPLE OF SMALL-AREA VARIATION AND SUPPLIER-INDUCED DEMAND

An area of study and research called *small-area variation* works toward understanding the relationships among the various components, motivations, and outcomes.

Supply, Costs, and Small-Area Variation

> Sandra is frustrated. A social worker with years of experience in a community health center, she is upset that there is so much that could be done for patients that simply is not happening. "Why can't people just get what they need?" she laments.

Sandra seems to be asking a simple question, and on the surface, the answer seems straightforward. Nevertheless, there is a great deal of uncertainty when attempting to dissect what constitutes "need," as well as an evolution in understanding the complexity of this construct. Culvyer (cited in Rodriguez Santana et al., 2023) described *need* as "arguably the most used and least properly comprehended word in discussions of health. The meanings that attach to it are legion" (p. 2).

Even the use of early models of health services differentiated between *perceived need* and *evaluated need* (Anderson, 1968), with evaluated need presumed to correlate with actual need. But this straightforward distinction conceals a complex reality. Eddy (1996) notes that need was once simply defined—it was whatever the physician said it was. Yet does the fact that it is named by clinician evaluation make it real, actual, or correct? Over time and many research studies, it has become increasingly clear that the answer is a resounding "No!" Different providers may offer different diagnoses for the same situation, or—even with the same diagnosis—order different amounts of tests or treatment.

Over time, groundbreaking work (Wennberg & Gittelsohn, 1973) led by Jack Wennberg at Dartmouth created a whole new area of investigation around this concept, called *small-area variation*. Small-area variation refers to differing patterns of health care utilization in one region as compared to another, even when controlling for differences in the patients. Small-area variation illustrates that services delivered in response to what is considered need in one part of the country would not be delivered in another. This is not driven by mistakes or incompetence. Instead, it flows from a phenomenon termed *supplier-induced demand* that is reinforced by the U.S. payment system and professional education.

WHAT IS SUPPLIER-INDUCED DEMAND?

Wennberg, a physician with a master's degree in public health studying for a doctorate in sociology, was working in rural Vermont, an ideal laboratory for health services research because of its relative homogeneity. Pioneering concepts in medical practice epidemiology, Wennberg noted that 70% of children from one Vermont community had tonsillectomies by age 15, whereas in a community 10 miles away, the proportion of children with tonsillectomies was 20%. On closer examination, there was no logical explanation for this variance. The children were not different in any way that could explain the large discrepancy in the apparent "need" for tonsillectomies.

Using increasingly complex analytic tools over time, one difference between high-utilization areas and low-utilization areas was evident: the numbers and types of providers. Areas with more internists, for example, had patients receiving more diagnostic tests, even when the patient profiles were similar. Areas with more cardiovascular surgeons, in general, had more patients receiving cardiovascular surgery. Thus, the concepts of small-area variation and supplier-induced demand became areas of ongoing scientific inquiry and policy application. Although better accepted today, the notion of overtreatment and anything less than objective clinical decision-making was very radical thinking when first introduced. Today the Dartmouth Atlas of Health Care documents "glaring variations" in the use of health services (see www.dartmouthatlas.org). In 2022, advanced methodologies enabled comparisons across Medicare, Medicaid, and commercial insurer payers for the first time (Dartmouth Atlas Project, 2023), finding payer-specific variation (Cooper et al., 2022) and further underscoring the lack of precision in the execution of care reflecting genuine need.

Unlike Health Care, in Traditional Markets Oversupply Decreases Demand

The importance of this concept is illustrated in contrast to a classic free market in the following scenario.

> Jannie is excited. She is going to her first farmers market selling her mother's homemade fudge. As she wheels into the parking area, she is thrilled by the number of vendors. "This should bring in a ton of customers," Jannie notes with glee. As she sets up her booth, however, her heart sinks. To her left, there is another booth selling fudge. She wheels around to the right. More fudge vendors. Marching to the aisle between rows of booths, she stands with arms akimbo. The farmers market is booth after booth of fudge vendors, 35 in all. Jannie is totally deflated. With the farmers market awash in fudge, why would anyone seek out her booth? Jannie knows that with so many people selling fudge, her sales will be almost nil . . . there is just too much competition!

In a classic free market, when supply is high, costs typically decrease due to market competition. If there is a glut of a product, similar to fudge at Jannie's farmers market, many items of the product simply will not sell at all. Supplier-induced demand in health care is exactly the opposite: the greater the supply, the greater the use—the more surgeons, for example, the more surgeries. Santerre and Neun describe the capacity for providers to induce demand for their services as follows:

> [C]onsumers are relatively ill-informed concerning the proper amount of medical care to consume because an asymmetry of information exists regarding the various healthcare options available. This asymmetry forces consumers to rely heavily on the advice of their physicians for guidance. This implies that physicians are not only providers of physician services but also play a major part in determining the level of demand for those services. For example, physicians advise patients about how frequently they should have office visits, medical tests, and appropriate treatments. This situation places physicians in a potentially exploitative position. Physicians may be able to manipulate the demand curves of patients to advance their own economic interests. (Santerre & Neun, 2009, p. 370)

The subsequent passage of time has done little to change this dynamic. Seyedin et al., for example, state: "Induced demand is a major challenge of financing health promotion, whereby providers exploit patients' information gap to manipulate their demand for healthcare" (Seyedin et al., 2021, p. 1). These researchers also find fee-for-service to be a contributing factor because, as previously detailed, providers are financially rewarded for providing more care, needed or not.

But, as already noted, there is also a growing body of data that does not consistently find better health outcomes with higher utilization. Rodriguez

Santana et al. note the tension between unmet real need and inappropriate demand and use. Their definition of *need* recognizes the importance of *value*, as follows:

> **Need** is the capacity to benefit from healthcare. Healthcare means treatment, prevention and supportive care that is effective—either alone or as part of a care pathway—in improving, maintaining, or slowing the deterioration of health now or in the future (or both). Need is for 'appropriate' healthcare: this excludes care that is known to be cost-ineffective and includes cost-effective care. For care of unknown cost-effectiveness, need is for the right care provided in the right place and at the right time. (2021, p. 3, bold in the original)

Taken as a whole, this suggests that the typical relationship among supply, quality, and cost containment that is considered basic in traditional economics simply cannot be transferred to health care, which has, among other effects, fueled the experimentation with new payment models as detailed in Chapter 4.

Hypotheses about regional differences in utilization as a result of supplier-induced demand have led to policy questions about differential payment by geographic regions to reward appropriate utilization and lower cost. However, as Wennberg et al. (1982) noted early on, these differences are likely due to differences in the way providers diagnose and treat. This hypothesis was further supported in a complex, broad Institute of Medicine (2013) study that included not only Medicare but also commercial insurance usage. This report further confirmed the presence of substantial geographic variation in treatment rates and costs, without a consistent relationship between these variables and quality of care or outcomes for the patients. They recommend that these be addressed by targeting clinical decision-making, clinical and financial integration, and coordination of services. Finally, information about the product, health care, is essential to economic decision-making. However, as Arrow noted in 1963:

> The value of information is frequently not known in any meaningful sense to the buyer; if, indeed, he knows enough to measure the value of information, he would know the information itself. But information, in the form of skilled care, is precisely what is being bought from most physicians, and, indeed, from most professionals. The elusive character of information as a commodity suggests that it departs considerably from the usual marketability assumptions about commodities. (p. 946)

This seminal statement remains sound, yet is even more complex and nuanced, given the explosion of information-sharing technology, processes, and contemporary policy initiatives. Thus, we will turn our focus to information, economics, and health care in Chapter 6.

Acknowledgement

The author acknowledges the helpful suggestions of Gina Upchurch in an earlier version of this chapter.

End-of-Chapter Resources

THOUGHT QUESTIONS

1. Imagine you are a healthy 30-year-old male. For you, what are the pros and cons of a lower monthly insurance premium with higher cost sharing versus a higher monthly premium with lower cost sharing?
2. Imagine you are a 62-year-old female with multiple chronic conditions. For you, what are the pros and cons of a lower monthly insurance premium with higher cost sharing versus a higher monthly premium with lower cost sharing?
3. To what extent should patients feel a financial impact when they seek care? How can needed care best be separated from unnecessary care? Provide a rationale for your answer.
4. To what extent should providers be accountable for the cost and outcomes of care that they recommend? Provide a rationale for your answer.
5. Define the following key terms:
   Maximum out-of-pocket limits
   Self-rationing
   Small-area variation
   Supplier-induced demand
   Third-party payer
   Moral hazard

EXERCISE

1. Develop a presentation for your peers that details the ways in which the decision to use health care is similar to other decisions and the ways it is different. Explain the relationship of these to the contemporary reform era.
2. A dearly beloved relative is turning 65 in 3 months and asks your advice on Medicare options. How do you proceed? Where do you go for information about Medicare products? What information do you need from your relative to help her make the best decisions? What do you advise her?

QUIZ

True or False

1. In a classic free market, consumers bear the financial consequences of their decision to purchase a product or use a service.
2. Insurance companies are also called third-party payers.

3. In fee-for-service reimbursement models, providers have little incentive to limit treatment or consider the cost of treatment.
4. In health insurance, a deductible is another term for a copayment.
5. One way health care markets differ from classic free markets is that in a classic free market, oversupply decreases demand and enhances cost and quality competition.
6. The term asymmetry of information means that consumers have less information about health care options than physicians, and physicians can therefore influence demand for health services.
7. Need for health care services is a clearly defined phenomenon.
8. Individuals with high-deductible health insurance plans uniformly have worse health outcomes than those with low-deductible health insurance plans.
9. The Affordable Care Act attempts to incentivize some care by removing the cost share for the service.
10. Cost sharing and cost shifting refer to the same phenomenon.

Multiple Choice

11. Cost sharing
    A. Includes copayment and deductibles
    B. Is a strategy to encourage consumers of health care to consider the cost and value of care when using/purchasing health care services
    C. Both A and B
    D. Neither A nor B
12. Small-area variation
    A. Refers to differing patterns of health care utilization in one region as compared to another, differences that occur even when controlling for differences in the patients
    B. Refers to different types of hospitals in rural versus urban settings
    C. Both A and B
    D. Neither A nor B
13. Maximum out-of-pocket limits
    A. Cap the amount of health care costs an individual or family pays in a single year
    B. Do not exist in traditional Medicare
    C. Both A and B
    D. Neither A nor B
14. Third-party payers
    A. Spread financial risk among individuals in the insurance pools
    B. Are called third parties because they are not the first or second party, that is, not the buyer or seller

C. Both A and B

D. Neither A nor B

15. The cost of health care

    A. Is borne by society in the financial form of taxes and insurance premiums

    B. Becomes revenue to the provider

    C. Both A and B

    D. Neither A nor B

16. The concept of supplier-induced demand

    A. Was heralded by the work of Jack Wennberg

    B. Suggests that the supply of health care providers, rather than genuine need for health care services, drives at least some use of health services

    C. Both A and B

    D. Neither A nor B

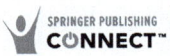

A robust set of instructor resources designed to supplement this text is located at http://connect.springerpub.com/content/book/978-0-8261-7236-5. Qualifying instructors may request access by emailing **textbook@springerpub.com**.

REFERENCES

Anderson, R. (1968). *A behavioral model of families' use of health services* (Research Series No. 25). University of Chicago Press.

Arrow, K. (1963). Uncertainty and the welfare economics of medical care. *American Economic Review, 53*(5), 941–973.

Artiga, S., Ubri, P., & Zur, J. (2017). *The effect of premiums and cost sharing on low-income populations: Updated review of findings*. Kaiser Family Foundation. https://www.kff.org/medicaid/issue-brief/the-effects-of-premiums-and-cost-sharing-on-low-income-populations-updated-review-of-research-findings/

ATI Advisory. (2022). *A profile of Medicare-Medicaid dual beneficiaries*. Author. https://atiadvisory.com/wp-content/uploads/2022/06/A-Profile-of-Medicare-Medicaid-Dual-Beneficiaries.pdf

Bouck, Z., Calzavara, A., Ivers, N., Keer, E., Chu, C., Ferguson, J., Martin, D., Tepper, J., Austin, P., Cram, P., Levinson, W., & Sacha Bhatia, R. (2020). Association of low-value testing with subsequent health care use and clinical outcomes among low-risk primary care outpatients undergoing an annual health examination. *Journal of the American Medical Association, 180*(7), 973–983. https://doi.org/10.1001/jamainternmed.2020.1611

Brenan, E. (2023). *Nurses retain top ethics rating in the U.S. but below 2020 high*. Gallup. https://news.gallup.com/poll/467804/nurses-retain-top-ethics-rating-below-2020-high.aspx

Brot-Goldberg, Z., Chandra, A., Handel, B., & Kolstad, J. (2017). What does a deductible do? The impact of cost-sharing on health care prices, quantities, and spending dynamics. *The Quarterly Journal of Economics, 132*(3), 1261–1318. https://doi.org/10.3386/w21632

Cassidy, A. (2013, June 20). *Health policy brief: Restructuring Medicare*. Health Affairs. http://www.healthaffairs.org/healthpolicybriefs/brief.php?brief_id=95

Chandra, A., Flack, E., & Obermeyer, Z. (2024). *The health costs of cost-sharing*. National Bureau of Economic Research. https://www.nber.org/papers/w28439

CMS.gov. (2023, November 2). *Hospital price transparency*. Author. https://www.cms.gov/priorities/key-initiatives/hospital-price-transparency

Commonwealth Foundation. (2023). *Tracking overtreatment and overspending in U.S. healthcare*. Author. https://www.commonwealthfund.org/publications/podcast/2023/nov/tackling-overtreatment-overspending-us-health-care

Commonwealth Foundation. (2024). *Medicare advantage: A policy primer*. Author. https://www.commonwealthfund.org/publications/explainer/2024/jan/medicare-advantage-policy-primer

Commonwealth Fund/New York Times/Harvard School of Public Health. (2019). *American's values and beliefs about National Health Insurance Reform*. https://www.hsph.harvard.edu/wp-content/uploads/sites/21/2019/10/CMWF-NYT-Harvard_Final-Report_Oct2019.pdf

Cooper, Z., Stiegman, O., Ndumele, C. D., Staiger, B., & Skinner, J. (2022). Geographical variation in health spending across the US among privately insured individuals and enrollees in Medicaid and Medicare. *JAMA Network Open, 5*(7), e2222138. https://doi.org/10.1001/jamanetworkopen.2022.22138

Cox, D., & Claxton, G. (2024). *Medical debt among new mothers*. Peterson-KFF Health System Tracker. https://www.healthsystemtracker.org/brief/medical-debt-among-new-mothers/

Dartmouth Atlas Project. (2023). *Geographic variations in spending and utilization across payer types*. Author. https://www.dartmouthatlas.org/spending-variation-3payers/

Eddy, D. (1996). *Clinical decision making: From theory to practice*. Jones & Bartlett.

Emanual, E. (2022). *The great Medicare rip off*. The Atlantic. https://www.theatlantic.com/ideas/archive/2022/12/medicare-advantage-private-insurance-overcharging-government-taxpayers/672549/

Emerson, J. (2023, December 14). *Hospitals are dropping Medicare Advantage right and left*. Becker's Hospital News. https://www.beckershospitalreview.com/finance/hospitals-are-dropping-medicare-advantage-left-and-right.html

Freed, M., Fuglesten Biniek, J., Damico, A., & Neuman, T. (2024, August 8). https://www.kff.org/medicaid/issue-brief/the-effects-of-premiums-and-cost-sharing-on-low-income-populations-updated-review-of-research-findings/. Kaiser Family Foundation. https://www.kff.org/medicare/issue-brief/medicare-advantage-in-2024-enrollment-update-and-key-trends/

Fusco, N., Sils, B., Graff, J. S., Kistler, K., & Ruiz, K. (2023). Cost-sharing and adherence, clinical outcomes, health care utilization, and costs: A systematic literature review. *Journal of Managed Care & Specialty Pharmacy, 29*(1), 4–16. https://doi.org/10.18553/jmcp.2022.21270

Galbraith, A., Ross-Degnan, D., Soumerai, S., Rosenthal, M., Gay, C., & Lieu, T. (2011). Nearly half of families in high-deductible health plans whose members have chronic conditions face substantial financial burden. *Health Affairs, 30*(2), 322–331. https://doi.org/10.1377/hlthaff.2010.0584

Glenn, J., Kleinhenz, G., Smith, J. M., Chaney, R., Moxley, V., Donoso Naranjo, P. G., Stone, S., Hanson, C., Redelfs, A., & Novilla, M. L. B. (2024). Do healthcare providers consider the social determinants of health? Results from a nationwide cross-sectional study in the United States. *BMC Health Services Research, 24*, 271. https://doi.org/10.1186/s12913-024-10656-2

Glied, S., Black, M., Lauerman, W., & Snowden, S. (2019, April 11). *Considering "single payer" proposals in the U.S.: Lessons from abroad*. The Commonwealth Fund. http://www.commonwealthfund.org/publications/2019/apr/considering-single-payer-proposals-lessons-from-abroad

Healthcare.gov. (n.d.). *Out-of-pocket maximum/limit*. Retrieved February 17, 2024, from https://www.healthcare.gov/glossary/out-of-pocket-maximum-limit

Himmelstein, D. U., Dickman, S. L., McCormick, D., Bor, D. H., Gaffney, A., & Woolhandler, S. (2022). Prevalence and risk factors for medical debt and subsequent changes in social determinants of health in the US. *JAMA Network Open, 5*(9), e2231898. https://doi.org/10.1001/jamanetworkopen.2022.31898

Institute of Medicine. (2013). *Variation in health care spending: Target decision making, not geography*. National Academies Press.

Jacobson, G., Leonard, F., Sciupac, E., & Rapoport, R. (2024, February 22). *What do Medicare beneficiaries value about their coverage*. The Commonwealth Fund. https://www.commonwealthfund.org/publications/surveys/2024/feb/what-do-medicare-beneficiaries-value-about-their-coverage

Kacik, A. (2024, April 4). *Higher fines compel most hospitals to disclose prices*. Modern Healthcare. https://www.modernhealthcare.com/providers/price-transparency-fines-cms

Kaiser Family Foundation. (2018). *In all but four states, seniors on Medicare can be denied a Medigap policy due to pre-existing conditions, except during specified windows of opportunity*. Author. https://www.kff.org/medicare/press-release/in-all-but-four-states-seniors-on-medicare-can-be-denied-a-medigap-policy-due-to-pre-existing-conditions-except-during-specified-windows-of-opportunity/

Keckley, P. (2023, October 16). *U.S. healthcare's existential threat: The loss of public trust*. The Keckley Report. https://paulkeckley.com/the-keckley-report/2023/10/16/u-s-healthcares-existential-threat-loss-of-public-trust/

Kherad, O., & Carneiro, A. V., & On behalf of Choosing wisely working group of the European Federation of Internal Medicine. (2023). General health checkups: To check or not to check? A question of choosing wisely. *European Journal of Internal Medicine, 109*, 1–3. https://doi.org/10.1016/j.ejim.2022.12.021

Krogsbøll, L. T., Jørgensen, K. J., Grønhøj Larsen, C., & Gøtzsche, P. C. (2012). General health checks in adults for reducing morbidity and mortality from disease: Cochrane systematic review and meta-analysis. *BMJ (Clinical research ed.), 345*, e7191. https://doi.org/10.1136/bmj.e7191

Krogsbøll, L. T., Jørgensen, K. J., & Gøtzsche, P. C. (2019). General health checks in adults for reducing morbidity and mortality from disease. *The Cochrane Database of Systematic Reviews, 1*(1), CD009009. https://doi.org/10.1002/14651858.CD009009.pub3

Liss, D. T., Uchida, T., Wilkes, C. L., Radakrishnan, A., & Linder, J. A. (2021). General health checks in adult primary care: A review. *Journal of the American Medical Association, 325*(22), 2294–2306. https://doi.org/10.1001/jama.2021.6524

Loehrer, A. P., Leech, M. M., Weiss, J. E., Markey, C., Wengle, E., Aarons, J., & Zuckerman, S. (2021). Association of cost sharing with delayed and complicated presentation of acute appendicitis or diverticulitis. *JAMA Health Forum, 2*(9), e212324. https://doi.org/10.1001/jamahealthforum.2021.2324

Medicare.gov. (2024). *Costs*. Author. https://www.medicare.gov/basics/costs/medicare-costs

Medicare Interactive. (2024). *Maximum out-of-pocket limit*. Author. https://www.medicareinteractive.org/get-answers/medicare-health-coverage-options/medicare-advantage-plan-overview/maximum-out-of-pocket-limit

MedPAC. (2023). *The Medicare Advantage program: Status repor*. MedPAC. https://www.medpac.gov/wp-content/uploads/2023/03/Ch11_Mar23_MedPAC_Report_To_Congress_SEC.pdf

Mortensen, K. (2010). Copayments did not reduce Medicaid enrollees' nonemergency use of emergency departments. *Health Affairs, 29*(9), 1643–1650. https://doi.org/10.1377/hlthaff.2009.0906

Newhouse, J. (1993). *Free for all? Lessons for the RAND health insurance experiment: RAND Corporation*. Harvard University Press.

Rakshit, S., Rae, M., Clazton, G., Amin, K., & Cox, C. (2024, February 12). *The burden of medical debt in the United States*. Peterson-KFF Health System Tracker. https://www.healthsystemtracker.org/brief/the-burden-of-medical-debt-in-the-united-states/

Rodriguez Santana, I., Mason, A., Gutacker, N., Kasteridis, P., Santos, R., & Rice, N. (2023). Need, demand, supply in health care: Working definitions, and their implications for defining access. *Health Economics, Policy, and Law, 18*(1), 1–13. https://doi.org/10.1017/S1744133121000293

Saad, L. (2023). *Americans sour on healthcare quality*. Gallup. https://news.gallup.com/poll/468176/americans-sour-healthcare-quality.aspx

Santerre, R., & Neun, S. (2009). *Health economics: Theories, insights, and industry studies*. South-Western Cengage Learning.

Segal, J. B., Sen, A. P., Glanzberg-Krainin, E., & Hutfless, S. (2022). Factors associated with overuse of health care within US health systems: A cross-sectional analysis of Medicare beneficiaries from 2016 to 2018. *JAMA Health Forum, 3*(1), e214543. https://doi.org/10.1001/jamahealthforum.2021.4543

Seyedin, H., Afshari, M., Isfahani, P., Hasanzadeh, E., Radinmanesh, M., & Bahador, R. C. (2021). The main factors of supplier-induced demand in health care: A qualitative study. *Journal of Education and Health Promotion, 10*, 49. https://doi.org/10.4103/jehp.jehp_68_20

Tong, N. (2023, December 11). *House price transparency legislation bill passes with bipartisan support*. Fierce Healthcare. https://www.fiercehealthcare.com/payers/house-price-transparency-legislation-bill-passes-two-thirds-vote

Welch, H. G., Schwartz, L. M., & Woloshin, S. (2011). *Overdiagnosed: Making people sick in the pursuit of health*. Beacon Press.

Wennberg, J., Barnes, B., & Zubkoff, M. (1982). Professional uncertainty and the problem of supplier-induced demand. *Social Science and Medicine, 16*(7), 811–824. https://doi.org/10.1016/0277-9536(82)90234-9

Wennberg, J., & Gittelsohn, A. (1973). Small area variations in health care delivery. *Science, 182*(4117), 1102–1108. https://doi.org/10.1126/science.182.4117.1102

Wong, M., Anderson, R., Sherbourne, C., Hays, R., & Shapiro, M. (2001). Effects of cost sharing on care seeking and health status: Results from the Medical Outcomes Study. *American Journal of Public Health, 91*(11), 1889–1894. https://doi.org/10.2105/ajph.91.11.1889

CHAPTER 6

Health Care Outcomes, Cost, Safety, and Value: The Critical Role of Information in Health Care Markets, Decision-Making, and Payments

CHAPTER 6 details how information is used by consumers to make decisions that, in aggregate, may enhance quality while reducing cost, in contrast to health care markets in which this information is more difficult to access and understand. The link between information and selected payment models is described. The evolution of emerging strategies and technologies to support information access and clinical applications is detailed. Following completion of this chapter, you will be able to:

- Describe the role of information in economic decision-making.
- Describe the relationship among information, clinical and patient decision-making, and digital transformation.
- Address persistent health care challenges such as price variability and the lack of price transparency.
- Describe legislative and regulatory strategies to address "surprise billing" and price opacity.
- Describe technological innovations shaping nursing and health care, including the Internet of Things, artificial intelligence, large language platforms, and blockchain.
- Consider new and emerging roles for RNs in a data-rich world striving to reduce unnecessary variation in health care delivery.

THE NEED FOR INFORMATION

Philip, a nurse, has a problem. He worked hard to save enough money for a down payment on his condo, picking up extra shifts at the hospital and using public transportation rather than getting a car. It has been worth it! Philip loves

> his new home. Settled in for 3 months, Philip was just finding financial breathing room, or so he thought. Now this!
>
> Three times in the past 3 weeks Philip has found water streaming out of his dishwasher and onto the floor. Now there is a stain in the basement ceiling, so Philip knows the leak is serious, and his attempts at home repair did not work. Philip considers his options: (a) Wash all dishes by hand in soapy water, (b) call a repair person, or (c) buy a new dishwasher.
>
> Philip needs more information to make a decision. He calls the repair shop, and the manager tells Philip that a visit by a repair technician will cost a minimum of $200. Moreover, there may be parts that are needed and a second visit, so the total cost is unclear. Philip then visits a local appliance shop as well as several discount stores and a warehouse. He compares the cost of the different models as well as the features. He then looks online for more product information and is surprised to find that one of the "off-brand" models is actually made by the same company as a highly rated brand name; in fact, it is the same dishwasher, just with a different label. Finally, Philip checks the different store policies on delivery and installation and finds that several of the stores offer these as a free service. Philip now feels confident he accurately knows the cost of the different options. Philip has all the information he needs to make the best decision possible, or at least the decision that is best for him.

Similarly,

> Arnett stops by the local grocer after her clinical rotation at a primary care office. She notices that the store brand of canned green beans is almost 30 cents cheaper than the name brand. "How bad can they be?" she asks herself as she picks up the store brand. In the next aisle, Arnett pauses in front of the coffee. There is a much cheaper brand than what she is using, but Arnett's boyfriend, Howard, likes Fancybrand, and Arnett decides to stick with it. Saturday morning coffee is just too precious to mess with, Arnett decides, as she puts Fancybrand coffee in her cart.

Classic free markets rest on a foundation of information. As Philip's experience exemplifies, the consumer knows about the product or knows how to obtain information. Information sources may include consumer guides, or stars and "thumbs up" ratings on websites, or may be rooted in past experience. Indeed, shoppers sort through information informed by their own experience on a daily basis, as Arnett's example illustrates. When purchasing green beans, for example, the shopper can sort out the pros and cons of the less expensive store brand and the one with the fancy label. Moreover, except for very large purchases, the impact of a choice with an undesirable outcome can be easily rectified. If Arnett buys the cheaper store brand and does not like it, she can toss it out and make a different decision next time without much financial or quality-of-life impact. Notably, the buying power is in the hand of the individual consumer, not the seller, because—after thinking about the pros and cons as well as the impact of the expense on the capacity to obtain other goods and services, as discussed in the previous chapter—the buyer can walk away.

Buying Power and Vulnerability

Health care is dramatically different. First, unlike the power a consumer has in a classic free market, as noted in the previous chapter, health care is a *vulnerable purchase*. A mother whose child has lost consciousness and cannot be roused after a hard fall in the playground, for example, does not have the option of taking time to review the treatment pros and cons, costs, and likely outcomes on the way to the emergency department. Moreover, the cost of inaction may prove life-threatening, unlike whether Philip decides to forego a dishwasher, which would result in a small investment from him of kitchen time with hands in soapy water each day.

Asymmetry of Information and Supplier-Induced Demand

Second, unlike a classic market in which the consumer has information about the product or knows how to obtain it, the consumer of health care usually goes to the provider to obtain information, for example, a diagnosis or prognosis. This *asymmetry of information* (Arrow, 1963) does not exist in classic free markets in which the power is in the hands of the consumer. Moreover, once a patient is seen, the provider can also control the *demand* for health care by ordering tests, offering referral or specialty services, surgery, and repeat visits, and the patient is not in a position to easily discern what is necessary and what is not. Instead, the patient trusts that what the provider states is right, necessary, and in the patient's best interest. As detailed in Chapter 5, there is consistent, substantial, and long-standing evidence (Dartmouth Atlas of Health Care, n.d.; Mulley, 2009; Jacobs et al, 2022) that this *supplier-induced demand* creates large variations in patterns of care, even when the differences among patients are controlled. As Atsma and colleagues note: "Typically, the variation is large, omnipresent, persistent and difficult to grasp (2000, p. 271). Moreover, natural experiments in nations changing provider remuneration systems have found that fee-for-service offers a powerful fuel for supplier-induced demand (van Dijk et al., 2012).

The magnitude of a health care provider's capacity to induce demand for services is largely unique among all U.S. goods and services. As Wennberg, cited as "the creator of modern evaluative science" (Mullan & Wennberg, 2004, VAR 73), states, "Lurking behind variations in patterns of care are often huge hospital investments in expensive technologies that are directly tied to their economic stability" (VAR 79). In other words, expensive investments in facilities and technologies must be paid for, and a "build it and they will come" orientation has prevailed. This sort of information is not readily accessible to a patient who is trying to determine what health services they need. At a broader level, resources like *The Dartmouth Atlas of Health Care* that documents "glaring variations in how medical resources are distributed and used in the United States" can be examined by health analysts to shape health policy. Over time, the *Atlas* has provided increasingly sophisticated analyses, inclusive of interactive, user-friendly portals and timely analyses of rapidly evolving challenges such as that presented by COVID-19. Although supplier-induced demand and its impact have been well recognized for decades, redressing the problem has been challenging. One particular challenge for health care stems from the lack of *price transparency*.

Price Transparency

A unique element of the health care system relates to a different piece of information a wise consumer needs: cost. Imagine a grocery store in which there are no prices listed on anything in the store, and when store workers are asked what things cost, they respond, "I don't know." Imagine if, when told you needed an injection, your first question was, "How much will it cost?" Yet this is an important question. What *do* individual health care services cost? What does the care you provide as a nurse cost the patient? The taxpayers?

This seemingly simple question is surprisingly complicated in health care and is at the heart of an issue called *price transparency*. Recall from Chapter 5 that buyers self-ration their own purchases in classic free markets because the buyer knows that they will bear the impact of the decision-making. Information is central to making that decision. Philip may decide to "self-ration" and not replace his dishwasher. Conversely, he may decide to go with one of the purchase options. In all cases, he has the opportunity to know the cost impact and weigh his decision accordingly. Similarly, imagine driving along a busy roadway hunting for a gas station. How would you decide which one to go to if prices were not posted? What would impel gas station owners to practice any type of price competition? Similarly, what would impel the owner to practice cost containment if both you and they thought you could pass those costs off to someone else? Yet there is a much greater difference in the cost of the same health care services in (a) different settings and (b) by payer type than there is in gas prices. This is termed *price variability*.

Price Variability

In health care, the situation is even more complicated because a second answer to the "How much does it cost?" question is, "It depends." Different employer groups negotiate to obtain discounted fees. Large employers, therefore, have an advantage in negotiating lower rates. In addition to different prices secondary to negotiated rates, different facilities charge dramatically different amounts for the same goods or services. In reflection, Dentzer (2013) notes:

> What does U.S. health care have in common with an exotic international bazaar? The prices at either one are almost never posted, whether for a heart bypass operation or an antique rug. And the final price will also most certainly have little to do with the seller's opening bid (para 1).

Despite hospital charges having been set prospectively via diagnosis-related groups (DRGs) since 1984 (see Box 6.1), dramatic differences in average hospital charges persist despite state and federal efforts for change. Pollock and colleagues (2023) report that the median price for an uncomplicaged major hip or knee joint arthroplasty at a sample of highly ranked orthopedic hospitals ranged from $39,927 to $195,264; charges for revisions ranged from $58,967 to $247,715. In this study, median household income was not correlated procedure cost and cost of living was only weakly correlated to procedure price, suggesting that the higher charges did not stem from overall higher cost of living in the hospital service area. Similarlly, Blue Cross and Blue Shield reports a 313% variation depending on where the knee and hip replacements are done, with some hospitals charging tens of thousands of dollars more, even within the same metropolitan statistical area. In Dallas, for example, hip replacement costs varied dramatically, with the most expensive being 267% the least expensive; in Boston, the difference was more than 300%

 BOX 6.1

REMINDER: WHAT ARE PROPSECTIVE PAYMENT DIAGNOSIS-RELATED GROUPS

Prior to the adoption of prospective payment for hospitalized Medicare patients in 1983, hospitals were reimbursed retrospectively for whatever they would decide to charge, including a per diem—meaning by the day—charge for each day of hospitalization. Reform was necessary to prevent insolvency, and the new model paid hospitals a fixed rate based on the diagnosis or combination of diagnoses (Mayes, 2007). In this manner, although the federal government via Medicare retained financial risk for the overall number of hospital admissions, the hospital assumed financial risk for the length of stay (Bodenheimer et al., 2023). Mayes notes that 'the change was nothing short of revolutionary. For the first time, the federal government gained the upper hand in its financial relationship with the hospital industry. Medicare's new prospective payment system with diagnosis-related groups triggered a shift in the balance of political and economic power between the providers of medical care (hospitals and physicians) and those who paid for it—power that providers had successfully accumulated for more than half a century" (2007, p. 21).

(Japsen, 2015). Adding to the confusion, higher charges may foster a higher payment, or may not. In response, the American Hospital Association notes:

The complex and bewildering interplay among "charges," "rates," "bills" and "payments" across dozens of payers, public and private, does not serve any stakeholder well, including hospitals. This is especially true when what is most important to a patient is knowing what his or her financial responsibility will be (cited in Castellucci, 2017, para 8).

There is a dramatic difference in cost of care by state as well. Adding to the confusion, these figures vary with the source reporting the information, the year, and the analytic lens. A 2018 report, for example, lists Colorado being 19% above average among those studied and Maryland—a state with all-payer hospital rate setting—being 20% below (Network for Regional Health Care Improvement, 2018). A 2020 Kaiser Family Foundation report states Utah has the lowest expenditures per capita (and also the youngest population) and District of Columbia the highest (KFF, 2020), while Forbes (Horton & Smith, 2024) reports North Carolina as being the most expensive and Hawaii the least, followed by Michigan, Washington, California, and Massachusetts. Despite this swirl of information, most agree that regardless of the exact rankings, U.S. health care is too expensive: Americans are concerned about health care affordability, with half of U.S. adults reporting that it is difficult to afford health care and one in four reporting problems paying for health care (Lopes et al., 2024).

In health care, price and quality are not only not easily discernible but may not even be related. Unruh et al. (2020), for example, found that the highest-priced physicians were paid more than twice as much per procedure as the lowest, but there was no difference in quality between these groups, including among high-need patient groups. Moreover, Issa and colleagues note the disconnection of prices to input costs, stating that spinal fusion "DRG prices remain widely variable with little to no correlation with practice cost or socioeconomic parameters" (2023, p. 677) even after the passage of price transparency laws. Finally, a comprehensive Congressional Budget Office (CBO) study illustrates the magnitude of price variability using vaginal birth, a fairly straightforward procedure, as an example (see Figure 6.1).

This analysis also reports price variability among different hospitals within the same metropolitan statistical area as well within a single hospital. Finally, in a study that included over 1 million patients, patients treated by female surgeons had lower 30-day, 90-day, and 1-year cost compared to those treated by male surgeons, for example, 1-year total costs of $24,882 for male surgeons and $18,519 for female surgeons. Analysis was procedure specific and accounted for covariates other than sex that could have contributed to or explained this difference, such as patient, surgeon, anesthesiologist, and hospital-level covariates (Wallis et al., 2024). In summary, U.S. health care is riddled with price variability and opacity. Halverson (cited in Meden, 2019) notes: "Providers who can demand the higher prices are the one who create a brand everyone wants. In some markets, the prestigious medical institutions can name their price" (para 8). Ponder the contrast with markets that are more familiar, such

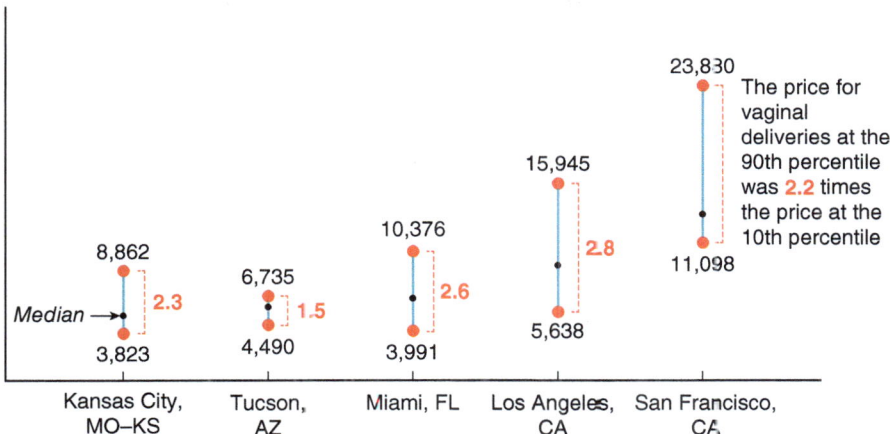

FIGURE 6.1: Vaginal delivery price variability in selected metropolitan areas.
Source: Congressional Budget Office. (2022, January). *The prices that commercial health insurers and Medicare pay for hospitals' and physicians' services.*

as a restaurant that charges much more for roughly the same meal, service, and ambience. This sort of difference would be easily discernible to the savvy diner but is very difficult for the consumer of health care to recognize. The challenges with transparency and variability have led to legislation to address two different but related things: transparency and surprise billing.

Surprise Billing

Have you ever ordered something and then been shocked at the sticker price? This happens in health care, but one troubling element has recently gained public attention, including in Congress. It is called *surprise billing*.

Surprise billing is the term used for an insured person who uses health care, only to later discover that the provider they saw was *out-of-network* and they are responsible for much more expense than they bargained for. There are two main categories of surprise billing (Pollitz, 2016).

1. *Cost-sharing surprise* billing: One category of surprise billing is when a patient is responsible for more *cost sharing*—deductible, copayments, and co-insurance—when they receive health services out-of-network. Recall that different providers charge markedly different prices for the same services, and payers and providers negotiate for rates; patients who use services only within a more narrow, previously defined "in-network" set of providers bear less cost sharing. The differences between in-network and out-of-network cost sharing can be substantial. A patient may be responsible for 40% of the cost, for example, rather than the 10% or 20% patient responsibility for care from in-network providers.

2. *Balance billing surprise billing*: The second category of surprise billing is *balance billing*. Here is how it works. As noted, in-network providers negotiate

with insurance companies to provide services at a discount from what they deem "full price." Typically, then, the providers are not allowed to bill patients for the difference between the discounted price and the full price. This is not true for out-of-network providers, who can bill for the full amount.

Both categories can happen for the same services, leaving the patient with a hefty, unexpected bill. So why aren't patients just more careful about staying in network? In the current system, it is almost impossible. Ambulance services—likely used when people are least prepared to consider costs—are well documented as culprits in surprise billing, with one study finding additional charges of $450/land ambulance and $21,698/air transport (Chharbra et al., 2020). Then, when hospitalized after an accident, a consult with a neurologist is not uncommon. Yet the neurologist may actually be out of network, even if providing services in the same facility that an in-network physician uses. Similarly, the anesthesiologist may be out-of-network as well. They, along with emergency medicine physicians, have been frequent sources of surprise billing because they are not hospital employees, but outside contractors. The variability state by state is also dramatic; for example, mean anesthesiology charges for the same services ranged from 4 times Medicare rates in Oklahoma to 11 times this rate in Wisconsin (Adler et al., 2019). Most people who use such services are not in the frame of mind to consider each member of the health care team and query them about their network status yet nevertheless bear costs they could not possibly have foreseen.

Over time, bipartisan members of Congress have proposed different bills to stop surprise billing; for example, HR 3502 Protecting People from Surprise Medical Bills Act of 2019 (introduced by a Democrat, with 110 cosponsors, both Republican and Democrat) and S.1531 Stopping the Outrageous Practice of Surprise Medical Bills Act of 2019 (introduced by a Republican with 30 cosponsors, both Republican and Democrat). Policy makers ensured that treatment for COVID-19 could not create surprise billing, with ongoing congressional consideration of ending surprise billing for all forms of care (Peterson & Bykowicz, 2020). In general, insurance companies, employer groups, and consumer groups support ending the practice of surprise billing. Many hospital groups and physician groups oppose it, saying it will harm patients (Luthi, 2019) even as they benefit financially from the practice. As the U.S. Congress dealt with COVID-19 and other complex policy and politics issues in late 2020, momentum on surprise billing appeared stalled. This changed when "The No Surprises Act" was included in the 2,124-page COVID-19 stimulus package signed into law on December 27, 2020, and went into effect in January 2022. This legislation aimed to protect people from

- surprise billing for emergency services received without prior authorization from an out-of-network provider;
- out-of-network cost sharing for emergency services and some nonemergency services (note, "some"); and

- balance billing and out-of-network charges for care by out-of-network providers who work at in-network facilities (Consumer Financial Protection Bureau, 2023).

There is also a process for dispute resolution (see the AMA summary of this law at https://www.ama-assn.org/system/files/2021-02/surprise-billing-provisions-guide.pdf) and price transparency, the latter of which has a much larger legislative history at both state and federal levels.

Price Transparency Legislation and Administrative Rules

Whaley and Bai (2023) note, "Unlike prices in nearly all other U.S. markets, U.S. health care prices are notoriously opaque" (para 2) and "High [health care] spending comes directly out of worker wages and tax dollars" (para 1). This should be a concern to all nurses, particularly given the relationship of these costs to equity. Hagar and colleagues (2024), for example, note the substantial wage stagnation stemming from the rising cost of employer-based health insurance and the differential impact this has on lower-wage workers. Efforts toward price transparency have evolved as one tool toward empowered health care consumers. Indeed, Pollock describes price transparency as an "ethical and policy imperative for American health care" (2022, para 1).

Hospital prices and third-party payer rates as well as pricing for 300 common health care services have been required since January 1, 2021 (see Code of Regulations, updated February 2024 for extensive details https://www.ecfr.gov/current/title-45/subtitle-A/subchapter-E/part-180#180.40). Yet there had been slow uptake of the requirements, and some organizations' were willing to pay the fine rather than comply with the rule. A 2022 report stated: "Hospitals have been slow to comply with transparency rules. Between July and September 2021, fewer than 6% of hospitals had disclosed prices as required. Hospitals with higher revenues and in highly consolidated markets were found to be more likely to flout the law. CMS had set a maximum fine of about $2 million a year for larger hospitals that fail to comply, but some of these hospitals have stated that they would rather pay the fines than forgo their competitive advantage" (Kona & Corlette, 2022, para 9). In the same vein, the Patient Rights Advocate Organization's semi-annual survey of hospitals found that, although increasing, less than a quarter of surveyed hospitals were compliant in 2023. Lo and colleagues highlight challenges with the transparency reports, stating "they are messy, inconsistent and confusing, making it challenging, if not impossible, for patients or researchers to use them for their intended purpose" (2023, para 2). The 2024 transparency rules became more stringent, including expanded information requirements and a greater likelihood an organization will be publicly cited if noncompliant (Hut, 2023). As this book goes to press, the much more stringent and expansive Lower Prices More Transparency Act has passed the

House of Representatives with bipartisan, bicameral support and is being considered in the Senate. Regardless of the fate of this particular bill, policy interest in greater transparency is likely to continue. Take a moment to check the websites of a few of your local hospitals. Are prices transparent? What about value transparency?

Recall that value includes not only the cost of care but also short- and long-term outcomes, which is sometimes termed quality but is much more expansive than that seemingly simple term. Thus, to understand the value of care, it is essential to understand the cost as well as the short- and long-term outcomes stemming from the care and how people experience those outcomes. An important element of this is what has meaning and importance to people. What do they wish? Recall supplier-induced demand and the vulnerability of a health care "purchase." People may not easily find themselves in a position to determine their own best interests. Thus, shared decision-making (SDM) remains an important, as of yet not fully realized opportunity to support informed patient choice in health care (recall from Chapter 3 that SDM is part of the Affordable Care Act). Moreover, Vasher et al. (2020) found that physicians perceive they do a better job in communication than they actually do and ". . . clinicians who lack communication skills endorsed in professional guidelines may also lack the metacognitive skills required to recognize their deficiencies" (para 3). Research has underscored the contribution of shared decision-making inclusive of price transparency for the well-being of older people with serious illness and their lack of familiarity with tools and processes that support such discernment (FAIR Health, 2023). Nurses can play a key role in supporting patient self-determination through more informed choice.

The Role of Patient Choice

Informed patient choice adds further complexity to the price transparency, cost, and value dynamic. Sommers et al. (2013), for example, found that patients tend to equate higher cost with higher quality, even when the higher-cost care is not higher in quality. Beauvais et al. (2020) state: "In most consumer markets, higher prices generally imply increased quality. For example, in the automobile, restaurant, hospitality, and airline industries, higher pricing generally conveys a signal of complexity and superiority of a service or product. However, in the healthcare industry there is room to challenge the price quality connection as both health prices and health quality can be difficult to interpret" (para 1). Although many Americans support shopping for better prices for care, the vast majority don't do so. Gordon (2022) reports that 65% of consumers have never tried to find health care prices, with variations by age (younger more likely), cost sharing (greater cost sharing more likely), and familiarity with social media applications. Additional reasons include fear of altering the relationship with their provider and the difficulty in actually obtaining price information (Methrotra et al., 2017). Other studies found that the creation of user-friendly price transparency tools was largely ineffective; people did not use the price transparency tools, and overall health care spending was not reduced in the study setting (Desai et al., 2017). And while online advertisements about provider price tools in New Hampshire resulted in a 600% increase in visits to the website, it did not result in the use of lower-price providers (Desai et al., 2021).

SDM inclusive of cost and value consideration could potentially redress this challenge; however, researchers identified substantial barriers to SDM (see Box 6.2) with reference to cost (see Box 6.3). They conclude that substantial efforts to broaden patient understanding will have to be complemented by greater provider preparation in being informed about the cost/value equation and provider capacity to discuss the cost of care with a patient. This provider learning curve is important. Espinoza Suarez and colleagues (2021), for example, found cost conversations with patients did not have a negative effect on decision-making, but instead was associated with a modest but measurable reduction in decisional conflict and an increase in patient engagement, particularly when cost conservations were supported with an

BOX 6.2

WHAT IS SHARED DECISION-MAKING?

The U.S. Agency for Healthcare Research and Quality defines SDM as "…a collaborative process in which patients and clinicians work together to make healthcare decisions informed by evidence, the care team's knowledge and experience, and the patient's values, goals, preferences, and circumstances. Family members and caregivers also play an important role in SDM (AHRQ, 2023, para 1). Introduced in 1982 by the President's Commission for the Study of Ethical Problems in Medicine and Biomedical Research, Lee and Emanuel (2013) submit that it is a "sleeper provision of the Affordable Care Act" (p. 6) and particularly useful for circumstances in which there is not a clear, single best treatment option, thus enabling optimal, informed alignment with the patient's values and wishes. Blumenthal-Barby et al. (2019) note challenges and potential unintended consequences that include

- SDM in events that unfold over time and include different providers;
- incenting hyper-individualism without accounting for family values, preferences, and involvement;
- providing information to patients without them then truly being partners in care decisions;
- implying that patients cannot or should not defer decision-making to the provider;
- assuming that physicians are or can be neutral in the decision; and
- ignoring public health implications.

BOX 6.3

BARRIERS TO SHARED DECISION-MAKING THAT IS INCLUSIVE OF COST

- Patients want what they perceive as the best care and assume that the most expensive care is the best possible care.
- Patients perceive that the most expensive is the best even when there are other available alternatives with acceptable outcomes that are less expensive. A patient, for example, may perceive an expensive highly advertised brand-name pharmaceutical to be more effective than a bioidentical generic medication.
- Patients have little experience in considering health cost trade-offs—what they are getting and what they are giving up by using the most expensive care.
- Patients have a lack of interest in lower-cost care when they perceive—or assume—that the costs are borne by insurers and society, even if this includes depletion of scarce resources.

Source: From Sommers, R., Dorr Gould, S., McGlunn, E., Pearson, S., & Danis, M. (2013). Focus groups highlight that many patients object to clinicians' focusing on costs. *Health Affairs*, *32*(2), 338–346. https://doi.org/10.1377/hlthaff.2012.0686

SDM tool. Do you feel comfortable talking to patients about cost? If not, how would you go about gaining those skills? What tools can assist you?

Your efforts in developing this skill can directly help the people you care for. Politi and colleagues (2023) detail the importance of cost conversations as part of SDM, as follows:

- "Financial toxicity (burden of high costs of care) is prevalent across conditions and countries
- Clinicians rarely bring up costs without prompts and training
- Patients want clinicians to bring up costs as part of treatment discussions, in some contexts finding clinicians trustworthy, honest, and transparent when they address costs
- Patients often worry that if they bring up cost, it will lead to biases and lower-quality care
- Patient decision aids and standards rarely include relative costs to compare options
- When costs are discussed, they rarely include downstream direct or indirect costs (e.g., costs that build over time, relating to frequent monitoring or ongoing morbidity)
- Making space to ask about costs supports broader care goal conversations and practical issues affecting implementation" (2023, para 9).

These authors also detail a scenario in which a nurse checked on the cost of cancer treatment and found a benefit card that enabled a dramatic reduction in cost, illustrating nurses' potentially pivotal role in such efforts and the tangible outcomes enabled when nurses are cost conscious.

DATA ON QUALITY

Clearly, transparency in pricing is just one element of the sort of information consumers need to make wise decisions. Another key element introduced in this chapter is meaningful information about quality. Finger states:

> We rate Uber drivers, restaurants, Amazon delivery, and much more, but when it comes to our own health experience, we often have little to no data. That's especially scary because the business model of the healthcare provider (e.g., Doctor) is to get money from the insurance company. The patient is actually not the customer. Knowing quality is, therefore, of utmost importance for each of us. (2023, para 1)

Public and private organizations have encouraged public reporting of quality, and payers increasingly link such metrics to payment. Although initially riddled with contradictory findings (see, e.g., Ryan et al., 2012; Smith et al., 2012), more recent research has demonstrated encouraging trends. Hoffman and Yakusheva (2020), for example, found hospitals with greater incentives for avoiding readmissions had larger decreases in them than those without such incentives. Financial incentives and disincentives are not the only effective strategy. Navathe et al. (2020) found peer comparisons to be an effective strategy for improving physician performance. Conversely, Agweyu and colleagues argue that to substantially improve quality information, systems with continuous and rapid feedback are essential, as are people who know how to use this information for performance improvements as skillful change managers (Agweyu et al., 2023). Lansky goes a step further and calls for a total redesign of health care quality measurement, stating, "The current retrospective, transactional system for measuring and rewarding improvement is ineffective, expensive, burdensome, no longer credible, and does not measure health or the outcomes of health care" (2022, para 1).

Many of the measures related to payment include *nurse-sensitive indicators*, measures that are directly related to nursing performance and, potentially, nursing staffing. Nurses who understand these dynamics are well positioned to positively influence not only the quality of care but also the economic vitality of their organization. This skill set is particularly important in the financial wake caused by COVID-19 (Yakusheva et al., 2020). The potential adoption of national provider indicators or unique nurse identifiers will also enable a quantification of each nurse's contribution to outcomes and cost (see Chan et al., 2023, for more information).

Programs linking outcomes to reimbursement abound. As noted in Chapter 3, some of these are permanent payment models. Hospital value-based purchasing, for example, cuts reimbursement to prospective payment system hospitals (those that use DRGs for payment and thus the majority in the United States) by 2%, with the opportunity to recoup some, all, or more than that 2% based on a composite measure that includes nurse-sensitive hospital-acquired conditions, among others (see Figure 6.2). Each of the four overall domains are worth 25% of the total score. The four

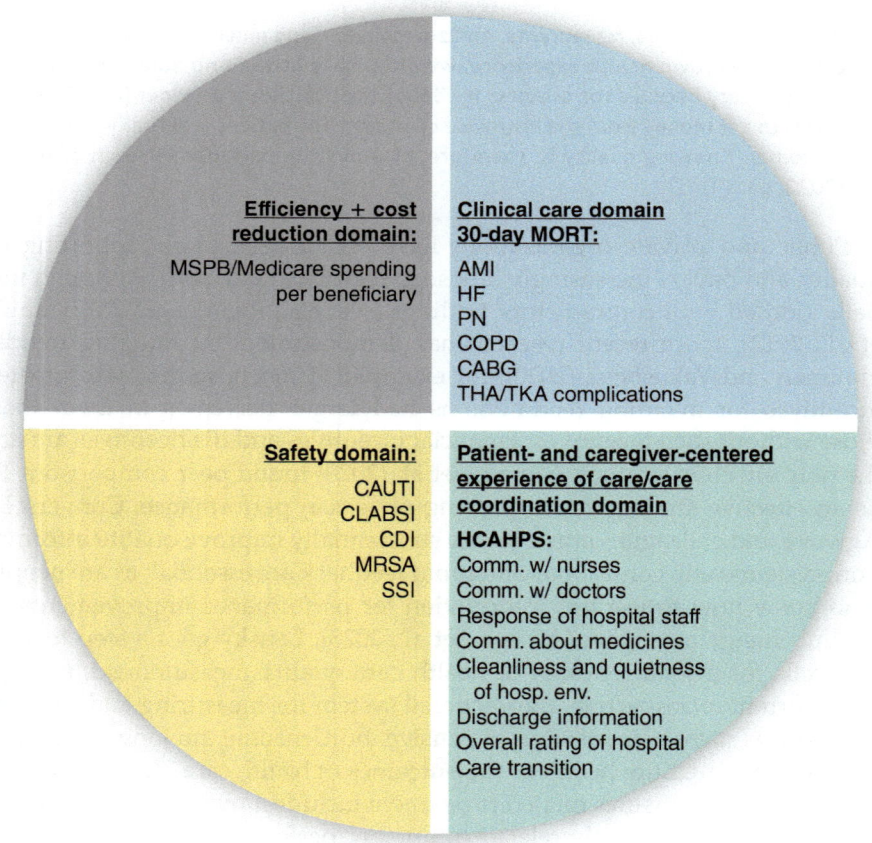

FIGURE 6.2: Domain weights and measures.

AMI, acute myocardial infarction; CABG, coronary artery bypass graft; CAUTI, catheter-associated urinary tract infection; CDI, *Clostridium difficile* infection; CLABSI, central line–associated bloodstream infection; COPD, chronic obstructive pulmonary disease; HCAHPS, Hospital Consumer Assessment of Healthcare Providers and Systems; HF, heart failure; MORT, morality measure; MRSA, methicillin-resistant *Staphylococcus aureus*; PN, pneumonia; SSI, surgical site infection; THA, total hip arthroplasty; TKA, total knee arthroplasty.

domains are safety, clinical care, efficiency and cost reduction, and person and community engagement. Importantly, either the overall score or the improvement score can be used, thus not penalizing high-performing organizations.

Other predominant programs linking quality to payment include the Merit-based Incentive Payment System, the Hospital Readmission Reduction Program, and Hospital-Acquired Condition Reduction Program described in Chapter 3.

Although these initiatives will evolve over time, the wise nurse will attend to the payment mechanisms in place in their employment setting and the quality metrics associated with them as organizations react and respond to financial incentives. Many nurses, when first learning about initiatives that link payment to quality, understand for the first time why their organization is focused on, for example, noise mitigation or reduction in catheter-related urinary tract infection. What quality improvement strategies have you witnessed in clinical practice? Were they linked to payment reform initiatives? Recall that prior to many of these initiatives, low-quality care was often reimbursed at higher rates than high-quality care; hospitals received additional reimbursement for managing complications they caused in the first place.

For nurses, these approaches linking quality to payment introduce a much more complicated picture than what has traditionally been identified as quality care and performance improvements. It requires an approach that uses a variety of analytic points and integrated methodologies to assess what constitutes quality, track changes, and plan corrective improvements. At the far extreme, it calls for analytic approaches reliant on new data strategies and skills with data science.

DATA SCIENCE

Technological and analytic innovations have dramatically changed the information landscape. Data science is an overarching term that refers to contemporary and emerging strategies to extract insights and meaning from data. Health care generates vast amounts of data, both numerical, for example, blood pressure, and free text, for example, classic nursing notes. In addition, unprecedented volumes of data are generated from social media sites, wearable devices, and other "smart" applications, all of which will be increasingly used in patient care. Key opportunities for nurses to expand their social and economic value include big data, data mining, natural language processing (NLP), blockchain, artificial intelligence (AI), and deep learning—a subset of machine learning. Each of these will be described briefly in turn. This landscape has dramatically exploded with the introduction of generative AI large language models such as ChatGPT introduced on November 30, 2022.

The Digital Transformation of Health Care

THE INTERNET OF THINGS AND THE INTERNET OF MEDICAL THINGS

Roberts defines the Internet of Things (IoT) as "a physical world where smart devices or *things* and computers are interconnected through wired or wireless networks to share and process information without human intervention" (2021, para 1). She notes the Health Internet of Things (HIoT) may be implanted, stationary, or wearable (see Table 6.1).

The Internet of Medical Things (IoMT) "encompasses a network of interconnected healthcare devices and systems that gather, analyze and transmit health data. This enables remote patient monitoring, diagnosis, and treatment, revolutionizing the way healthcare is delivered" (Huang et al., 2023, para 3). Dwivedi and colleagues (2022) visualize IMoT as central to many health care applications and innovations (Figure 6.3).

Yesmin et al. (2022) explored use of IoT to enhance hospital patient safety and, in qualitative interviews with nurses, found perceptions of more time spent with patients and fewer patient falls, while Arora (2020) details potential for better care at a lower cost. In summary, IoMT offers an area of rich opportunities for nurse scientists and innovators.

BIG DATA

A quickly evolving area both within and beyond health care is the use of multiple data sets together to create a more nuanced understanding than

TABLE 6.1 HEALTH INTERNET OF THINGS

Category	Example	Characteristics
Implanted	Pacemakers Defibrillators Nerve stimulators	Carefully monitored by health care personnel
Stationary	X-ray and mammography MRI scanners Nuclear imaging machines	Integrate with other applications such as electronic medical records and transmit to providers
Wearable	Smartwatches Wristbands that track activity Hearables Head-mounted displays Smart clothing Smart patches	Growing availability of products that offer fitness monitoring and personalized care; estimated at $100 billion in 2023, with 15% annual compounded increase expected through 2030 (Health Economics Times, 2023)

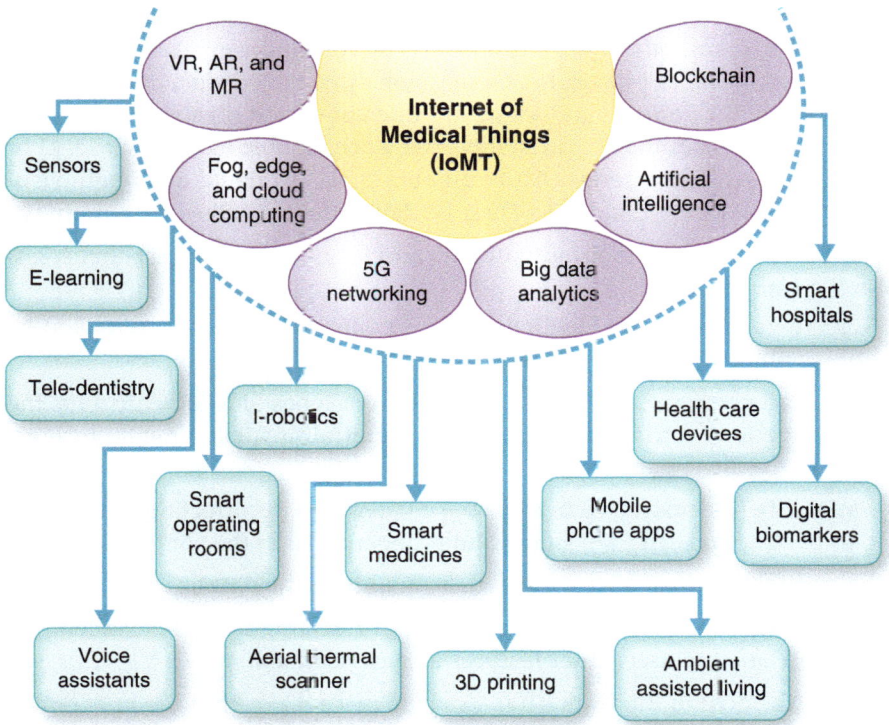

FIGURE 6.3: Internet of Medical Things.

could be gleaned by any one data set. Termed *big data*, such approaches have been broadly used in industries outside of health care to decrease cost and increase quality. As early as 2014, Keenan stated an urgent plea for nursing big data, and Rambur and Fitzpatrick (2018) voiced a similarly urgent plea, calling for big data use to be foundational knowledge in all nursing programs.

Big data was initially conceptualized as *the three Vs: volume, variety,* and *velocity* (Baro et al., 2015). Big data has massive amounts (volume) of data, potentially straining traditional data management systems. It uses many different data types (variety), which may range from diagnostic images to social media streaming and mobile applications, as well as structured and free text fields of electronic health records (EHRs). Thus, big data synthesizes and links divergent data sources to enable clinical, research, and policy questions to be answered in unprecedented ways. Big data's massive information is processed rapidly (velocity). This velocity is a necessary element. Consider the case in which an accountable care organization wants to understand emergency department utilization by payer type in those with congestive heart failure to see if additional care management is necessary for any one segment of their population. Data that are 2 years old would not be helpful.

Over time, more *Vs* were added: *veracity*, meaning the data are correct and free from error, and *value*, meaning the data can contribute in meaningful ways by offering clinical or practical value. Obviously, to have value, the data must be correct. Thus, veracity and value are interconnected attributes. A sixth *v* has been suggested, that of variability, that is, being able to track seasonal or other variable disease trends (Audreu-Perez et al., 2015) and a seventh, visualization (Batko & Ślęzak, 2022). These authors offer the following summary:

- "Volume (refers to the amount of data and is one of the biggest challenges in Big Data Analytics),
- Velocity (speed with which new data is generated, the challenge is to be able to manage data effectively and in real time),
- Variety (heterogeneity of data, many different types of healthcare data, the challenge is to derive insights by looking at all available heterogeneous data in a holistic manner),
- Variability (inconsistency of data, the challenge is to correct the interpretation of data that can vary significantly depending on the context),
- Veracity (how trustworthy the data is, quality of the data),
- Visualization (ability to interpret data and resulting insights, challenging for Big Data due to its other features as described above),
- Value (the goal of Big Data Analytics is to discover the hidden knowledge from huge amounts of data)." (para 20)

Taken as a whole, big data enables comprehensive analyses and discovery of patterns and potentials that could not be discerned with traditional methods and data sets.

Data Visualization

The product of effective data visualization is well known to nurses. A chart or diagram that quickly shares a complex story in an understandable, appealing, powerful manner represents effective data visualization. The massive amount of information generated by big data can obscure meaning without effective data visualization to illustrate trends or other patterns. Data visualization uses graphic design and human–computer interactions to translate information to understanding and "sits right in the middle of analysis and visual storytelling" (Tableau, n.d., para 9). It offers substantial opportunities to integrate visualization into health care systems that nurses can use for individual and population health management (Topaz & Pruinelli, 2017). Austin and colleagues (2022), for example, deployed data visualization to detect "whole person" patterns in adults 64 and older, noting that "wholeperson health examines a person's environmental, psychosocial and physical health, as well as their health-related behaviours; and assesses their strengths, challenges and needs" (para 1), illustrating the alignment with this approach and nurses' domain of interests and expertise.

Data Mining

Data mining offers an underutilized tool in nursing practice. Data mining, as the term implies, is the exploration of data sets to identify novel patterns and create new understanding. Nurses regularly rely on pattern discernment in clinical practice, for example, "Is Mr. Gonzalez's respiration becoming more labored?" Data mining offers key opportunities to enhance this skill to positively impact patient care. Topaz and Pruinelli (2017) describe two major categories in which data mining strategies are used in health care: predictive modeling, and descriptive tasks. Nurse-led research using the tools provided by data mining includes discernment of patterns associated with improvement in patient mobility among those receiving home care (Dey et al., cited in Topaz & Pruinelli, 2017) and nurses' post–acute care referral patterns (Bowles et al., cited in Topaz & Pruinelli, 2017). Data mining was also used to efficiently and reliability predict the possibility of recovery from COVID-19 (Muhammad et al., 2020).

Artificial Intelligence

The explosion in AI applications has been termed everything from an existential threat to humanity to a "great equalizer" for employees as it trims mundane, routine tasks (Rometty, 2024). A 2024 *Economist* article details the hope: "Better diagnoses. Personalised support for patients. Faster drug discovery. Greater efficiency. Artificial intelligence (AI) is generating excitement and hyperbole everywhere, but in the field of health care it has the potential to be transformational." (2024, para 1).

The health care promise of AI is illustrated in findings like Gallo et al. (2024), who found that an AI model to support recognition of patient deterioration reduced risk of care escalations in hospitalized adults. Some providers are using generative AI to craft empathetic provider–patient interactions scripts, and at least one study found ChatGPT-generated dialogue to be more empathetic than a physician's (Ayers et al., 2023). Naturally, the explosion in position use cases of AI raises ethical, regulatory, and malpractice accountability questions (Mello & Guha, 2023).

Although the term AI is off-putting to some, invoking images of a world driven by heartless robots, AI is simply a more sophisticated form of something nurses are familiar with: algorithmic-driven decision-making. AI can assist clinical decision-making and diagnoses and is part of health care, particularly as voice and image recognition become refined. The Healthcare Information and Management Systems Society (2019) aptly details how AI can and will meet the needs of both patients and nurses, improving quality and decreasing cost through reallocation of menial tasks to enhance productivity. Their clarion call for nurses' embrace of AI states: "The need for nurses' comprehension of the foundations of AI and the symbiotic nature of it with nursing practice is essential with its increased use in practice in today's value-based care environment" (para 1). Further, they note that AI will lead nurses to "serve the Quadruple Aim by adding value through expedited, more precise, enriched decision making" (para 8). Generative AI's most common use as this text goes to print is documentation assistance, clinical decision support, and patient-facing chatbots. This list will expand. The Institute for Healthcare Improvement's safety-focused entity, the Lucian Leape Institute (2024), has developed broad parameters that emphasize the need for informed patient consent, rigorous testing, and strict oversight. Nurses' broad and deep involvement in these efforts is critical to nursing's future and our patients' safety.

MACHINE LEARNING AND ITS SUBSET, DEEP LEARNING

Machine learning. Machine learning is a subset of AI. It focuses on the development and use of computer programs that can access data and then learn from it without additional human intervention. It generally relies on structured data to create algorithms that can modify themselves ("learn") in response to additional new information.

Deep learning. Deep learning is also grounded in artificial neural networks that can learn without human supervision. These networks, however, are able to process vast amounts of structured *and* unstructured data. Such volumes would take humans decades or even a lifetime to process or understand. Instead of traditional linear artificial neural networks, deep learning depends on layered hierarchical networks to process information. Hargrave (2019) notes: "The artificial neural networks are built like the human brain, with neuron nodes connected together like a web" (para 7). Deep learning is sometimes called *deep neural learning* or *deep neural network*.

Natural Language Processing

Comprehension of the full range and dimensions of human communication—termed *natural language*—is a challenging adaptation for computers, yet an important one in health care as well as other segments of society. NLP is being used with machine learning to enable complex tasks such as emotion detection and enhanced human–computer interaction. Gupta and Gupta (2019) suggest that NLP in health care is particularly valuable because of the vast amounts of data health care produces each day and the potential for NLP to streamline documentation and reporting. Other applications include claims processing, cost reduction, and quality improvement (Olaronke & Olaleke, 2015). Topaz and Pruinelli (2017) note that NLP is particularly critical because 80% of EHR data is stored as free text and other data sources are 100% free text, with only a few NLP systems focusing on nursing data explicitly; analysis of "nursing-relevant" narrative data will require that nurses understand machine learning methods and collaborate with computer science and computational linguistics. There is a great deal of opportunity for nurses in this area. Scharp et al.'s (2024) scoping review of NLP, for example, notes that NLP applications in the postacute setting are "nascent" (p. 63), yet NLP integrated with predictive models could help identify patients who are at risk for negative outcomes. Such inquiries and applications illustrate a broad avenue for nursing practice and leadership.

Blockchain

Interest in blockchain's promise for health care was reignited during the COVID-19 pandemic as one strategy for ensuring supplies of needed goods, including medical equipment and devices. This potential for better *supply chain management* was complemented with blockchain's potential to ensure the origin and monitor migration of goods as well as its potential for widely accessible public health records and immunity certificates, if or when such immunity is certain (Cohen, 2020). But what is blockchain?

In blockchain, a block of information is chained to the next block in chronological order. Each data block, or *ledger*, contains a unique identifier (sometimes called a digital fingerprint or "hash") that is time stamped and cannot be changed without changing all of the subsequent blocks at the exact same time, which is virtually impossible (Yoon, 2019) because the blocks are stored on thousands of computers, not on a central computer. Thus, the data are not only immutable, they are held within a network of information that is very difficult to hack. This offers both security and potential access to medical records. Daley (2020), for example, notes:

> while blockchain is transparent it is also private, concealing the identity of any individual with complex and secure codes that can protect the sensitivity of medical data. The decentralized nature of the technology also allows patients, doctors and healthcare providers to share the same information quickly and safely. (para 6)

This author further notes that decentralization of information illustrates blockchain's potential to address the $11 billion/year in waste that results from miscommunication among providers because it creates "one ecosystem [of] patient data" that can be efficiently referenced to lead to timely, personalized plans of care. Blockchain also offers solutions to the challenges and cost of professional credentialing, including nursing credentialing (Buiser Schnur, 2020).

Blockchain was also deployed during COVID-19 for surveillance, vaccine passport monitoring, and contact tracing. A systematic review also found non–COVID-19–specific applications that include electronic medical record and supply chain monitoring and IoT applications such as remote monitoring or mobile health (Ng et al., 2021). Ghosh and colleagues (2023) offer an expansive vision, based on their review of 144 articles and reflecting the dramatic acceleration of research articles since 2020. They map blockchain uses in health care as illustrated in Figure 6.4.

They also note the considerable interest in blockchain technology but that it is still in development. It is likely that blockchain will become much more familiar to nurses than it is at the time of this writing. Tsang et al. (2021), for example, has detailed a blockchain approach to staffing long-term care settings to ensure adequate nursing talent. Kim and colleagues' review of nursing-specific research on blockchain identified only eight articles, but

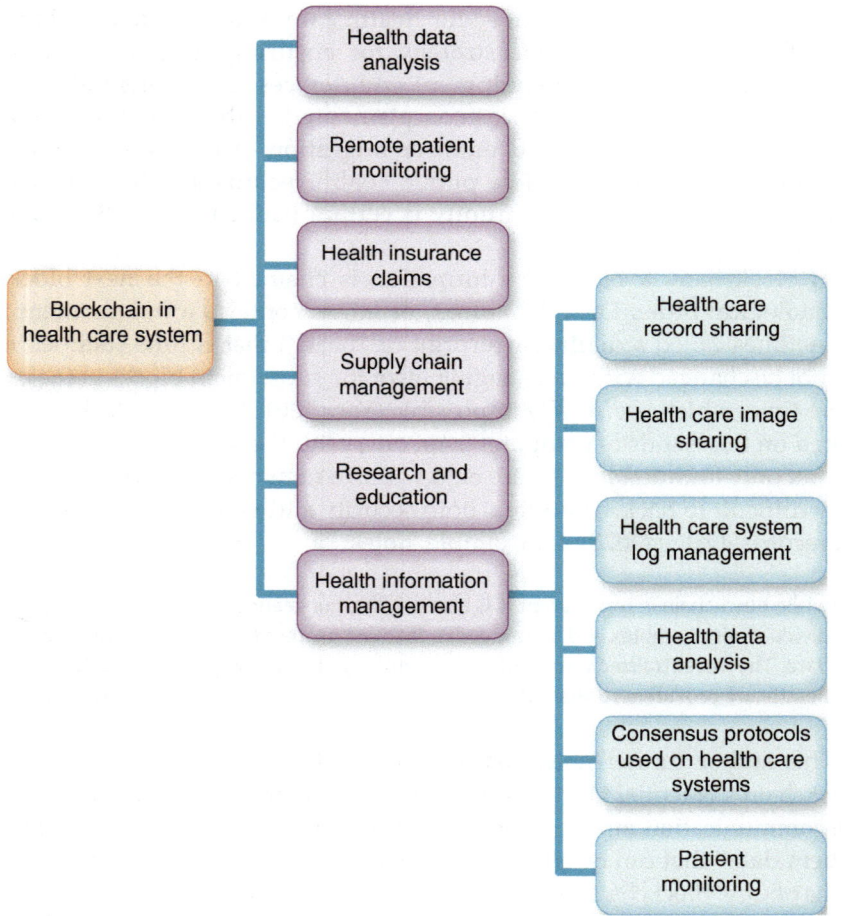

FIGURE 6.4: Applications of blockchain in health care.

they conclude there is the potential for improved patient care (2024). Online incubator FasterCapital suggests blockchain benefits that include greater efficiency and trust, care coordination, potential to decrease errors, and optimization of resource allocation. They suggest that nurses

> "[e]ducate yourself and others about the basics of blockchain and its implications for nursing care. Blockchain is a complex and evolving technology that requires a certain level of understanding and awareness to be used effectively. Nursing care stakeholders should seek reliable sources of information and education on blockchain, such as online courses, webinars, podcasts, books, and articles. They should also share their knowledge and insights with their colleagues, patients, and partners, and foster a culture of learning and innovation in their organizations" (2024, para 20).

What's Next for Data Science and Nursing?

Information is central to the creation of a safe, effective, affordable health system, and the digital age has created—and will continue to create—a cascading crescendo of new tools and strategies. Professional nurses must be armed with these tools in order to serve not only their patients and society writ large but also their careers. A lifelong strategy for continuous education and mastery of progressively more nuanced tools is a daunting, yet necessary, professional obligation.

INFORMATION SCIENCE, QUALITY SCIENCE, AND DATA

What does the future hold for information science, quality science, data, and nursing? As health care cost concerns continue and the public feels more financial impact when seeking services due to cost sharing, it is likely that there will be accelerating attention to the value equation, that is, "What am I getting for my money?" Thus, it is likely that there will be increased attention to how valid information is defined, collected, and analyzed to determine the cost and value of health care. Increasingly sophisticated electronic medical record systems may link clinical information with financial information, such as the EHR–insurance claims data linkages illustrated in Figure 6.4. Easily accessible quality data will enable patients and employer groups to quickly scan options for health care. In-home monitoring of a patient's health status provides yet a different form of information—patient-monitoring information—which will revolutionize the nature of the patient–provider interaction. Moreover, the explosion of telehealth during the COVID-19 pandemic has forever changed the face of health care delivery.

In summary, Therese Fitzpatrick, PhD, MS, RN, FAAN, senior vice president of performance improvement at Kaufman Hall, states:

Artificial Intelligence may seem to many as unprecedented and quite revolutionary, however it is simply the next evolution of machine intelligence. We might think of it as the next chapter in the ongoing history of information. We are observing a similar evolution of analytics whereas we are no longer able to solve complex problems with simple descriptive statistics but through the use of predictive analytics where we study the likelihood of events happening in the future. And optimization science takes the analysis one step further by determining the best choice of action out of a myriad of possible solutions when confronting that event. Imagine the implications for our industry.

I like to think of generative AI and advanced analytics as the accelerant for nursing's elevated ambitions. Social, clinical, and business problems are becoming increasingly complex and requiring a higher level of thinking suggesting that we free our experts from mundane operations and allow them to focus on higher value work which aligns with tomorrow's imperatives. We might approach AI and advanced analytics as a force multiplier for our imaginations as the future belongs to those that ask better questions and have more exciting ideas and options to amplify. (Therese Fitzpatrick, May 27, 2024)

This chapter opened by illustrating the role of information in classic free markets, for example, the purchase of an appliance or coffee. It then detailed the historic challenges in "information" as it appears in health care markets, for example, asymmetry of information, and the phenomenon of supplier-induced demand. The role of data in discerning value, both cost and outcomes, was described, including emerging trends such as AI. In health care, the information revolution is just beginning. The savvy nurse understands the role of information in accountability for both cost and outcomes, continually expands skills to use complex data sources in clinical practice, and embraces a spirit of adventure in exploring new technological applications.

End-of-Chapter Resources

THOUGHT QUESTIONS

1. Recall your first cell phone or the oldest cell phone you have seen. Then reflect on the most up-to-date phone you have seen. What features do you notice on the new phone? These features can be called functionalities. Now, describe health care cost and quality information you have seen. Has it been helpful? What functionalities would add further value to your use of your personal health data? What functionalities do you use in clinical practice? What aspects are useful, and which would benefit from enhancement?

2. Your neighbor is considering an elective surgery and notices that the available price information suggests that the procedure is nearly three times as expensive in Setting A than in Setting B. The neighbor then asks you what to do. What other information is needed to make a recommendation to your neighbor? Do considerations change if your neighbor has a low-deductible plan versus a high-deductible plan?
3. What sorts of data would be useful to plan care strategies for a selected population of patients? How does planning for the population differ from planning for the individual? What sorts of data are useful for both individual and population approaches?
4. What knowledge and skills prepare you to understand and apply big data in clinically relevant ways? What additional skills do you need? Develop a plan to obtain them.
5. You are responsible for developing a data science and AI learning agenda for yourself and your peers. What skills do you define as essential? Develop a plan to obtain them.
6. Define the following key terms:
   AI
   Asymmetry of information
   Big data
   Data mining
   Data visualization
   Deep learning
   Hospital value-based purchasing
   Informed decision-making
   Machine learning
   Natural language processing
   Price transparency
   Price variability

EXERCISES

1. Describe ways you have seen information used in the health care system. What recommendations would you offer to improve the flow and accuracy of health information?
2. Prepare a presentation for your peers that provides information on how to talk to patients about the cost of care within a framework of quality and overall value. Include opportunities for role-playing.
3. Consider quality metrics you have seen in your practice settings. Are they connected to a payment model? If so, which one or ones?

QUIZ

True or False

1. One characteristic of a classic free market is that the consumer knows about the product or, alternatively, how to obtain information about the product.
2. The term price transparency refers to the degree to which the price of a product or service is readily evident.
3. The same health care service provided by different providers always costs the patient the exact same amount.
4. A weakness of shared decision-making models is the exclusion of patients' values and wishes when planning a therapeutic approach to their care.
5. Health care data and the use of quality metrics consistently improve the quality of care while decreasing cost.
6. High patient satisfaction has consistently been associated with high-quality patient outcomes.
7. Big data is characterized by volume, variety, velocity, veracity, variability, visualization, and value.
8. In health care, consumers can easily obtain information about the price and value of proposed treatments.
9. One potential use of big data is to address clinical, research, and policy questions.
10. One ethical consideration in the use of patients' personal health information in big data analyses is the protection of patient privacy.

Multiple Choice

11. Barriers to considering cost in shared decision-making between providers and patients include
    A. Patients may perceive the most expensive care as the best care
    B. Patients and providers are skilled in discussing cost within the context of health care
    C. Both A and B
    D. Neither A nor B
12. Shared decision-making is
    A. A provision of the Affordable Care Act
    B. Defined as a collaborative process that allows patients and their provider to make health decisions together
    C. Both A and B
    D. Neither A nor B

13. The use of quality metrics and measurement targets for reimbursement is an element of
    A. Fee-for-service reimbursement
    B. Accountable care shared savings programs
    C. Both A and B
    D. Neither A nor B
14. Big data
    A. Enables comprehensive analyses and discovery of patterns that could not be discerned with a single data set
    B. Consistently includes nursing data entries
    C. Both A and B
    D. Neither A nor B
15. Potentially, big data can support
    A. Comparative effectiveness research
    B. Personalized health care
    C. Both A and B
    D. Neither A nor B

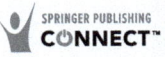

A robust set of instructor resources designed to supplement this text is located at http://connect.springerpub.com/content/book/978-0-8261-7236-5. Qualifying instructors may request access by emailing textbook@springerpub.com.

REFERENCES

Adler, L., Lee, S., Hannick, K., & Duffy, E. (2019, December 5). *Provider charges relative to Medicare rates, 2012–2017*. Brookings Institute. https://www.brookings.edu/blog/usc-brookings-schaeffer-on-health-policy/2019/12/05/provider-charges-relative-to-medicare-rates-2012-2017/

Agency for Healthcare Research and Quality. (2023). *About shared decision making*. http://www.ahrq.gov/sdm/about/index.html

Agweyu, A., Hill, K., Diaz, T., Jackson, D., Hailu, B. G., & Muzigaba, M. (2023). Regular measurement is essential but insufficient to improve quality of healthcare. *British Medical Journal, 380*, e073412. https://doi.org/10.1136/bmj-2022-073412

Arora, S. (2020). IoMT (Internet of Medical Things): Reducing cost while improving patient care. *IEEE Pulse, 11*(5), 24–27. https://doi.org/10.1109/MPULS.2020.3022143

Arrow, K. (1963). Uncertainty and the welfare economics of medical care. *The American Economic Review, 53*(5), 941–973.

Atsma, F., Elwyn, G., & Westert, G. (2020). Understanding unwarranted variation in clinical practice: a focus on network effects, reflective medicine and learning health systems. *International journal for quality in health care: journal of the International Society for Quality in Health Care, 32*(4), 271–274. https://doi.org/10.1093/intqhc/mzaa023

Audreu-Perez, J., Poon, C., Merrifield, R., Wong, S., & Yang, G. (2015). Big data for health. *IEEE Journal of Biomedical Health Information, 19*(4), 1193–1208. https://doi.org/10.1109/JBHI.2015.2450362

Austin, R. R., Mathiason, M. A., & Monsen, K. A. (2022). Using data visualization to detect patterns in whole-person health data. *Research in Nursing & Health, 45*(4), 466–476. https://doi.org/10.1002/nur.22248

Ayers, J. W., Poliak, A., Dredze, M., Leas, E., Zhu, Z., Kelley, J., Faix, D., Goodman, A., Longhurst, C., Hogarth, M., & Smith, D. (2023). Comparing physician and artificial intelligence chatbot responses to patient questions posted to a public social media forum. *JAMA Internal Medicine, 183*(6):589–596. https://doi.org/10.1001/jamainternmed.2023.1838

Baro, E., Degoul, S., Beuscart, R., & Chazard, E. (2015). Toward a literature-driven definition of big data in healthcare. *BioMed Research International, 2015*, 639021. https://doi.org/10.1155/2015/639021

Batko, K., & Ślęzak, A. (2022). The use of big data analytics in healthcare. *Journal of Big Data, 9*(1), 3. https://doi.org/10.1186/s40537-021-00553-4

Beauvais, B., Gilson, G., Schwab, S., Jaccaud, B., Pearce, T., & Holmes, T. (2020). Overpriced? Are hospital prices associated with the quality of are? *Healthcare (Basel), 2020*(2), 135. https://doi.org/10.3390/healthcare8020135

Blumenthal-Barby, J., Opel, D. J., Dickert, N. W., Kramer, D. B., Edmonds, B. T., Ladin, K., Peek, M. E., Peppercorn, J., & Tilburt, J. (2019). Potential unintended consequences of recent shared decision making policy initiatives. *Health Affairs, 38*(11), 1876–1881. https://doi.org/10.1377/hlthaff.2019.00243

Bodenheimer, T., Grumbach, K., & Willard-Grace, R. (2023). *Understanding health policy: A clinical approach*. 9th ed. Lange Medical Books.

Buiser Schnur, M. (2020, March 10). *Is blockchain the new pathway to credentialing?* Lippincott Nursing Center Blog. https://www.nursingcenter.com/ncblog/march-2020/blockchain-credentialing

Castellucci, M. (2017, August 31). *Variation in charges and payments for hospitals persists in new Medicare data*. Modern Healthcare. https://www.modernhealthcare.com/article/20170831/NEWS/170839968/variation-in-charges-and-payments-for-hospitals-persists-in-new-medicare-data

Chan, G. K., Cummins, M. R., Taylor, C. S., Rambur, B., Auerbach, D. I., Meadows-Oliver, M., Cooke, C., Turek, E. A., & Pittman, P. P. (2023). An overview and policy implications of national nurse identifier systems: A call for unity and integration. *Nursing Outlook, 71*(2), 101892. https://doi.org/10.1016/j.outlook.2022.10.005

Chharbra, K., McGuire, K., Sheetz, K., Scott, J., Nuliyalu, U., & Ryan, A. (2020). Most patient undergoing ground and air ambulance transportation receive sizable out-of-network bills. *Health Affairs, 38*(5), 777–782. https://doi-org.uri.idm.oclc.org/10.1377/hlthaff.2019.01484

Cohen, L. (2020, May 17). *COVID-19 might be the best thing to happen to the blockchain industry*. CTech. https://www.calcalistech.com/ctech/articles/0,7340,L-3823871,00.html

Consumer Financial Protection Bureau. (2023, December 7), *What is a "surprise medical bill" and what should I know about the No Surprised Act*. Author. https://www.consumerfinance.gov/ask-cfpb/what-is-a-surprise-medical-bill-and-what-should-i-know-about-the-no-surprises-act-en-2123/

Daley, S. (2020, March 25). *15 examples of how blockchain is reviving healthcare*. Built In. https://builtin.com/blockchain/blockchain-healthcare-applications-companies

Dartmouth Atlas of Health Care. (n.d.). *Understanding of the efficiency and effectiveness of the health care system*. http://www.dartmouthatlas.org

Dentzer, S. (2013, May 21). *Sorting out the meaning of hospital pricing disparities* [Blog post]. http://www.rwjf.org/en/blogs/culture-of-health/2013/05/sorting_out_the_mean.html

Desai, S., Hatfield, L., Hicks, A., Sinaiko, A., Chernew, M., Cowling, D., Gautam, S., Wu, S.-J., & Mehrotra, A. (2017). Offering a price transparency tool did not reduce overall spending among California public employees and retirees. *Health Affairs, 36*(8), 1401–1407. https://doi.org/10.1377/hlthaff.2016.1636

Desai, S., Shambhu, S., & Mehrotra, A. (2021). Online advertising increased New Hampshire residents' use of provider price tool but not use of lower-price providers. *Health Affairs, 40*, 3, 521–528. https://doi.org/10.1377/hlthaff.2020.01039

Dwivedi, R., Mehrotra, D., & Chandra, S. (2022). Potential of Internet of Medical Things (IoMT) applications in building a smart healthcare system: A systematic review. *Journal of Oral Biology and Craniofacial Research, 12*(2), 302–318. https://doi.org/10.1016/j.jobcr.2021.11.010

Espinoza Suarez, N. R., LaVecchia, C. M., Fischer, K. M., Kamath, C. C., & Brito, J. P. (2021). Impact of cost conversation on decision-making outcomes. *Mayo Clinic Proceedings: Innovations, Quality & Outcomes, 5*(4), 802–810. https://doi.org/10.1016/j.mayocpiqo.2021.05.006

FAIR Health. (2023, February 22). *Advancing shared decision making among older adults with serious health conditions.* Author. https://s3.amazonaws.com/media2.fairhealth.org/brief/asset/Advancing%20Shared%20Decision%20Making%20among%20Older%20Adults%20with%20Serious%20Health%20Conditions%20-%20A%20FAIR%20Health%20Brief.pdf

FasterCapital. (2024, March 10). *Nursing care blockchain: Building trust in nursing care: The role of blockchain technology.* Author. https://fastercapital.com/content/Nursing-care-blockchain--Building-Trust-in-Nursing-Care--The-Role-of-Blockchain-Technology.html

Gallo, R. J., Shieh, L., Smith, M., Marafino, B. J., Geldsetzer, P., Asch, S. M., Shum, K., Lin, S., Westphal, J., Hong, G., & Li, R. C. (2024). Effectiveness of an artificial intelligence-enabled intervention for detecting clinical deterioration. *JAMA Internal Medicine, 184*(5), 557–562. https://doi.org/10.1001/jamainternmed.2024.0084

Ghosh, P. K., Chakraborty, A., Hasan, M., Rashid, K., & Siddique, A. H. (2023). Blockchain application in healthcare systems: A review. *Systems, 11*(1):38. https://doi.org/10.3390/systems11010038

Gordon, D. (2022, October 11). *64% of consumers have never tried to find healthcare prices, new survey shows.* Forbes. https://www.forbes.com/sites/debgordon/2022/10/11/64-of-consumers-have-never-tried-to-find-healthcare-prices-new-survey-shows/?sh=391275da67d5

Gupta, S., & Gupta, S. K. (2019). Natural language processing in mining unstructured data from software repositories: A review. *Sādhanā, 44*, 244. https://doi.org/10.1007/s12046-019-1223-9

Hager, K., Emanuel, E., & Mozaffarian, D. (2024). Employer-sponsored health insurance premium cost growth and its association with earnings inequality among US families. *JAMA Network Open, 7*(1), e2351644. https://doi.org/10.1001/jamanetworkopen.2023.51644

Hargrave, M. (2019, April 30). *Deep learning.* Investopedia. https://www.investopedia.com/terms/d/deep-learning.asp

Health Economics Times. (2023, November 21). *Wearable technology in medical market to exceed $100 billion in 2023: GlobalData.* Author.

https://health.economictimes.indiatimes.com/news/medical-devices/wearable-technology-in-medical-market-to-exceed-100-billion-in-2023-globaldata/105378828

Healthcare Information and Management Systems Society. (2019, February 6). *Artificial intelligence, critical thinking and the nursing process.* https://www.himss.org/resources/artificial-intelligence-critical-thinking-and-nursing-process

Hoffman, G., & Yakusheva, O. (2020). Association between financial incentives in Medicare's Hospital Readmission Reduction Program and hospital readmission performance. *JAMA Network Open, 3*(4), e202044. https://doi.org/10.1001/jamanetworkopen.2020.2044

Horton, C., & Smith, K, A. (2024). *The most (and least) expensive states for healthcare 2024.* Forbes. https://www.forbes.com/advisor/health-insurance/most-and-least-expensive-states-for-health-care-ranked/

Huang, C., Wang, J., Wang, S., & Zhang, Y. (2023). Internet of medical things: A systematic review. *Neurocomputing, 557*(3), 126719. https://doi.org/10.1016/j.neucom.2023.126719

Hut, N. (2023, November). *CMS finalizes enhanced hospital price transparency requirements for 2024.* Healthcare Financial Management Association. https://www.hfma.org/price-transparency/cms-finalizes-enhanced-hospital-price-transparency-requirements-for-2024/

Issa, T. Z., Lee, Y., Mazmudar, A. S., Padovano, R., Lambrechts, M. J., Canseco, J. A., Hilibrand, A. S., Vaccaro, A. R., Kepler, C. K., & Schroeder, G. D. (2023). Evaluation of hospital compliance with federal price transparency regulations and variability of negotiated rates for spinal fusion. *The Journal of the American Academy of Orthopaedic Surgeons, 31*(13), 677–686. https://doi.org/10.5435/JAAOS-D-23-00053

Jacobs, K., Roman, E., Lambert, J., Moke, L., Scheys, L., Kesteloot, K., Roodhooft, F., & Cardoen, B. (2022). Variability drivers of treatment costs in hospitals: A systematic review. *Health Policy (Amsterdam, Netherlands), 126*(2), 75–86. https://doi.org/10.1016/j.healthpol.2021.12.004

Japsen, B. (2015). *Hip, knee surgery cost vary by $40000 from Anchorage to Manhattan.* Forbes. https://www.forbes.com/sites/brucejapsen/2015/01/21/knee-hip-surgery-costs-vary-by-40000-from-anchorage-to-manhattan/

Kaiser Family Foundation. (2020). *State Health Facts: Health care expenditures per capita by state of residence.* Author. https://www.kff.org/other/state-indicator/health-spending-per-capita/?currentTimeframe=0&sortModel=%7B%22colId%22:%22Location%22,%22sort%22:%22asc%22%7D

Keenan, G. (2014). Big data in health care: An urgent mandate to CHANGE nursing EHRs! *Online Journal of Nursing Informatics (OJNI), 18*(1). http://ojni.org/issues/?p=3081

Kim, H., Lee, C., Pendyala, D., Ng, A., & Kuo, T. T. (2024). A comparative study for blockchain applications in nursing informatics. *medRxiv: The Preprint Server for Health Sciences.* https://doi.org/10.1101/2024.02.24.24301619

Kona, M., & Corlette, S. (2022, September 12). Hospital and insurer price transparency rules now in effect but compliance is still far away. *Health Affairs Forefront.* https://doi.org/10.1377/forefront.20220909.326193

Lansky, D. (2022, January 25). Reimagining a quality information system for US health care, *Health Affairs Forefront.* https://doi.org/10.1377/forefront.20220120.301087

Lee, E., & Emanuel, E. (2013). Shared decision making to improve care and reduce cost. *New England Journal of Medicine, 368*(1), 6–8. https://doi.org/10.1056/NEJMp1209500

Lo, J., Claxton, G., Wager, E., Cox, C., & Amin, K. (2023, February 10). *Ongoing challenges with hospital price transparency*. Kaiser Family Foundation. https://www.kff.org/health-costs/issue-brief/ongoing-challenges-with-hospital-price-transparency/

Lopes, L., Nontero, A., Presiado, M., & Hamel, L. (2024, March 1), *American's challenges with health care costs*. Kaiser Family Foundation. https://www.kff.org/health-costs/issue-brief/americans-challenges-with-health-care-costs/

Lucian Leape Institute. (2024). *Patient safety and artificial intelligence: Opportunities and challenges for care delivery*. Institute for Healthcare Improvement; https://www.modernhealthcare.com/safety-quality/ai-healthcare-oversight-testing-ihi

Luthi, S. (2019, June 11). *Physician, hospital groups gear up for fight on surprise billing*. Modern Healthcare. https://www.modernhealthcare.com/politics-policy/physician-hospital-groups-gear-up-fight-surprise-medical-bills

Mayes, R. (2007). The origins, development, and passage of Medicare's revolutionary prospective payment system. *Journal of the History of Medicine and Allied Sciences*, 62(1), 21–55. https://doi.org/10.1093/jhmas/jrj038

Meden, K. (2019, October 16). *The health care cost-quality quandary*. Motiv health. www.motivhealth.com/es/2019/10/16/the-healthcare-cost-quality-quandray/

Mello, M. M., & Guha, N. (2023). ChatGPT and physicians' malpractice risk. *JAMA Health Forum*, 4(5), e231938. https://doi.org/10.1001/jamahealthforum.2023.1938

Methrotra, A., Dean, K., Sinaiko, A., & Sood, N. (2017). Americans support price shopping for health care, but few actually seek out price information. *Health Affairs*, 36(8), 1392–1400. https://doi.org/10.1377/hlthaff.2016.1471

Modern Healthcare. (2020, May 11). *Finding answers in the data*. p. 11.

Muhammad, L. J., Islam, M. M., Usman, S. S., & Ayor, S. I. (2020). Predictive data mining models for novel coronavirus (COVID-19) infected patients' recovery. *SN Computer Science*, 1(4), 206. https://doi.org/10.1007/s42979-020-00216-w

Mullan, F., & Wennberg, J. (2004). Wrestling with variation: An interview with Jack Wennberg. *Health Affairs*, 23(Suppl. 2). VAR73-80. https://www.healthaffairs.org/doi/abs/10.1377/hlthaff.var.73

Mulley, A. (2009). Inconvenient truths about supplier induced demand and unwarranted variation in medical practice. *British Medical Journal*, 339, b4073. https://doi.org/10.1136/bmj.b4073/

Navathe, A., Volpp, K., Bond, A., Linn, K., Caldarella, K., Troxel, A., Zhu, J., Yang, L., Mathloubieh, S., Drye, E., Bernheim, S., Oshima Lee, E., Mugiishi, M., Takata Endo, K., Yoshimoto, J., & Emanuel, E. (2020). Assessing the effectiveness of peer comparisons as a way to improve health care quality. *Health Affairs*, 39(5), 852–861. https://doi.org/10.1377/hlthaff.2019.01061

Network for Regional Health Care Improvement. (2018). *Healthcare affordability. Data is the spark, collaboration is the fuel*. https://civhc.org/wp-content/uploads/2018/11/NRHI-and-CIVHC-Total-Cost-of-Care.pdf

Ng, W. Y., Tan, T. E., Movva, P. V. H., Fang, A. H. S., Yeo, K. K., Ho, D., Foo, F. S. S., Xiao, Z., Sun, K., Wong, T. Y., Sia, A. T., & Ting, D. S. W. (2021). Blockchain applications in health care for COVID-19 and beyond: A systematic review. *The Lancet Digital Health*, 3(12), e819–e829. https://doi.org/10.1016/S2589-7500(21)00210-7

Olaronke, I., & Olaleke, I. (2015). A systematic review of natural language processing in healthcare. *International Journal of Information Technology and Computer Science, 8*(8), 44–50. https://doi.org/10.5815/ijitcs.2015.08.07

Patient Rights Advocate. (2023, February). *Fourth semi-annual hospital price transparency report*. Author. https://static1.squarespace.com/static/60065b8fc8cd610112ab89a7/t/63dfc34f156b45423beb87b7/1675608912170/PatientRightsAdvocate.org+Feb+2023+Price+Transparency+Compliance+Report.pdf

Peterson, K., & Bykowicz, J. (2020, May 14). Congress debates push to end surprise billing. *The Wall Street Journal*. https://www.wsj.com/articles/congress-debates-push-to-end-surprise-medical-billing-11589448603

Politi, M. C., Housten, A. J., Forcino, R. C., Jansen, J., & Elwyn, G. (2023). Discussing cost and value in patient decision aids and shared decision making: A call to action. *MDM Policy & Practice, 8*(1), 23814683221148651. https://doi.org/10.1177/23814683221148651

Pollitz, K. (2016). *Surprise medical bills*. Kaiser Family Foundation. https://www.kff.org/private-insurance/issue-brief/surprise-medical-bills/

Pollock, H. (2022, November). Necessity for and limitations of price transparency in American health care. *AMA Journal of Ethics*. https://journalofethics.ama-assn.org/article/necessity-and-limitations-price-transparency-american-health-care/2022-11

Pollock, J. R., Doan, M. K., Moore, M. L., Haglin, J. M., Arthur, J. R., Deckey, D. G., Patel, K. A., & Bingham, J. S. (2023). Large variation in listed chargemaster price for total joint arthroplasty among top orthopaedic hospitals in the United States. *Journal of the American Academy of Orthopaedic Surgeons. Global research & reviews, 7*(9), e23.00052. https://doi.org/10.5435/JAAOSGlobal-D-23-00052

Rambur, B., & Fitzpatrick, T. (2018). A plea to nurse educators: Incorporate big data use as a foundational skill for undergraduate and graduate nurses. *Journal of Professional Nursing, 34*(3), 176–181. https://doi.org/10.1016/j.profnurs.2017.10.005

Robert, N. J. (2021, September 30). The promise and perils of health internet of things (HIoT). *OJIN: The Online Journal of Issues in Nursing, 26*(3). https://doi.org/10.3912/OJIN.Vol26No03Man01

Ryan, A., Nallamouthu, B., & Dimick, J. (2012). Medicare's public reporting initiative on https://doi.org/10.3912/OJIN.Vol26No03Man01 hospital quality had modest or no impact on mortality from three key conditions. *Health Affairs, 31*, 585–592. https://doi.org/10.1377/hlthaff.2011.0719

Scharp, D., Hobensack, M., Davoudi, A., & Topaz, M. (2024). Natural language processing applied to clinical documentation in post-acute care settings: A scoping review. *Journal of the American Medical Directors Association, 25*(1), 69–83. https://doi.org/10.1016/j.jamda.2023.09.006

Smith, M., Wright, A., Queram, C., & Lamb, G. (2012). Public reporting helped drive quality improvements in outpatient diabetes care among Wisconsin physician groups. *Health Affairs, 31*, (3), 570–570. https://doi.org/10.1377/hlthaff.2011.0853

Sommers, R., Dorr Gould, S., McGlunn, E., Pearson, S., & Danis, M. (2013). Focus groups highlight that many patients object to clinicians' focusing on costs. *Health Affairs, 32*(2), 338–346. https://doi.org/10.1377/hlthaff.2012.0686

Tableau. (n.d.). *Data visualization beginner's guide: A definition, examples, and learning resources.* www.tableau.com/learn/articles/data-visualization

The Economist. (2024, March 27). *The AI doctor will see you…eventually.* Author. https://www.economist.com/leaders/2024/03/27/the-ai-doctor-will-see-youeventually

Topaz, M., & Pruinelli, L. (2017). *Big data and nursing: Implications for the future.* IMIA and IOS Press. https://doi.org/10.3233/978-1-61499-738-2-165

Tsang, Y. P., Wu, C. H., Leung, P. P. L., Ip, W. H., & Ching, W. K. (2021). Blockchain-IoT-Driven nursing workforce planning for effective long-term care management in nursing homes. *Journal of Healthcare Engineering, 2021,* 9974059. https://doi.org/10.1155/2021/9974059

Unruh, M., Zhang, Y., Jung, H., Zjang, M., Li, J., O'Donnell, E., Toscano, F., & Casalino, L. (2020). Physician prices and the cost and quality of care for commercially insured patients. *Health Affairs, 39*(5), 800–808. https://www.healthaffairs.org/doi/10.1377/hlthaff.2019.00237

van Dijk, C., van den Berg, B., Verheij, R., Spreeuwerberg, P., Groenewegen, P., & de Bakker, D. (2012). Moral hazard and supplier-induced demand: Empirical evidence in general practice. *Health Economics, 22*(3). https://doi.org/10.1002/hec.2801

Vasher, S., Oppenheimer, I., Sharma Basyal, P., Lee, E., Hayes, M., & Turnbull, A. (2020). Physician self-assessment of shared decision-making in simulated intensive care unit family meetings. *JAMA Network Open, 3*(5), e205188. https://doi.org/10.1001/jamanetworkopen.2020.5188

Wallis, C. J. D., Jerath, A., Aminoltejari, K., Kaneshwaran, K., Salles, A., Buntin, M. B., Coburn, N. G., Wright, F. C., Gotlib Conn, L., Heybati, K., Luckenbaugh, A. N., Ranganathan, S., Riveros, C., McCartney, C., Armstrong, K. A., Bass, B. L., Detsky, A. S., & Satkunasivam, R. (2024). Surgeon sex and health care costs for patients undergoing common surgical procedures. *JAMA Surgery, 159*(2), 151–159. https://doi.org/10.1001/jamasurg.2023.6031

Whaley, C., & Bai, G. (2023, September 8). *Health care price transparency legislation: How can Congress help employers and workers* Health Affairs Forefront. https://www.healthaffairs.org/content/forefront/health-care-price-transparency-legislation-can-congress-help-employers-and-workers

Yakusheva, O., Rambur, B., & Buerhaus, P. I. (2020). Value-informed nursing practice can help reset the hospital-nurse relationship. *JAMA Health Forum, 1*(8), e200931. https://doi.org/10.1001/jamahealthforum.2020.0931

Yesmin, T., Carter, M. W., & Gladman, A. S. (2022). Internet of things in healthcare for patient safety: An empirical study. *BMC Health Services Research, 22*(1), 278. https://doi.org/10.1186/s12913-022-07620-3

Yoon, H.-J. (2019). Blockchain technology and healthcare. *Healthcare Informatics Research, 25*(2), 59–60. https://doi.org/10.4258/hir.2019.25.2.59

CHAPTER 7

Market Entry, Exit, and Antitrust Law—Why It Matters to Nurses

CHAPTERS 5 AND 6 detailed two key ways in which health care markets differ from classic free markets as an organizing framework for understanding health care economics and to illuminate emerging health care trends. These first two principles—(a) buyers bear the consequences of their decision-making and (b) buyers have information about the product or know how to obtain information—are complemented by two additional principles: (c) Sellers are free to enter and exit the market and (d) no one buyer or seller is large enough to influence the market. This chapter now details these two additional ways in which health care markets differ from classic free markets to further explicate contemporary issues in health care reform. Recall, however, that the goal of the comparison between health care markets and classic free markets is to illuminate complex issues rather than to suggest that health care markets can or should function like classic free markets. Many contemporary reforms, however, represent attempts to address health care market imperfections and make health care markets function within the sorts of checks and balances that characterize free markets. These are often invisible to nurses yet have dramatic impact on their salaries and career opportunities. Thus, mastering these concepts represents time well spent.

Following completion of this chapter, you will be able to:

- Explain the rationale for Certificate of Need (CON) legislation.
- Consider nurse licensure regulations and rules from the perspective of markets.
- Describe the basic elements of antitrust law.
- Discuss contemporary trends in health care mergers and acquisitions and their impact on costs and quality.
- Consider the impact of antitrust law on health care and on nurses' careers.

ENTERING AND EXITING THE MARKET

Heidi has always enjoyed baking. Typically, she uses the finest ingredients—real butter, rich cream, and the best chocolate. Inheriting a bit of money after her father died, Heidi decides to open a small bakery specializing in traditional

> Italian and German pastries. After an initially rocky start and nearly losing all of her start-up capital, Germalian, as she named her bakery, was doing fairly well. The 12-hour-plus workdays notwithstanding, Heidi was enjoying her work and her life as an entrepreneur. Near the end of her third year in business, Heidi was dismayed to learn that Big Company Health Food Store was opening just up the block from her bakery. Big Company not only includes a high-end bakery but also has a coffee shop where customers can sample and enjoy the baked goods... and almost always buy something to take home. Heidi notes that Big Company's high-end pastries are less expensive than hers... much less expensive, and they also have a middle-of-the-line set of baked products. As a large chain, Big Company benefits from lower cost of ingredients due to bulk buying. Also, with over 149 stores in all states, they can simply undercut Heidi on cost until she loses her market share. Heidi contemplates using less expensive ingredients or smaller portions to compete on price, but also worries she will then lose on quality. She tries both strategies. Nevertheless, in less than a year after Big Company opened, Heidi's business was bankrupt and she lost all of her initial investment and most of her savings.

In this example, Heidi was free to enter the market. So was Big Company. In classic free markets, companies compete with each other on the basis of price, quality, and public demand. Consumers "decide with their feet," purchasing what they want and when and where they want it. Businesses must meet zoning and safety regulations. They also must come up with the capital—the funds to start the business—either through personal money, loans, or some other mechanism. With exceptions (e.g., regulations to limit the density of liquor establishments or other issues for public safety), entry into the market is typically not rigidly regulated. Such *laissez-faire* enterprise is guided by an overall doctrine that opposes governmental interference or oversight and is characterized by a conscious, deliberate absence of governmental involvement beyond that necessary for peace, property rights, and public safety. Individuals are free to enter the market but also—as in Heidi's case when her business could not withstand the competition from Big Company—to exit. While Heidi was perfectly free to enter the market, she was also, unfortunately for her, free to fail.

How Are Health Care Markets Different From This Example?

In a typical health care case, providers do not raise the capital for their enterprise, nor are they personally financially liable for financial failure. A group of hospital-employed physicians who wish to do robotic-assisted surgery, for example, do not raise the money for the purchase of the equipment that will enable them to charge for new services and potentially charge more for the service than that it is replacing. Instead, the hospital purchases the equipment, the cost of which is diffusely passed on to the consumer in the form of higher hospital rates and correspondingly higher insurance rates. Thus, some of the typical market checks are not in place. Recall also that the phenomena of supplier-induced demand and asymmetry of information described in the previous two chapters are also in play. The purchase of a new piece of equipment means some demand for that equipment will be created, even if care outcomes would be the same without it.

Are Health Care Organizations Free to Fail or Exit the Market?

Some health care organizations that would not be financially viable under typical free market principles and practices are subsidized or differently reimbursed to ensure that they do not exit the market. Examples include critical access hospitals, discussed in Chapter 9, and *federally qualified health centers (FQHCs)*. FQHCs are safety-net providers that offer outpatient services and receive enhanced reimbursement from Medicare and Medicaid and must serve an underserved population or area. Categories of FQHCs include community health centers, health care for the homeless centers, migrant health centers, public housing care centers and health center service "lookalikes" (Centers for Medicare & Medicaid Services, 2019), with a lookalike being an organization that meets FQHC criteria and many of the benefits but does not receive US Public Health Service funding (FQHC Associates, n.d.). Additional examples of subsidies to help prop up care delivery that may not be financially viable without that extra help are *disproportionate share subsidies* provided to *disproportional share hospitals* (DSH, pronounced "dish"). These funds are provided to organizations that treat a higher proportion of Medicare or Medicaid patients. Recall that commercial insurance reimburses at higher rates than these two governmental payers. Thus, organizations with a payer mix that is disproportionally governmental may face financial difficulties, an issue that DSH payments are attempting to address.

Another way health care provides directed funding is through the tax-exempt status nonprofit organizations enjoy. Although not a subsidy per se, there has been increasing scrutiny of the tax breaks given to nonprofit health care organizations (see Box 7.1).

Despite differential financial support, many safety net providers are financially challenged. From 2005 to 2023, for example, 191 U.S. rural hospitals closed (105 complete closures, 86 converted to a different type of facility; Sheps Center Report, 2023). Of those that remain, more than 600 (30%) are at risk of closing (Center for Healthcare Quality and Payment Reform, 2023). Maternity services are particularly scarce in rural areas, creating "maternity care deserts" (Sonenberg & Mason, 2023). A comparatively new designation, Rural Emergency Hospital (REH), has enabled some communities to retain emergencies (see Box 7.2).

BOX 7.1

TAX-EXEMPT STATUS

The tax-exempt status of nonprofit health care has drawn increasing congressional and public scrutiny. Roughly 75% of U.S. hospitals are governmentally owned or nonprofit and thus exempt from income taxes, property taxes, and sales taxes. In turn they must provide "community benefit," a condition that—despite clearer parameters outlined in the Affordable Care Act (ACA)—remains "vaguely defined" (Pope, 2024a, para 5). Pope (2024b) notes that although these subsidies are to fund emergency health for indigent people, the tax exemption costs far exceed the care provided and are unequally distributed. The state of New Hampshire, for example, received $2,123 per poor resident, the state of Wyoming $4. Bai et al. (2021) report that for-profit hospitals provided 65% more charity care than nonprofit hospitals did. They conclude that the charity care provided is not well aligned with the favorable tax treatment and that corrective policy initiatives are warranted. Indeed, in August 2023 a bipartisan group of U.S. senators joined to demand more accountability for these funds and their expenditures (Makary, 2024). As this book goes to press the issue remains unresolved, but will likely continue to undergo scrutiny and eventual policy changes.

BOX 7.2

WHAT IS A RURAL EMERGENCY HOSPITAL?

In response to rural hospital closures, the Rural Emergency Hospital (REH) designation was signed into law with the Consolidated Appropriations Act of 2020. Effective January 1, 2023, eligible facilities could convert to this status and provide emergency department services and observation but are prohibited from providing inpatient services (CMS 2024).

Challenges With Volume-Based Payment When Volumes Drop or in Low-Volume Regions

The COVID-19 pandemic further underscored foundational flaws in the U.S. health system that depends on volumes of services, for example, hospitals dependent on elective procedures to ensure cash flow. As volumes dropped, record numbers of health care workers were laid off or furloughed (Gooch, 2020), leading some to conclude that COVID-19 boosted the shift to value-based care (Livingston, 2020) as well as other innovations. Phillion, for example, notes: "Value-based payment models were not only good for business during the pandemic, but also ushered in a new acceptance of telehealth" (Phillion, 2021, para 3).

Rural areas, particularly frontier counties (remote, sparsely populated areas with a population density of fewer than six individuals per square mile), have inherent challenges in a volume-driven payment scheme. In response, different states have adopted different innovations (recall the Pennsylvania rural hospital example detailed in Chapter 4). Another example of an innovative response is the state of North Dakota's Rough Rider High Value Network, a collaboration among 23 independent critical access hospitals designed to strengthen the availability, quality, and affordability of care in rural areas (Raths, 2023). Unlike an REH, this model retains inpatient capacity.

What About Freedom to Enter the Market?

To better align health care investments with societal need, *Certificate of Need (CON, pronounced see-oh-n)* legislation was passed, and CON programs were implemented to restrain the growth of facilities and the cost of such growth. A second goal of CON legislation is to better coordinate new construction and services, rather than allowing them to develop unchecked. Initially developed on a state-by-state basis, the 1974 *Health Planning Resources Development Act* required all states to have processes by which all capital projects—for example, the purchase of high-tech equipment or the construction of new buildings—would be reviewed and approval required before any action to purchase or construct was taken. In theory, purchase or construction that did not meet true societal need would not be approved. Adoption of this approach was incentivized with federal funding, yet both the act and the funding were repealed in 1987. Modifications to state CON laws then proceeded on a state-by-state basis, with some states rescinding the CON process and others retaining CON. At the time of this writing, 35 states and Washington, DC, retain some sort of CON, although the exact provisions and *threshold triggers* vary widely by state. The term *threshold trigger* refers to the conditions or situations that set off a CON review. Some states have CON only for elements of the health care industry, for example, long-term care (National Conference of State Legislatures, 2024). Take a moment to review the CON details in your home and nearby states (https://www.ncsl.org/health/certificate-of-need-state-laws and https://nashp.org/state-tracker/50-state-scan-of-state-certificate-of-need-programs/).

DOES CON WORK?

Perceptions of the effectiveness of CON vary, with some analyses finding the process to be more influenced by politics than policy (Yee et al., 2011). An early study concluded that the CON process helped prevent duplication of services in the scenarios they analyzed (Lucas et al., 2011), while others

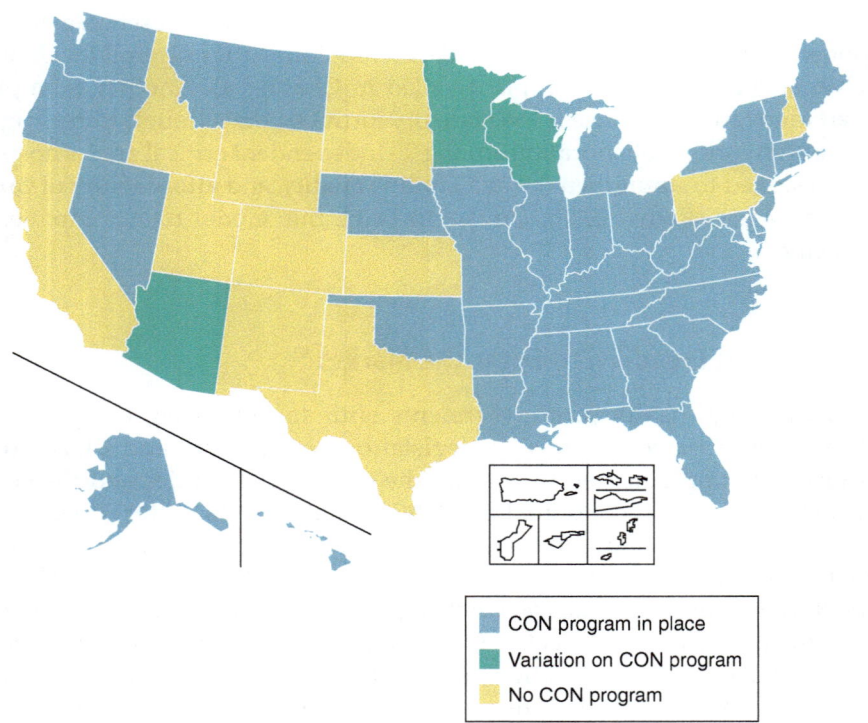

FIGURE 7.1: Certificate of need state laws.

conclude that CON is associated with higher per-unit costs and greater total cost expenditures (Mitchell, 2019). Conflicting evidence is also found by type of service. Gaines and Cagle (2023), for example, found CON to have a modest but positive association with hospice quality, and Cancienne et al. (2020) found reduced expenditure and rate of complications in Medicare beneficiaries undergoing knee arthroscopy. Conversely, Yuce et al. (2020) found no difference in volumes or quality of 10 procedures (including knee arthroscopy) between states with or without CON. Conover and Bailey's (2020) systematic review on cost-effectiveness notes that the evidence (90 articles) is mixed and without a definitive conclusion. Thus, they note that their estimates are "uncertain" but tentatively conclude that existing evidence suggests costs of CON exceed its benefits; they also conclude that more and stronger evidence is needed for a definitive conclusion.

The National Conference of State Legislatures (2019) notes that, while the value of CON law continues to be debated, many states consider CON to be one way to increase access and control costs. Their analysis of pros and cons is detailed on their website and may be found at www.ncsl.org/research/health/con-certificate-of-need-state-laws.aspx. What do you think?

CON AND PAYMENT REFORM

Payment reform is also impacting both market entry of new services and market exit. The extent to which new payment models that embrace provider risk sharing modify or replace CON intentions is unclear. Recall, for example, the payment reform models described in Chapter 4. In a fee-for-service environment, new equipment can catalyze a demand for new services and create new revenue for the hospital, even though this action represents an overall cost to society. Would a hospital under a global budget be more prudent about expansion of services or creation of new buildings? This is likely, as these are the very sorts of incentives global budgets are designed to create. Thus, the evolution, application, and usefulness of CON laws in a reformed payment environment are unclear at this time.

Licensing Laws

CON programs are one way that health care markets differ from classic free markets. Licensing laws are another. A professional license is a form of monopoly on services; an RN, for example, cannot legally offer physical therapy services, nor can a physical therapist dispense medications as a pharmacist. Although licenses provide some level of information about what a provider can do and what a patient can expect, the monopolist power of organized medicine is associated with difficulty containing cost. To illustrate this complex idea, ponder, for example, if when the first McDonald's restaurant opened, they had a situation similar to medicine's scope of practice in which no other entity could sell hamburgers. Such monopolies are not allowed in free markets, and competition among different hamburger sellers helps to control cost and spur innovation and quality. Group and Roberts (2001) argue that physicians have created that monopoly in part through the subordination of nurses, who could provide a legitimate, quality-enhancing form of competition—a perspective that has some powerful allies, which is the focus of the next section.

NURSES AND THE MONOPOLISTIC POWER OF MEDICAL LICENSES

The regulation of advanced practice nurses pointedly illustrates the dilemma of unnecessary restriction of nurses' scope of practice. Renowned health economist Uwe Reinhardt (cited in Henderson, 2013) notes that "Organized medicine invariably opposes wider scopes of practice and independent practice of nonphysician health professionals. ... Not many economists today are buying the medical profession's position on this issue" (para 1). Instead, they view it as an issue of "monopolistic market power" (para 2).
Although progress has been made, physicians retain control of NPs' practice in many U.S. states, despite consistent evidence of NPs' quality and

cost-effectiveness. Indeed, staff of the powerful Federal Trade Commission (FTC), which exists to promote market competition to enhance quality and contain costs, urges states to remove barriers to NP practice, stating:

> Physician supervision requirements may raise competition concerns because they effectively give one group of health care professionals the ability to restrict access to the market by another, competing group of health care professionals, thereby denying healthcare consumers the benefits of greater competition. In addition, APRNs play a critical role in alleviating provider shortages and expanding access to healthcare services for medically underserved populations. For these reasons, the FTC staff has consistently urged state legislators to avoid imposing restrictions on APRN scope of practice unless those restrictions are necessary to address well-founded patient safety concerns. Based on substantial evidence and experience, expert bodies have concluded that ARPNs are safe and effective as independent providers of many health care services within the scope of their training, licensure, certification, and current practice. Therefore, new or extended layers of mandatory physician supervision may not be justified. (FTC, 2014, pp. 1–2)

The FTC continues to provide supports to states upon request and occasionally files an amicus (friend of the court) brief in support of eliminating restrictive occupational laws for nurses as well as other professions (see https://www.ftc.gov/policy/advocacy-research/advocacy/economic-liberty/selected-advocacy-relating-occupational-licensing).

In summary, the manner in which classic free markets continually refine cost and quality—through high-value products and services gaining market share while low-value products lose market share—is dramatically altered in health care. Removal of barriers that prevent nurses and NPs from functioning within their full scope of practice is one valuable step toward quality enhancement and access within an environment of cost containment. This was dramatically illustrated in 2020 in response to the COVID-19 pandemic. The U.S. Centers for Medicare and Medicaid Services relaxed NP regulations, as did some states through temporary executive orders. Ongoing efforts to maintain or enhance nurses' capacity to practice to the full extent of their preparation as demonstrated during these temporary measures continues, although there continues to be opposition from some physician groups. Nurse Licensure Compact laws, whereby a nurse can hold one license yet practice in all Compact states, are another mechanism for facilitating nurses' entry into the health care market.

MERGE, CONSOLIDATE, OR STAND ALONE: AN OVERVIEW OF ANTITRUST LAW

U.S. *antitrust law* was created to ensure that no one buyer or seller is large enough to dominate the market. Rooted in concerns about potentially monopolist control of key industries in the late 1800s, the foundational

Sherman Antitrust Act of 1880 protects competition by making it illegal to restrain free trade. Augmented by amendments and additional laws such as the Clayton Antitrust Act of 1914 and the Federal Trade Commission Act of 1914, the fundamental principle behind antitrust law is to support market competition to enhance quality, contain costs, and—importantly—drive innovation. The heretofore-mentioned FTC serves as the nation's antitrust watchdog. They state: "Free and open markets are the foundation of a vibrant economy. Aggressive competition among sellers in an open marketplace gives consumers—both individuals and businesses—the benefits of lower prices, higher quality products and services, more choices, and greater innovation. The FTC's competition mission is to enforce the rules of the competitive marketplace—the antitrust laws" (FTC, n.d., para 1). At the federal level, the FTC works with the U.S. Department of Justice to monitor anticompetitive behavior. States typically have an antitrust mechanism in place as well, typically through the state attorneys general (AGs). Federal antitrust law gives the AG antitrust enforcement authority, and some state statutes are more expansive than federal law (Hulver & Levinson, 2023).

Perhaps nurses view the term *competition* negatively, instead espousing *cooperation*. This nation is based on a free market economy in which *market competition* is a central feature. Thus, nurses need to understand health care markets, threats to positive competition, and the basic rationale behind contemporary antitrust issues. This is particularly important because of the impact of mergers and acquisitions (leading to market concentration) on nurses' salaries and career opportunities. But first, let's review basic antitrust terms and concepts.

Antitrust law aims to address anticompetitive behavior that can distort a market's propensity to spur innovation, lower costs, and enhance quality. Market concentration, meaning one buyer or seller has a large hold on a market, is one concern. Market concentration is usually measured by the Herfindahl–Hirschman Index or HHI (see Box 7.3).

Search the website for recent mergers and acquisitions in your region. Was there an FTC review? Is an HHI listed?

Market concentration in health care typically follows mergers and acquisitions, termed *M and A*. A merger is a combination of two or more firms or organizations to create a new legal entity, while an acquisition is a purchase or takeover of one firm or organization by another. In describing M and A activity, the terms *consolidation* and *integration* are often used interchangeability. Two broad categories are recognized: *horizontal integration* and *vertical integration* (or consolidation). Providers of a similar service type under a common organizational and legal structure reflect *horizontal integration*, for example, the merger of two or more hospitals. Providers of different service types, such as hospitals, nursing homes, and home health care agencies within a common organizational structure, reflect *vertical integration*. Examples of

BOX 7.3

HOW IS MARKET CONCENTRATION MEASURED?

"The HHI is calculated by squaring the market share of each firm competing in the market and then summing the resulting numbers. For example, for a market consisting of four firms with shares of 30%, 30%, 20%, and 20%, the HHI is 2,600 ($30^2 + 30^2 + 20^2 + 20^2 = 2,600$)" (U.S. Department of Justice [DOJ], 2024, para 1). The HHI can range from 0 (no market concentration) to 10,000, with 10,000 being market control by a single company. Moderately concentrated markets are defined as holding an HHI between 1,000 and 1,800 points, and highly concentrated markets are those in excess of 1,800 points. Mergers and acquisitions that lead to increase in HHIs of more than 200 points and an overall HHI of greater than 2,500 typically received DOJ and FTC review for potential anticompetitive effects (Holmes et al., 2024).

vertical integration include the acquisition of a provider organization like an MD/NP practice by a hospital or a joint venture by an insurance company and a pharmacy chain.

In general, the FTC has greater authority over horizontal integration than vertical integration. This is, in part, because market concentration is easier to measure in horizontal integration. Moreover, until relatively recently, many health care mergers went unchallenged (Holmes et al., 2024). However, growing health care price pressures and mounting evidence of the negative impact of market concentration has fueled greater antitrust regulatory activity.

Relevant History

Market concentration has dramatically increased in the 21st century, fueled in part by the passage of the ACA. Dafny (2014), for example, notes that health reform efforts, specifically the ACA, "unleashed a merger frenzy, with hospitals scrambling to shore up their market positions, improve operational efficiency, and create organizations capable of managing population health" (p. 198). Theoretically, market concentration could be beneficial if it reduces duplication of service and generates efficiencies (Holmes et al., 2024). At the same time, there is substantial evidence that such mergers do not improve quality, access, or affordability. These data are long-standing. Over a decade ago, Gaynor and Town (2012), for example, examined hospital consolidations and reported that:

1. Hospital market consolidation increases the cost of care—costs which in turn are passed on to citizens in the form of higher insurance premiums, fewer benefits, and lower wages for employees.

2. Hospital competition (not consolidation) is associated with increased quality.
3. Physician–hospital consolidation has not led to an increase in quality or to a decrease in cost.

Moreover, when physicians move from being independent physicians to becoming hospital-employed physicians, the charge to the consumer is higher for the same services due to the additional billing of *facility fees* associated with hospital-employed physician practices even if that physician remains in the same outpatient setting. This issue is entwined with another policy issue: *site-neutral billing* (see Box 7.4).

The cost impact of consolidation extends beyond ambulatory visits; Baker et al. (2014) found higher hospital prices and spending in markets where hospitals had ownership of physician practices. Data from 2019 suggest higher health care prices and insurance premiums in markets with little competition, that is, in concentrated markets (Boozary et al., 2019; Cooper et al., 2019). Liu et al. (2023) found horizontal consolidation of commercial insurers to be associated with lower prices paid to providers, but these savings were not passed on to the consumers. Paradoxically, premiums actually increased! In summary, Goodwin and colleagues state: "A growing body of evidence shows that consolidation in healthcare provider markets has led to increases in prices without clear evidence of increases in quality" (2023, para 1).

What Has This to Do With You? The Impact of Market Concentration on Nurses' Salaries

Mergers and acquisitions that create a consolidated market can create a situation in which there is not only monopolistic power (one seller of health care

BOX 7.4

WHAT IS SITE-NEUTRAL BILLING?

Site-neutral billing refers to providers receiving the same level of reimbursement regardless of where the service is delivered. Currently, a service performed in a hospital outpatient department is more handsomely reimbursed than the same service performed in a physician's office or ambulatory surgery center. Site-neutral billing is strongly opposed by the American Hospital Association, and one study suggested that under site-neutral billing, 2021 Medicare spending would have been $201 million lower, with corollary reductions in patient cost sharing and premiums (Bulat & Brake, 2024). Although site-neutral billing has bipartisan support, only limited policies have passed to date, specifically, site neutrality for new off-campus hospital outpayment departments. There is concern that the lack of site-neutral billing has fueled hospital acquisition of physician practices, creating more market consolidation (MedPAC, 2023).

BOX 7.5

WHAT IS THE DIFFERENCE BETWEEN A MONOPOLY AND A MONOPSONY?

A monopoliy removes competators for thier product, including substitutions for it. A complete monopoly prevents others from entering the market. As a result, the monopolistic company can set it prices and buyers have no choice, removing the consumers buying power. The monopolistic company typically also has higher profits

Conversely, a monopsony occurs when there is only one buyer for a product or the monopsonic company is the sole purchaser of a product. The purchased "product" can include people. Specifically a monopsony can be "common in labor markets when a single employer has an advantage over the workforce . . . the suppliers—in this case, the potential employees—agree to a lower wage . . . (Anderson, 2022, para 7). The employee may not consciously perceive they are "agreeing" to a lower wage, it is simply the salary offered and the potenital employee does not perceive other, higher wage options. In sum, a monopsony results in lower wages for those working in the setting and higher profits for the employer.

An organization can have both a monopoly and monopsony. Both represent market imperfections, whereby the supply and demand dynamics that lead to better outputs and products at a lower price is disrupted.

---

services in an area, for example, a regionally dominant system) but also only one "buyer" of health care workers, including nurses. The term for this is *monopsony* (see Box 7.5). In other words, the employer can keep salaries low because the nurses have no other employers competing for the workforce and the nurse has no other, more highly compensated options.

Research supports the monopsonic wage compression resulting from health care mergers. Allegretto and Graham-Squire (2023a), for example, found that for every 0.1 increase in consolidation (HHI), real hourly nurse wage growth decreased by $.70 (*p*-value of .038) and real hourly wages (adjusted for inflation, thus representing real buying power) of nurses grew less than that of comparable workers by $4.08. They state: ". . . labor shortages among hospital-based nurses, which may be a symptom of monopsony, have been endemic in the industry for many years. The wages of nurses were stagnant between 1995 and 2015 despite increasing demand for healthcare over the same timeframe even as it was the only sector that added employment during the Great Recession. Explanations for the stagnation of nurse wages—in one of the more highly unionized professional occupations in the country—are not readily apparent" (Allegretto & Graham-Squire, 2023b, para 3), underscoring that monopsony was a likely culprit.

Similarly, Prager and Schmitt (2021) found negative wage impacts following consolidation, with effects somewhat mitigated by unionization status. They also found that mergers that leave local employer concentration unchanged—mergers between two entities not in the same geography and not direct competitors (also termed cross-market mergers)—did not have the magnitude of wage impacts. Goodwin et al. note that cross-market mergers may benefit patients when hospital and health systems are able to be more efficient when combined and share clinical wisdom, but such mergers may also increase prices. They report price increases ranging from 6% to 17%; however, there are relatively few studies on cross-market mergers (Goodwin et al., 2023).

Other Mechanisms That Negatively Impact Nurses by Restraining Healthy Market Competition

Organizations have still other ways they can suppress healthy market dynamics. Have you ever noticed that nursing salaries are often largely the same among similar organizations? "Is it possible that those organizations are *colluding* and have formal or informal *price fixing* and/or *no poaching agreements*?" Both of these practices represent anticompetitive behavior because they violate the principles that make healthy markets function. These behaviors riddle the U.S. health care system and impact nurses. Take a moment to familiarize yourself with the antitrust terms in Box 7.6.

Such anticompetitive behavior has likely impacted health care markets and nurses for decades, but only now, with increased antitrust activity and

BOX 7.6

HOW ABOUT ANTITRUST TERMS

Collusion—competitors secretly agree to practices that will limit market competition in their favor and at the expense of consumers and, in some cases, employees. The agreement may be written, verbal, or inferred from conduct. Examples of collusion include:

Price fixing—an agreement among competitors to raise, lower, or maintain or stabilize prices at a certain level
Bid rigging—an agreement among competitors regarding who the winning bidder will be
Customer allocation (also called market diversion or market allocation)—competitors conspire to divide up customers or geography, including workers
No poaching agreements—competitors agree to not hire each other's employees or match offers
Wage fixing—competitors agree to keep employees' salaries below the market rate

enforcement, are emerging from the shadows. In a 2022 Department of Justice (DOJ) antitrust investigation, for example, a health care staffing company pleaded guilty to engaging with a competitor to allocate employee school nurses and fix the wages of the nurses, thus undercutting their salary potential as well as career mobility. In a DOJ antitrust press release, Assistant Attorney General Jonathan Kanter of the Justice Department's Antitrust Division stated, "Free and open labor markets are a cornerstone of the American dream. Today's guilty plea demonstrates our commitment to ensuring that workers receive competitive wages and a fair chance to pursue better work and that criminals who conspire to deprive them of those rights are held accountable. The court's sentence will compensate the hardworking healthcare workers who were victims of this crime" (cited in U.S. DOJ, 2022a, para 3).

Another criminal antitrust prosecution resulted from no poaching agreements whereby four owners/managers of home health agencies agreed to fix the rates paid to workers and also agreed to not hire each other's employees. Again, this type of behavior stifles healthy market competition and artificially holds salaries low. The DOJ noted that this indictment is part of a "larger ongoing federal antitrust investigation into wage fixing and worker allocation in the home health industry" (U.S. DOJ, 2022b, para 8).

Finally, in April 2024 the FTC announced a sweeping crackdown on noncompete clauses (see Box 7.7).

An illustration of the behavior now prohibited would be an NP who wanted to leave their primary care or hospital employment to start their own nurse-run business or concierge service. Prior to this recent FTC action, if the NP had signed a noncompete clause, they would not be able to start their own business for a certain period of time or in a particular geographic region, as stated in the clause. The FTC notes that, overall, one in five American workers is bound by a noncompete clause (FTC, 2023). Physicians and hospitals have been in marked conflict over the FTC's prohibition of noncompete clauses, with physicians supporting the FTC's action and hospitals opposing (Southwick, 2024). The American Nurses Association (ANA) strongly supports the FTC action, particularly as it pertains to nurses. The FTC projects that elimination of noncompete clauses will reduce health care costs by $194 billion

BOX 7.7

WHAT IS A NONCOMPETE CLAUSE?

The FTC defines a noncompete clause as a "contractual term [agreement] between an employer and a worker that blocks the worker from working for a competing employer, or starting a competing business, typically within a certain geographic area and period of time after the worker's employment ends" (FTC, 2023, para 1). They are considered anti-competitive because they prevent an individual from seeking better opportunities and/or potentially increasing market competition.

over 10 years. The director of at the ANA, Lisa Stand, was pleased with the FTC ruling and its strength. She stated: "It absolutely will make job mobility easier. We're nurses, and we think that ultimately this is good for patients as well, as there is more sort of robust competition for clinical talent and an expanded access to more choices of provider and provider setting" (Stand, cited in Choi, 2024).

The author believes that nurses who are informed about antitrust issues will be able to see what has been right in front of them and be prepared to take action. In summary, understanding the nation's mechanisms to foster market competition is central to nurses' salary and career mobility. Spread the word!

End-of-Chapter Resources

THOUGHT QUESTIONS

1. Why do some states retain CON regulation and others do not?
2. Using an economic and market perspective, how would you argue for removal of state restrictions that stop nurses from practicing to the full extent of their preparation?
3. Define the following key terms:
   Antitrust law
   Certificate of Need
   Collusion
   Disproportionate share hospital
   Facility fee
   Federal Trade Commission
   Federally qualified health center
   Horizontal integration
   Noncompete clause
   Price fixing
   Vertical integration
   Wage fixing

EXERCISE

1. Prepare a list of hospitals or health systems that have recently reorganized in your area. What patterns do you see? What forces served as an impetus? What has been the impact on nursing? What has been the impact on the patient experience?

2. Develop a presentation of the role of the Federal Trade Commission and why their activities are important to nurses and their patients.
3. A colleague who has not studied health economics and policy states: "Competition is always bad. Why can't we all just cooperate?" What is your response? Be sure to tease out market competition from interpersonal conflict.
4. Have you or a colleague been impacted by noncompetitive behavior? Defend your answer.

QUIZ

True or False

1. Disproportionate share subsidies are provided to some health care organizations that treat a high proportion of individuals with commercial insurance.
2. Medical licenses are a form of monopoly.
3. In 2014, the U.S. Federal Trade Commission staff published a report critical of states' restriction of nurse practitioner scope of practice because it is an inappropriate restraint of appropriate market competition.
4. The passage of the ACA has led to mergers among hospitals and other health care organizations.
5. When an independent physician becomes a hospital-employed physician, the charge for that physician's care may be higher due to the inclusion of an additional facility fee.
6. Antitrust law exists to ensure that no one buyer or seller is large enough to dominate the market and therefore disable the potential for market competition.
7. Consolidation of health care organizations consistently eliminates unnecessary duplication of services and decreases costs.
8. In health care, some facilities that would not be financially viable are subsidized to prevent their exit from the marketplace.

Multiple Choice

9. CON legislation
   A. Attempts to restrain unnecessary growth of health care facilities
   B. Has been rescinded in all U.S. states to comply with provisions in the ACA
   C. Both A and B
   D. Neither A nor B

10. Hospital consolidations
    A. Have consistently decreased the cost of health care
    B. Have decreased competition among hospitals and, as a result, increased quality of care
    C. Both A and B
    D. Neither A nor B
11. Federally qualified health centers
    A. Receive enhanced reimbursement from Medicare and Medicaid
    B. Must serve an otherwise underserved population
    C. Both A and B
    D. Neither A nor B
12. In a classic free market, buyers and sellers are free to
    A. Enter the marketplace
    B. Exit the marketplace
    C. Both A and B
    D. Neither A nor B
13. Noncompete clauses
    A. Can decrease career mobility of nurses
    B. Are strongly supported by the FTC
    C. Are strongly opposed by hospital organizations
    D. All of the above

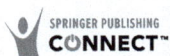

A robust set of instructor resources designed to supplement this text is located at http://connect.springerpub.com/content/book/978-0-8261-7236-5. Qualifying instructors may request access by emailing **textbook@springerpub.com**.

REFERENCES

Allegretto, S., & Graham-Squire, D. (2023a, January 5). *Monopsony in professional labor markets: Hospital system concentration and nurses' wages*. Institute for New Economic Thinking, Working Paper, Series No. 197, https://www.ineteconomics.org/uploads/papers/WP_197-Allegretto-HospCons.pdf

Allegretto, S., & Graham-Squire, D. (2023b, January 19). *Monopsony in professional labor markets: Hospital system concentration and nurse wage growth*. Institute for New Economic Thinking. https://www.ineteconomics.org/perspectives/blog/monopsony-in-professional-labor-markets-hospital-system-concentration-and-nurse-wage-growth

Anderson, S. (2022, December 22). *What's the difference between a monopoly and a monopsony?* Investopedia. https://www.investopedia.com/ask/answers/032415/whats-difference-between-monopoly-and-monopsony.asp

Bai, G., Zare, H., Eisenberg, M. D., Polsky, D., & Anderson, G. F. (2021). Analysis suggests government and nonprofit hospitals' charity care is not aligned with their favorable tax treatment. *Health Affairs (Project Hope), 40*(4), 629–636. https://doi.org/10.1377/hlthaff.2020.01627

Baker, L., Bundorf, M., & Kessler, D. (2014). Vertical integration: Hospital ownership of physician practices is associated with higher prices and spending. *Health Affairs, 33*(5), 756–765. https://doi.org/10.1377/hlthaff.2013.1279

Boozary, A., Feyman, Y., Reinhardt, U., & Jha, A. (2019). The association between hospital concentration and insurance premiums in ACA marketplaces. *Health Affairs, 38*(4), 668–674. https://doi.org/10.1377/hlthaff.2018.05491

Bulat, T., & Brake, R. (2024, January 3). *Potential impacts of Medicare site neutrality on off-campus drug administration costs*. Actuarial Research Corporation. https://craftmediabucket.s3.amazonaws.com/uploads/Sizing-Medicare-Off-Campus-HOPD-Site-Neutrality-Proposals-2024.01.03.pdf

Cancienne, J. M., Browning, R., Haug, E., Browne, J. A., & Werner, B. C. (2020). Certificate-of-Need Programs are associated with a reduced incidence, expenditure, and rate of complications with respect to knee arthroscopy in the Medicare population. *HSS Journal: The Musculoskeletal Journal of Hospital for Special Surgery, 16*(Suppl. 2), 264–271. https://doi.org/10.1007/s11420-019-09693-z

Centers for Medicare & Medicaid Services. (2019). *Federally qualified health center*. https://www.hhs.gov/guidance/sites/default/files/hhs-guidance-documents/FQHC-Text-Only-Factsheet.pdf

Centers for Medicare and Medicaid Services. (2024). *Rural Emergency Hospitals*. Author. https://www.cms.gov/files/document/rural-emergency-hospitals-factsheet-september-2024.pdf

Center for Healthcare Quality and Payment Reform. (2023). *Rural hospitals at risk of closure*. Author. https://ruralhospitals.chqpr/downloads/Rural_Hospitals_at_Risk_of_Closing.pdf

Choi, J. (2024, May 23). *How noncompete ban could shake up health care landscape*. The Hill. https://fox40.com/news/national-and-world-news/how-noncompete-ban-could-shake-up-health-care-landscape/

Clayton Antitrust Act. (1914). 15 U.S.C. §§ 12–27, 29 U.S.C. §§ 52–53.

Conover, C. J., & Bailey, J. (2020). Certificate of need laws: A systematic review and cost-effectiveness analysis. *BMC Health Services Research, 20*(1), 748. https://doi.org/10.1186/s12913-020-05563-1

Cooper, Z., Craig, S., Gaynor, M., & Van Reenen, R. (2019). The price ain't right? Hospital prices and health spending on the privately insured. *Quarterly Journal of Economics, 134*(1), 51–107. https://doi.org/10.1093/qje/qjy020

Dafny, L. (2014). Hospital industry consolidation—Still more to come? *New England Journal of Medicine, 370*(3), 198–199. https://doi.org/10.1056/NEJMp1313948

Federal Trade Commission. (n.d.). *Guide to antitrust laws*. Author. https://www.ftc.gov/advice-guidance/competition-guidance/guide-antitrust-laws#:~:text=Competition%20Guidance%20The%20FTC's%20competition%20mission%20is,consumers%20from%20anticompetitive%20mergers%20and%20business%20practices.

Federal Trade Commission. (2014). *Policy perspectives: Competition and the regulation of advanced practice nurses*. Author.

Federal Trade Commission. (2023, January 5). *Non-compete clause rulemaking*. Author. https://www.ftc.gov/legal-library/browse/federal-register-notices/non-compete-clause-rulemaking

FQHC Associates. (n.d.). *What is a look-alike and what benefits does one receive?* https://www.fqhc.org/fqhc-look-alike-info#:~ text=What%20is%20an%20FQHC%20Look%2DAlike%20and%20what%20benefits%20does,does%20not%20receive%20grant%20funding.

Gaines, A. G., & Cagle, J. G. (2023). Associations between certificate of need policies and hospice quality outcomes. *The American Journal of Hospice & Palliative Care, 41*(5), 471–478. https://doi.org/10.1177/10499091231180613

Gaynor, M., & Town, R. (2012). *The impact of hospital consolidation—Update.* The Synthesis Project (Policy Brief No. #9). The Robert Wood Johnson Foundation.

Gooch, K. (2020, June 5). *Record number of healthcare workers laid off, furloughed during pandemic.* Becker's Hospital Review. https://www.beckershospitalreview.com/workforce/record-number-of-healthcare-workers-laid-off-furloughed-during-pandemic.html

Goodwin, J., Leviņson, Z., & Hulver, S. (2023, August 23). *Understanding mergers between hospitals and health systems in different markets.* Kaiser Family Foundation. https://www.kff.org/health-costs/issue-brief/understanding-mergers-between-hospitals-and-health-systems-in-different-markets/

Group, T., & Roberts, J. (2001). *Nursing, physician control, and the medical monopoly: Historical perspectives on gender inequality in roles, rights, and range of practice.* Indiana University Press.

Henderson, D. (2013, October 17). *Reinhardt on doctor's monopoly.* Library of Economics and Liberty. Retrieved March 23, 2014, from https://www.econlib.org/archives/2013/10/reinhardt_on_do.html

Holmes, J., Lunge, R., & Rambur, B. (2024). *Mastering healthcare regulation*: A comprehensive case study approach. Health Administration Press.

Hulver, S., & Leviņson, Z. (2023, August 7). *Understanding the role of the FTC, DOJ, and states in challenging anticompetitive practices of hospital and other health care providers.* Kaiser Family Foundation. https://www.kff.org/health-costs/issue-brief/understanding-the-role-of-the-ftc-doj-and-states-in-challenging-anticompetitive-practices-of-hospitals-and-other-health-care-providers/

Liu, J., Levinson, Z., Zhou, A., Zhao, X., Nguyen, P., & Qureshi, N. (2023). Environmental scan on consolidation trends and impacts in health care markets. *Rand Health Quarterly, 10*(3), 2. https://pubmed.ncbi.nlm.nih.gov/37333669/

Livingston, S. (2020, June 13). *COVID-19 may end up boosting value based payments.* Modern Healthcare. https://www.modernhealthcare.com/insurance/covid-19-may-en-up-boosting-value-based-payments

Lucas, F., Siewers, A., Goodman, D., Wang, D., & Wennberg, D. (2011). New cardiac surgery programs established from 1993 to 2004 led to little increased access, substantial duplication of services. *Health Affairs, 30*(8), 1569–1574. https://doi.org/10.1377/hlthaff.2010.0210

Makary, M. (2024, April 14). *Hospitals that make profits should pay taxes.* Stat News. https://statenews.com/2024/04/14/nonprofit-hospitals-turn-profit-charity-care-tax-exempt-status/

MedPAC. (2023, June). *Aligning fee-for-service payment rates across ambulatory settings.* https://www.medpac.gov/recommendation/ambulatory-surgical-center-services/

Mitchell, M. (2019, September 3). *Do certificate-of-need laws still make sense in 2019?* Managed Healthcare Executive. https://www.managedhealthcareexecutive.com/view/do-certificate-need-laws-still-make-sense-2019

National Conference of State Legislatures. (2019, December 1). *Certificate of Need: State health laws and programs.* http://www.ncsl.org/research/health/con-certificate-of-need-state-laws.aspx

National Conference of State Legislatures. (2024). *Certificate of need state laws.* https://www.ncsl.org/health/certificate-of-need-state-laws

Phillion, M. (2021, August 9). *Value-based healthcare: How it expanded during COVID-19.* Patient Safety and Quality Healthcare. https://www.psqh.com/analysis/value-based-healthcare-how-it-expanded-during-covid-19/

Pope, C. (2024a). *US hospitals receive billions in funding—but where does it actually go?* The Hill. https://thehill.com/opinion/healthcare/4424372-us-hospitals-receive-billions-in-funding-but-where-does-it-actually-go/

Pope, C. (2024b). *Untangling the hospital safety net.* Manhattan Institute. https://manhattan.institute/article/untangling-the-hospital-safety-net

Prager, E., & Schmitt, M. (2021). Employer consolidation and wages: Evidence from hospitals. *American Economic Review, 111*(2), 397–427. https://doi.org/10.1257/aer.20190690

Raths, D. (2023, October 13). *North Dakota critical access hospitals form network.* Healthcare Innovation. https://www.hcinnovationgroup.com/clinical-it/digital-health-innovation/news/53075111/north-dakota-critical-access-hospitals-form-network

Sheps Center Report. (2023). *Rural hospitals closures.* https://www.shepscenter.unc.edu/programs-projects/rural-health/rural-hospital-closures/

Sonenberg, A., & Mason, D. J. (2023). Maternity care deserts in the US. *JAMA Health Forum, 4*(1), e225541. https://doi.org/10.1001/jamahealthforum.2022.5541

Southwick, R. (2024). *Hospitals, physicians class over FTC rule banning non-compete agreements.* Chief Healthcare Executive. https://www.chiefhealthcareexecutive.com/view/hospitals-physicians-clash-over-ftc-rule-banning-non-compete-clauses

U.S. Department of Justice. (2022a, October 27). *Health care company pleads guilty and is sentenced for conspiring to suppress wages of school nurses.* Author. https://www.justice.gov/opa/pr/health-care-company-pleads-guilty-and-sentenced-conspiring-suppress-wages-school-nurses

U.S. Department of Justice. (2022b, January 28). *Four individuals indicted on wage fixing and labor market allocation charges.* https://www.justice.gov/opa/pr/four-individuals-indicted-wage-fixing-and-labor-market-allocation-charges

U.S. Department of Justice. (2024). *Herfindahl-Hirschman index.* https://www.justice.gov/atr/herfindahl-hirschman-index#:~:text=The%20HHI%20is%20calculated%20by,%2B%20202%20%3D%202%2C600

Yee, T., Stark, L., Bond, A., & Carrier, E. (2011). *Health care certificate-of-need laws: Policy or politics?* Issues Brief No. 4. National Institute for Health Care Reform.

Yuce, T. K., Chung, J. W., Barnard, C., & Bilimoria, K. Y. (2020). Association of State Certificate of Need regulation with procedural volume, market share, and outcomes among Medicare beneficiaries. *Journal of the American Medical Association, 324*(20), 2058–2068. https://doi.org/10.1001/jama.2020.21115

SECTION III

Ethics and Economics in an Age of Reform: Demographic Shifts, Political Tensions, and Recognition of Increasingly Scarce Resources

Unlike you, individuals who are not aware of the cost and harm of overtreatment may consider ensuring a lot of treatment to be the most ethical approach to health reform efforts. Many nurses and other providers see the flaws in the current system but do not have the background in health economics that enables them to dissect the issues, consider the ethical implications, and use moral reasoning to create better systems of care and a better society. You now possess an economic and financial background for further discernment. The first two sections of this text have provided the foundation that now enables us to layer on yet another important dimension of finance, economics, and policy in an age of reform: ethics.

Chapter 8 presents an orientation in which ethics and economics are not at odds but merely different sides of the same coin. This orientation is purposely chosen to counter the notion that considerations of economics are bad or unethical in health care, rather than essential to both individual patients and society at large.

Chapter 9 then reviews different models for ethical decision-making that you can use in daily practice as well as in broader systems redesign and reform efforts.

Let us start first with Chapter 8, to ensure that you can lace together ethical and economic considerations in your decision-making actions and inactions.

Ethics and Economics in an Age of Reform: Demographic Shifts, Points of Tensions, and Recognition of Increasingly Scarce Resources

CHAPTER 8

What Is Ethinomics?

CHAPTER 8 provides an overview of classic principles of health care ethics such as beneficence and nonmaleficence. It illustrates the interconnections among ethics, economics, and social determinants of health and tensions nurses may experience when shifting from a focus on the individual to more inclusive population-based perspectives.

Following completion of this chapter, you will be able to:

- Describe classic principles of health care ethics.
- Consider the relationship between individually focused ethical perspectives and population-based perspectives.
- Detail the relationship between health care ethics and health care economics.

> Peter, a high school senior, is not sure what he wants to study in college. He enjoys science and math and considers a career in engineering. Pondering his favorite playtime activities at age 5, playing superhero, Peter recalls that what he has most wanted to do is to "do good," to help. Peter decides to look more closely at a nursing career.

CAN ECONOMICS COEXIST WITH THE INTENTION OF "DOING GOOD"?

The intention of doing good, or *beneficence*, is not only central to professional nursing's code of ethics but also is at the heart of many nurses' attraction to the profession in the first place. Avoidance of doing harm, known as *nonmaleficence*, is the obverse principle of health care ethics rooted in the wisdom of the ancient Greek physician Hippocrates, who said, "Above all else, do no harm." For many nurses, "doing good" and "not harming" seem like simple, uncomplicated responsibilities with easily aligned tasks; you do what you can for the patient before you, working hard to avoid errors or mistakes. Certainly, one might argue, none of these should seem constrained by issues of economics. Such a view, however, belies the complexity of ethical decision-making and also incorrectly suggests that economics is a counterforce to ethics. The premise underlying this chapter is that ethics and economics are different faces of the same coin, specifically, you can't "do good" and avoid harm without the resources and information to do so. Moreover, health providers often feel more comfortable articulating the principles of ethics than economics or may actually be uneasy with either. Yet both are foundational nursing knowledge in the age of reform.

Schaller's (2008) observation remains apt today. Schaller notes that many issues are shaped by the underlying economics of the situation, yet Americans are not willing to speak about economic realities because to do so appears to dehumanize people. Schaller states:

> In reality, public policy decisions that are made legitimately for economic reasons are often clothed in other garb. . . . [I]t is not uncommon for vital economic concerns that actually drive the dispute to be unspoken and unacknowledged. . . . It would be far better for the underlying backgrounds to be openly disclosed and discussed during the policy debate rather than concealed (p. 4).

More recently, Mauro, writing for the International Monetary Fund, noted that "Policy decisions on taxation and public expenditures *intrinsically reflect moral choices*" (2022, para 1, emphasis added). Thus, it is essential that moral concerns rooted in economic realities be openly disclosed and discussed. Ranked for decades as America's most trusted professionals, highest in honesty and ethics (Brenen, 2023), nurses have a key opportunity to lead the articulation of ethics and economics in health care. Moreover, nurses were ranked as the group with the greatest proportion of the public trust to improve the health care system, with 58% of respondents citing their trust in nurses to improve the system, nearly twice that of the group ranked second, "doctors," at 30%. The state and federal government were each in the single digits (see Table 8.1).

TABLE 8.1 PUBLIC TRUST IN GROUPS TO IMPROVE THE U.S. HEALTH CARE SYSTEM

	Total
"A great deal" of public trust in. . . .	
Nurses	58%
Doctors	30%
Hospitals	18%
Labor unions	14%
State governments	6%
The federal government	6%
Congress	5%
Business leaders	5%
Health insurance companies	4%
Pharmaceutical companies	4%

Source: The Commonwealth Fund, New York Times, & Harvard School of Public Health. *Americans' values and beliefs about National Health Insurance Reform*. https://www.hsph.harvard.edu/wp-content/uploads/sites/21/2019/10/CMWF-NYT-Harvard_Final-Report_Oct2019.pdf.

Ethinomics

Medical ethicist Merrill Mathews suggests that the term *ethinomics* can be used to describe the area in which economics and ethics converge in public policy (Mathews, 1999, as cited in Tay, 2004/2005). This notion is useful because it reflects the conjoined nature of economic and ethical issues as different sides of the same coin and invites both underlying elements to be open to public debate in policy formation. Such an orientation offers valuable tools for the nurse and offers a conceptual orientation that holds both economics and ethics in the forefront. This remains a fresh perspective. Indeed, principles of health care ethics historically have not brought the economic impact of decision-making into focus. Instead, the *universal principles of health care ethics* have focused on care of the individual, with little attention to the impact of clinical decision-making on overall population health. Moreover, although universal principles have guided practice, they can conflict with each other in actual application. A therapy, for example, may be prescribed to benefit a patient but instead result in harm, and thus, beneficence and nonmaleficence are in conflict. Moreover, conflict can exist between autonomy—the patient's right to self-determination to make an informed choice—and nonmaleficence, and each of these with population-based justice.

> *Mr. Greenfield has recently been diagnosed with colon cancer. His surgeon, Dr. Knife, is pleased with how well Mr. Greenfield, at age 86, tolerated the surgery. One small node was found, but Dr. Knife is confident that Mr. Greenfield will die with the cancer rather than of it. He talks to Mr. Greenfield, suggesting no further treatment. Mr. Greenfield, however, seems reluctant to forgo more treatment. He states that chemotherapy might be a good idea because "everyone needs a good flushing out once in a while." Dr. Knife laughs, stating, "This isn't an enema, Mr. Greenfield, it is chemotherapy." Mr. Greenfield is insistent, however, and is not willing to hear about the potential risks in relation to benefits of chemotherapy for this particular type of cancer at his age. Finally, Dr. Knife reluctantly orders an oncology consult. As the patient walks out the door, Dr. Knife mutters to himself, "I know where this will go." Mr. Greenfield starts chemotherapy a week later.*

In the United States, the principle of autonomy has been applied in a manner that reflects an individual's right to make their own decisions. In practice, it often trumps other principles. Dr. Knife is legitimately concerned that chemotherapy will not help Mr. Greenfield and instead has great potential to do harm. In this scenario, autonomy is in direct conflict with beneficence and nonmaleficence. Note that cost is not part of this decision, yet the cost—financial, emotional, and social—is real. Overtreatment of Mr. Greenfield—treatment that is unlikely to help—harms not only Mr. Greenfield but also the society at large because the resources used in his care are not available for other societal needs.

Recall that health care is largely paid for through taxes (Medicare and Medicaid), and employer-based commercial insurance functions as a reduction in real wages and thus forms a hidden tax. Historically, the ethical decision-making lens has focused on maximizing the care of the individual without consideration of the broader implications of the cumulative impact of clinical decisions on the population at large or over time. This tension between individual autonomy and the overall population benefits is not easily visible to providers seeing patients in a clinical setting. Yet this tension has long been recognized by some. Physician David Eddy (1996), for example, stated:

> **Well intentioned attempts to maximize the care of individual patients can harm other people. The sense of harm is lessened by depersonalizing these other people and seeing them only through statistics. But in reality, they are just as real as the individual patients we see face to face. (pp. 109–110)**

At the same time, such maximization of care, even without benefit, has been enormously lucrative to many providers. Providers have viewed their accountability as being limited to the person right in front of them, largely blinded to the impact on others in the society (horizontal effects) and impacts over intergenerational time (temporal or longitudinal effects). As such, the accountability horizon for clinical decision-making in fee-for-service systems has not served the society well. Newacheck and Benjamin (2004), for example, argued that *entitlement funding* for Medicare, health care that you are "entitled to" simply because you are over 65, differentially places societal resources in the hands of older adults at the expense of younger generations and thus represents intergenerational injustice. Providers such as Dr. Knife, as well as the oncologist and oncology nurses later treating Mr. Greenfield, do not see themselves as violating principles of justice and fairness; they are simply doing the work before them. Nevertheless, seen or unseen, overtreatment removes finances from the pool of resources potentially available to treat others. Professional accountability horizons have simply been too narrow and short-term to account for these broader effects of clinical decision-making. Bambad and Englesbe (2020), both physicians in a department of surgery, noted that although surgery represents one-fourteenth of the U.S. gross domestic product, its impact on mortality and quality of life is minimal, leaving a "humbling assessment of our contribution as surgeons to health" (para 2). Indeed, the time and resources the oncology nurse and oncologist devote to Mr. Greenfield, for example, do take treatment resources away from another patient who could really benefit and, in addition, raise the cost of care for all. The shift from fee-for-service to population-based global budgets or bundled payments discussed in earlier chapters begins to better align these overlapping responsibilities.

SOCIAL DETERMINANTS OF HEALTH, HEALTH DISPARITIES, ETHICS, AND ECONOMICS

The intersection of economics and the ethics of societal good can also be understood from the perspective of social determinants of health. Although an enormous amount of the nation's resources goes into medical care, this care makes a relatively small contribution to the overall health status (review Figure 1.1), with the best predictor of health status being lifestyle and the environment, both of which are affected by socioeconomic status (SES). Adler and Newman (2002) note, "The most fundamental causes of health disparities are socioeconomic disparities" (p. 61). SES, although not identical to, is well correlated with educational attainment. Thus, it might be argued that to enhance *health*, resources now used for *health care* might be redirected to education to defray the cost of college and reduce student debt load (another national goal), given that—in general—the better the education of the person, the better the health status. As Adler and Newman note:

> Education is perhaps the most basic SES component since it shapes future occupational opportunities and earning potential. It also provides knowledge and life skills that allow better-educated persons to gain more ready access to information and resources to promote health. . . . To the extent that education is key to health inequalities, policies encouraging more years of schooling and supporting early childhood education may have health benefits. . . . When policy makers debate the merits of increasing access to education, they rarely consider improvement in the health of the population . . . collateral benefits such as decreasing health care costs also might emerge from increasing investment in education. (pp. 61–62)

Two decades later, there is evidence of too little progress in linking these domains. The Lancet Public Health (2020), for example, suggests that education is the "neglected social determinant." They state: "Education and health and wellbeing are intrinsically linked. The evidence behind the importance of education as a determinant of health is amongst the most compelling. Education is strongly associated with life expectancy, morbidity, [and] health behaviours, and educational attainment plays an important role in health by shaping opportunities, employment, and income" (para 1).

Excessive resources directed to health care could be redirected to the sort of job creation that can enhance the SES of individuals and their families. Indeed, the U.S. Centers for Disease Control and Prevention identify "work as a key social determinant" (Steege et al., 2023, para 1). These sorts of policy trade-offs are not always fully visible to the nurse or the general public, but are trade-offs nonetheless. Thus, as an informed nurse, you can more broadly consider the impact of your work, including the effects of overtreatment, and understand it as an ethical issue with broad range. The pernicious arch of disparities was dramatically revealed during the COVID-19 pandemic and will be detailed in later chapters.

Much of the increase in life expectancy over the past century is due to improvements in living conditions and a reduction in overcrowding, as well as reduction in deaths from infectious diseases. The former represents a standard-of-living issue, not a health care issue, and the latter, a public health initiative. In the United States, health expenditures in 2022 reached $4.5 trillion, $13, 493 per person, and 17.3% of the gross domestic product (Centers for Medicare & Medicaid Services [CMS], 2024). This means that of all the money spent on goods and services in the United States, over 17 cents on every dollar goes into health care; hence, those dollars are not available for other goods and services such as education, housing, entertainment, and childcare. Overtreatment harms individuals and society and therefore violates principles of health care ethics. Moreover, there is evidence that Black and Hispanic patients are more likely to receive low-value care than White patients (Schpero et al., 2017).

Ethinomics, Autonomy, and Justice

Ethinomics is concerned with such issues. It recognizes that economic forces interact with principles like autonomy and intergenerational justice. Should Mr. Greenfield, for example, be able to have any services he wishes, particularly given that although he paid taxes into Medicare, others are also paying for these services through their taxes? Or should there be limits on what Mr. Greenfield can demand? If so, who should define those limits? When do autonomy and right to self-determination become illogical and damaging? An emphasis on the wishes of the individual as a primary determinant of what constitutes perceived ethical conduct is a distinctive part of contemporary U.S. culture but is not universal.

> *Sylvain, a Canadian, is chatting with Paula, an American, regarding public testing for a novel sexually transmitted virus. Paula believes that everyone should be tested. After all, she reasons, the test is free through the public health clinic. Sylvain is bewildered. "This test is expensive, Paula, and it needs to be done in a thoughtful, strategic, and focused manner," he states. Who is correct?*

Paula and Sylvain are simply looking at this issue at different levels and at different levels of comprehensiveness. Paula perceives that this testing is free simply because *she* can get it for free. Paula is failing to look at the overall costs. The test is not free. In a publicly funded clinic, the costs of the test are picked up by the public through taxes. Sylvain, reared in a very different health system and culture, is aware that the test is expensive even though the test—like most of his health care—does not include an out-of-pocket charge at the time of the visit.

The issue of where the cost is borne along the scale from the individual to society at large is only one end of the continuum. The other issue addresses this question: "Who benefits financially?" In health care, one person's or group's cost is another's gain.

> Edward Jones, chief executive officer (CEO) of Cityville Hospital, is pleased! The hospital has had a banner year. Revenues have shot through the roof in almost every service line. Surgical revenues were up 9%, medical revenues up 4%, and emergency service revenues up a whopping 12%. CEO Jones is excited that the hospital just may finally be creating the financial reserves needed to undertake a highly anticipated capital project: a new entrance to the emergency department. He also thinks they can bump the nursing salary pool increase an additional 0.5% above the level requested by the union. He excitedly calls Cityville's chief nursing officer, Nicco Boyd, to share the good news.
>
> Jennifer Wells, CEO of a large company in Cityville, is perplexed and worried. As a large employer, she has been able to negotiate lower insurance rates for her employees through a preferred provider arrangement that requires employees to use Cityville Hospital or pay large out-of-pocket copayments and co-insurance. Because the insurance pool is so large, the financial expense of any one employee has been spread over many people. This risk sharing over such a large group, coupled with the discounted rates she was able to negotiate with Cityville Hospital in exchange for the arrangement in which her employees use Cityville services only, has meant the lowest insurance premium in the region. Jennifer knows this has been one of the reasons she has been able to attract such a talented workforce. Now her human resources director shares this information: "Employee utilization of health care services has been off the charts. Insurance rates may almost double for our employees, even with the discounted rates with Cityville, if we can get them again." Jennifer braces herself to notify her employees of the options. The business has done well this year, and she had hoped to give well-deserved raises. Now, she will either (a) need to put that money into covering the higher cost of the insurance premiums, reflecting higher utilization by the employees—meaning no raises again this year—or (b) switch to a different plan in which the employees need to contribute much more to their premium, which actually functions as a cut in overall take-home pay.
>
> Nicco and Jennifer meet for coffee after work. "What a terrible day!" Jennifer laments, "I am going to need to give my employees the equivalent of a pay cut, one way or another, due to the increase in premiums." "What a wonderful day," Nicco beams, "I am going to be able to give my staff a raise due to the increased utilization of the hospital."

These scenarios, although simplistic, illustrate that one group's cash is another group's cost. In fee-for-service health care, there is a misalignment between (a) the hospital's business case to maximize consumption of services used by paying customers and (b) the economic case of other businesses, which instead have an incentive to hold down health care use, and thus cost, so that money is available for other aspects of their industry or for direct compensation to employees. The individual business case for the hospital is also at odds with the overall social case, in which the costs of products made in the United States compete with products in a global market, where non-U.S. labor and health care costs are much lower. So, what is good for American hospitals and other health providers in fee-for-service is not necessarily good for Americans in general. The foundational flaws in the model were dramatically exposed during the COVID-19 pandemic, during which elective procedures were curtailed, resulting in dramatic cash flow problems for hospitals and health systems, issues that will be detailed in Chapter 13. In summary, the strain on employers (and thus employees) is growing, with employer-based insurance costing an average of nearly $24,000 for family coverage in 2023, a 7% increase from the previous year and an increase of 22% since 2018 and 47% since 2013 (Kaiser Family Foundation [KFF], 2023). Although these costs are shared between employer and employee, they are ultimately borne by the employee as a reduction in real wages because they are part of employees' total compensation package.

The equation is even more complicated, however, in that the drugs and equipment used in hospitals may be manufactured by U.S. companies that do gain financially when health care use increases. Recall that nonprofit insurance companies are the middlemen between employers and health care, gathering the money from individuals and the organization to have it spread across individuals as needed. There is a great deal of rhetoric and occasional venom against insurance companies and a level of salaries for insurance company executives some consider exorbitant. Although there is a level of administrative costs associated with insurance companies, insurance rates reflect the cost of the use of services by those in the insurance pool. On the surface, these may seem like economic issues. They are also ethical issues nurses can influence. Nurses, however, may get caught in situations in which they feel powerless to enact change or even to understand all the dynamics at play.

> *Simon is a 28-year-old male with a history of substance abuse and ensuing pericarditis, resulting in mitral valve prolapse. He had a mitral valve replaced in August, and following a 1-month hospitalization due to surgical complications, he was discharged on antibiotic therapy. Six months later, Simon returns, in need of repeat surgery. Simon did not complete his antibiotic therapy as prescribed and has returned to his drug habit. The surgeon states that he will not do repeat surgery on Simon. Gloria, the RN, cannot decide what she thinks about this. Is the refusal to treat just? Is it unjust? Was Simon merely bearing the consequences of his actions and inactions, or did the health system have a moral obligation to treat Simon? Simon has insurance coverage through Medicaid, yet*

> *Gloria also understands that others bear the financial consequences of Simon's behaviors, as well as that of the surgeons should Simon have expensive complications with—or without—surgery. Gloria wishes she had some system to help her think through the moral twists and turns so that she could come to a resolution and to feel that the right thing was done.*

What is Gloria to do in this case? How can she discern which action is morally sound? We turn to these issues in the next section.

MORAL CONDUCT OF NURSES IN CONTEMPORARY COMPLEXITY

As detailed in the opening section of this text, nurses have a contract with society. In return for the privilege of being professionals, professionals must place the best interests of those they serve at the center of their actions and decisions. Similarly, nurses, physicians, and other health professionals have special privileges in society, including being privy to some of the most intimate and vulnerable times in an individual's or family's life. In exchange, health professionals have the responsibility to serve the best interests of individual *and* societal health. Yet what constitutes best interest can be difficult to discern. As early as 2013 the Institute of Medicine (IOM) (now called National Academy of Sciences) reported roughly one-third of what is done in health care does not make a difference at all. At that time, Fineberg (2012; also cited in Redberg, 2012) suggested that hundreds of billions of dollars, up to a whopping trillion dollars, are spent on care that does not make a difference. This figure has remained remarkably stable over time, despite efforts to decrease the waste stemming from overtreatment, with Shrank et al. (2019) reporting 25% of health care representing waste or overtreatment, a figure that excluded costs related to administrative complexity. Similarly, the Peter G. Peterson Foundation reports waste at roughly one-quarter of all care (2023). Worse yet, some health care actions harm rather than heal. Hospital-based preventable harm is estimated at epidemic proportions of over 400,000 patients/year (James, 2013), with other studies suggesting that adverse events occur in one-third of hospitalizations (Classen et al., 2011). Looking at medication-related harm only, Hodkinson and colleagues' (2020) systematic review and metanalysis of 31 studies involving 285,687 people found that 1 in 30 patient encounters had preventable medication harm, and in more than a quarter this harm was severe or life threatening. Other studies exploring harm more broadly suggest that preventable harm is pervasive, occurring in 1 in every 20 patients and creates an estimated $9.3 billion in excessive charges in the United States (Panagioti et al., 2019). These findings suggest that some care creates not only economic harm but also bodily and/or emotional injury. The *more is better* ethical goalpost is clearly misplaced, and new, more robust ethical models to guide health care are necessary.

Emerging Ethical Systems

Classic "universal principles" of health care, such as autonomy, beneficence, and nonmaleficence, have not incorporated patients' ethical obligations, nor have they easily held a creative synergistic balance between the individual and the population that discernibly serves both simultaneously. Similarly, classical ethical systems do not easily enable the clinician to incorporate population and financial considerations in their moral guideposts. In response, a new moral framework has been proffered by Faden et al. (2013). This framework is grounded in the National Academy of Science's (previously IOM) call for a *health care learning system* in which the generation of new knowledge for the improvement of care is an explicit value. Such improvement includes cost, quality, and sustainability as foundational to fairness. These authors note, "Securing just health care requires a constantly updated body of evidence about the effectiveness and value of health care interventions and of alternative ways to deliver and finance health care" (p. S17). This inclusion of finance and testing of alternative delivery models as moral obligations offers additional reasons for nurses to be full participants in care redesign. It also underscores the importance of the evidence-based practice movement as an ethical obligation.

Health Care Learning System Ethical Framework Elements

The framework of Faden et al. (2013) delineates seven *fundamental obligations*—again, note that these are *moral obligations*—as follows:

- The obligation to respect patients
- The obligation to respect clinician judgment
- The obligation to provide optimal care to each patient
- The obligation to avoid imposing nonclinical risks and burdens
- The obligation to address unjust inequalities
- The obligation to conduct continuous learning activities that improve the quality of clinical care and health care systems
- The obligation of patients to contribute to the common purpose of improving the quality and value of clinical care and the health care system

Unlike some other ethical schema, patient autonomy (embedded in item 1) does not supersede all other considerations; all obligations must be held in concert. This framework demands accountability for a new set of precepts from the nurse and also asks that patients participate in heretofore unprecedented ways. One example considers patient privacy issues in the era of big data. The policy tension revolves around controversy regarding whether or not patients should be able to opt out of having their personal data included in all payer claims databases. These databases are ultimately used in cost containment and quality tracking and improvement. One argument would hold that the patient's right to autonomy and self-determination supports the idea that every patient has the right to refuse inclusion in the database. Conversely, Bates et al. (2014) reference Faden and colleagues and note that "patients have a moral obligation to contribute to the common purpose of improving the quality and value of clinical care" (p. 1129). The magnitude of this difference—the difference between a stance in which moral conduct consists of following patient wishes and one in which the patient has a moral obligation to the common good and the population as a whole—cannot be overstated. To this author's knowledge, An Ethics Framework for a Learning Health Care System (Faden et al., 2013) is the first definitively population-inclusive moral code offered for health and health care. More recently, research by Pauly et al. (2021) delineates ethical tensions that emerge when promoting health equity due to the oppositional nature of public health values and traditional medical care: (a) public health values focus on social determinants of health and system change and (b) biomedical models focused on situational care, with associated stigma in the context of mental health promotion and prevention of substance use harm. These ethical and pragmatic tensions were on full display during the COVID-19 pandemic and will be further discussed in later chapters.

Ethics and the Role of the Nurse: Role Fidelity

Yet another universal principle of health care ethics is that of *role fidelity*. This principle means that professionals must be responsible to and function within their role. An example might be an airline pilot. The pilot is responsible for the role of flying the plane safely. She must arrange her life and time to be faithful to the responsibilities of the role. Prior to the flight, she must rest appropriately and avoid any substances that might cloud her judgment. What if the pilot has hemorrhoids, is upset about a child or partner, or is just plain grumpy? It does not matter. The pilot must fly the plane impeccably; many lives depend on it. Similarly, nurses have an ethical obligation to the role of nurse. So, what is the nurse's obligation in Simon's case? Conversely, what is Simon's obligation to the situation, given that his behavior likely was an antecedent to his condition? To what extent does it matter that his behavior may be related to or have a societal etiology of anything from poverty to adverse childhood events?

More information about Simon would be necessary to fully resolve the moral dilemma about his care. It is likely, however, that the present system is designed to fail Simon. Perhaps he did not have the social support to ensure compliance with his postsurgical regimen. Perhaps he is homeless and recovering from surgery seemed less pressing than surviving the night. Perhaps he did not have transportation to obtain his medication, and the public transportation system was simply too daunting. Systems redesigned to ensure that Simon had the social support for the transition out of the hospital should be an essential nursing skill set, given nurses' knowledge of what is necessary in postacute care as well as nursing's community-inclusive education. Consistent with the model of Faden et al. (2013), nurse engagement with system redesign to ensure that the system does not fail Simon and others is as essential to nurses' moral code as is patient confidentiality. Chapter 9 details several additional models that can support nurses' development as moral agents and offer additional perspectives on the complexity, promise, and perils of clinical decision-making in an era of reform.

End-of-Chapter Resources

THOUGHT QUESTIONS

1. What forms of care do you see that make a tangible, substantive, long-term difference? What forms of care do you see as futile?
2. What is the cost–benefit ratio of these forms of care? In other words, when you see care that makes a difference, what is given up for the cost of that care?
3. Have you seen patients harmed by care? What system, policy, or practice changes could have prevented that harm?
4. What does it mean for a nurse to be part of a learning health care system? What sort of learning and knowledge should they have? What sorts of contributions are essential?
5. Should patients be obligated to contribute to health care in the ways envisioned in the ethical model of Faden and colleagues? Justify your answer.

EXERCISE

1. Prepare a presentation for your peers that details the pros and cons of considering economics in the ethics of health care.

QUIZ

True or False

1. One limitation of traditional *universal principles of health care ethics* is that they have focused on the impact of clinical decision-making on population health.
2. The term *beneficence* refers to the avoidance of doing harm.

3. Nurses are consistently rated as the most trusted professionals in the United States.
4. An Ethics Framework for a Learning Health Care System, offered by Faden and colleagues, is similar to traditional universal principles of health care ethics because both include a moral obligation for individual patients to contribute to the common purpose of improving the quality of care, the value of clinical care, and the health care system.
5. The term *role fidelity* refers to a professional's moral obligation to be faithful to the responsibilities of the role.
6. In general, socioeconomic status is associated with educational attainment.
7. Overtreatment and overutilization of health care may worsen population health disparities because the cost of these services erodes the social capacity to invest in other segments of the economy such as education and job creation.
8. In general, health care providers have had little accountability for the broader impacts of their clinical decision-making on population health.
9. The term *nonmaleficence* refers to "doing good."
10. In fee-for-service reimbursement models, the hospital business case to maximize the amount of services used is generally at odds with the social need for lower health care costs.

Multiple Choice

11. Ethinomics
    A. Is a term coined by medical ethicist Merrill Mathews
    B. Refers to the convergence of economics and ethics in public policy
    C. Both A and B
    D. Neither A nor B
12. Classic universal principles of health care ethics include
    A. Autonomy
    B. Beneficence and nonmaleficence
    C. Both A and B
    D. Neither A nor B
13. Ethical tensions can exist when ethical principles suggest competing approaches: For example, a patient insists on a particular treatment that the provider feels will not benefit the patient but will instead cause harm. This example illustrates tensions between
    A. Justice and autonomy
    B. Autonomy and nonmaleficence
    C. Confidentiality and autonomy
    D. Confidentiality and justice

14. Hospital-based preventable harm
    A. Over the past decade has dramatically diminished in the U.S. health care system
    B. Has both cost and ethical dimensions
    C. Both A and B
    D. Neither A nor B
15. Intergenerational justice
    A. May be negatively impacted when one U.S. age cohort receives health care and other services at the expense of another
    B. May be negatively impacted when women receive health care and other services and men do not
    C. Both A and B
    D. Neither A nor B

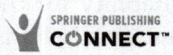

A robust set of instructor resources designed to supplement this text is located at http://connect.springerpub.com/content/book/978-0-8261-7236-5. Qualifying instructors may request access by emailing **textbook@springerpub.com**.

REFERENCES

Adler, N., & Newman, K. (2002). Socioeconomic disparities in health: Pathways and policies. *Health Affairs*, 21(2), 60–76. https://doi.org/10.1377/hlthaff.21.2.60

Bambad, M., & Englesbe, M. (2020, June 24). Surgery and population health: Redesigning surgical quality for greater impact. *JAMA Surgery*, 159(9), 799–800. https://doi.org/10.1001/jamasurg.2020.0808

Bates, D., Saria, S., Ohno-Machado, L., Shah, A., & Escobar, G. (2014). Big data in health care: Using analytics to identify and manage high-risk and high cost health care. *Health Affairs*, 33(7), 1123–1131. https://doi.org/10.1377/hlthaff.2014.0041

Brenen, M. (2023, January 10). *Nurses retain top ethics rating in U.S., but below 2020 high*. Gallop. https://news.gallup.com/poll/467804/nurses-retain-top-ethics-rating-below-2020-high.aspx

Centers for Medicare & Medicaid Services. (2024, September 10). *National health expenditures data: Historical*. https://www.cms.gov/data-research/statistics-trends-and-reports/national-health-expenditure-data/historical

Classen, D., Resar, R., Griffin, F., Federico, F., Frankel, T., Kimmel, N., Whittington, J. C., Frankel, A., Seger A., & James, B. (2011). "Global trigger tool" shows that adverse events in hospitals may be ten times greater than previously measured. *Health Affairs*, 30(4), 581–589. https://doi.org/10.1377/hlthaff.2011.0190

Eddy, D. (1996). *Clinical decision making: From theory to practice*. Jones & Bartlett.

Faden, R., Kass, N., Goodman, S., Pronovost, P., Tunis, S., & Beauchamp, T. (2013). An ethics framework for a learning health care system: A departure from traditional research ethics and clinical ethics. *Hastings Center Report*, 42(s1), S16–S27. https://doi.org/10.1002/hast.134

Fineberg, H. (2012). A successful and sustainable health system—How to get there from here. *New England Journal of Medicine, 366*, 1020–1027. https://doi.org/10.1056/NEJMsa1114777

Hodkinson, A., Tyler, N., Ashcroft, D. M., Keers, R. N., Khan, K., Phipps, D., Abuzour, A., Bower, P., Avery, A., Campbell, S., & Panagioti, M. (2020). Preventable medication harm across health care settings: A systematic review and meta-analysis. *BMC Medicine, 18*(1), 313. https://doi.org/10.1186/s12916-020-01774-9

Institute of Medicine. (2013). *Best care at lower cost: The path to continuously learning health care in America*. National Academies Press.

James, J. (2013). A new, evidence-based estimate of patient harms associated with hospital care. *Journal of Patient Safety, 9*(3), 122–128. https://doi.org/10.1097/PTS.0b013e3182948a69

Kaiser Family Foundation. (2023, October 18). *Section 1: Cost of health insurance*. https://www.kff.org/report-section/ehbs-2023-section-1-cost-of-health-insurance/

The Lancet Public Health. (2020). Education: A neglected social determinant of health. *The Lancet Public Health, 5*(7), e361. https://doi.org/10.1016/S2468-2667(20)30144-4

Mauro, P. (2022). *Adding ethics to public finance*. International Monetary Fund. https://www.imf.org/en/Publications/fandd/issues/2022/03/Adding-ethics-to-public-finance-Mauro

Newacheck, R., & Benjamin, A. (2004). Intergenerational equity and public spending. *Health Affairs, 23*(5), 142–146. https://doi.org/10.1377/hlthaff.23.5.142

Panagioti, M., Khan, K., Keers, R., Abuzour, A., Philips, D., Kontopantelis, E., Bower, P., Cmapbell, S., Haneef, R., Avery, A., & Ashcroft, D. (2019). Prevalence, severity, and nature of preventable patient harm across medical care settings; systemic review and meta-analysis. *British Journal of Medicine, 366*, l4185. https://doi.org/10.1136/bmj.l4185

Pauly, B., Revai, T., Marcellus, L., Martin, W., Easton, K., & MacDonald, M. (2021). "The health equity curse": Ethical tensions in promoting health equity. *BMC Public Health, 21*(1), 1567. https://doi.org/10.1186/s12889-021-11594-y

Peter Peterson Foundation. (2023, April 3). *Almost 25% of healthcare spending is considered wasteful. Here's why*. https://www.pgpf.org/blog/2023/04/almost-25-percent-of-healthcare-spending-is-considered-wasteful-heres-why

Redberg, R. (2012). Less is more. *NAM Perspectives*. Commentary, National Academy of Medicine. Washington, DC. https://doi.org/10.31478/201209cLessIsMore.aspx

Schaller, B. (2008). *Understanding bioethics and the law: The promise and perils of the brave new world of biotechnology*. Greenwood.

Schpero, W. L., Morden, N. E., Sequist, T. D., Rosenthal, M. B., Gottlieb, D. J., & Colla, C. H. (2017). For selected services, Blacks and Hispanics more likely to receive low-value care than Whites. *Health Affairs (Project Hope), 36*(6), 1065–1069. https://doi.org/10.1377/hlthaff.2016.1416

Shrank, W., Rogstad, T., & Parekh, N. (2019). Waste in the U.S. health care system: Estimated costs and potential for savings. *The Journal of the American Medical Association, 322*(15), 1501–1509. https://doi.org/10.1001/jama.2019.13978

Steege, A., Silver, S., Mobley, A., & Haring Sweeney, M. (2023, February 16). *Work as a key social determinant of health: the case for including work in all health data collections*. Centers for Disease Control and Prevention. https://blogs.cdc.gov/niosh-science-blog/2023/02/16/sdoh/

Tay, M. (2004/2005). *Ethics, economics and EQ in health care*. Hong Kong Society of Helath Services Executives. https://www.hkchse.org/database/newsletter/hkchse2004052.pdf

CHAPTER 9

Models to Guide Ethical Decision-Making

CHAPTER 8 detailed some of the complex interactions that can make it difficult to understand the full ethical dimensions of health care decision-making in contemporary culture. The limitations and often conflicting nature of the very principles that guide ethical decision-making were also illustrated. This chapter builds on this knowledge, detailing overarching models of ethical decision-making that take yet a different approach and can assist you when facing moral challenges. Three overarching models are reviewed as well as major branches within these models. These are

- consequence-based ethical decision-making (utilitarianism);
- rule-based ethical decision-making (deontology), with an emphasis on Rawls's theory of justice; and
- virtue-based ethics and an ethic of caring.

Following completion of this chapter, you will be able to:

- Compare and contrast utilitarianism, deontology, and virtue ethics.
- Describe Rawls's theory of justice.
- Discuss an ethic of caring.
- Describe considerations during times of scarcity or crisis.
- Consider the impact of ethical decision-making models on health care.
- Discern moral distress.

CONSEQUENCE-BASED DECISION-MAKING

Consequence-based decision-making is grounded in the idea that decisions should be made so that the greatest good can happen for the greatest number of people. In the most extreme version of this model, the consequences—ends—justify the means, no matter how extreme. The American Nurses Association's (ANA's) Code of Ethics for Nurses (2015) offers an example of consequence-oriented decision-making that is very familiar to nurses: triage in a disaster situation. Rather than place extensive resources to treat just one person, in crisis situations, triage deploys resources—both human and material—to maximize the number of people who survive, even at the expense of the few. A more dramatic, more controversial example is the dropping of the first atomic bombs in Hiroshima and Nagasaki, which effectively brought an end to World War II. The British Broadcasting Company estimates that between 60,000 and 80,000 people died instantly, with the heat so intense that some simply vanished in the explosion, thus making an exact count difficult. Many more died of the long-term effects of radiation sickness, with the final death toll calculated at 135,000 (British Broadcasting Corporation [BBC], 2012). Other sources suggest that the total number of casualties was 135,000 at Hiroshima alone, with another 64,000 at Nagasaki; again, a precise number is difficult to determine because of the mass confusion after the bombing and the fires that consumed many bodies (Atomic Archive, n.d.). The overall death toll for World War II is suggested to be roughly 50 to 70 million people. The war ended within a week of the bombing. Did the perceived good, the end of the war, outweigh the deaths of innocent civilians? This example illustrates the painful trade-offs that bookend a consequence-oriented approach, as an attempt is made to maximize the good of the many, even when individuals are trampled on along the way.

Nurses and Consequence-Oriented Decision-Making

Consequence-oriented decision-making is also called *utilitarianism*. Nurses may use consequence-oriented decision-making, often without being aware that there is an ethical dilemma, even though it may be on a microscale compared to the World War II example.

> Ruth, an RN, is working on a short-staffed night. She is concerned that Mr. Smith needs extra time and attention right now, but she has five other patients and knows that spending the time with Mr. Smith means the others will not have as much of her time and attention. Walking past Mr. Smith's room, she hears him calling for her. She feels a pang of discomfort as she hurries to the next room, but feels it is the right thing to do, given the demands of the other patients.[1]

Limitations of consequence-oriented decision-making include the impossibility of imagining and tracing forward all the consequences of actions and inactions. Moreover, if actions are to be directed toward consequences that increase "the good," how is "the good" defined, and by whom? Finally, if the focus is entirely on consequences, any act can conceivably be justified, no matter how harmful to the few. For many people, this focus does not meet a criterion of ethical decision-making, no matter how many people are ultimately positively impacted. Nevertheless, the ANA Code of Ethics (2015) notes that in complex, extreme, or extraordinary practice settings, "A utilitarian framework usually guides decision and actions with special emphasis on transparency, protection of the public, proportional restrictions of individual liberty, and fair stewardship of resources" (p. 33).

DEONTOLOGY: RULE-BASED DECISION-MAKING

In contrast, the orientation in rule-based decision-making is that the ethical or moral stance is determined by adherence to a rule, principle, or duty. Rule-based ethical decision-making is also called *deontological ethics* or *deontology*, from the Greek term for *duty*. In this moral schema, the ends cannot justify the means, and instead, an entirely different criterion is used, specifically the aforementioned rule. In the strictest conceptualization of such decision-making, the rule must be followed, regardless of the consequences. If, for example, the rule is "thou shall not kill," there can be no taking of another's life, regardless of the consequence. Rooted in the work of Immanuel Kant, deontology includes the principle of *universalizability*, whereby an action or inaction is morally acceptable only if it is acceptable under universal law. This means that if you can do it, everyone and anyone can. As an example, if you are trying to decide if it is morally acceptable to cheat on an exam, it would have to be morally acceptable for everyone and anyone to cheat on exams. This includes your airline pilot, your banker, and the engineer who designs the bridges you drive over. Applying this principle, it is not only easy to see that it is not morally acceptable to cheat on exams—it is an imperative not to cheat. The term *categorical imperative* is used to describe these types of circumstances.

Rawls's Theory of Justice

John Rawls offers a fresh perspective on deontology in his highly influential texts *A Theory of Justice* (Rawls, 1999) and *Justice as Fairness* (Rawls, 2001). Rawls suggests, among other things, that in a just society, all individuals have the same claim on basic liberties. To achieve this, he suggests that social systems should be organized from the *original position*. This original position refers to a sort of thought experiment in which the basic organization of society is viewed from what Rawls termed a *veil of ignorance*, in which participants do not know their position, status, race, and gender. Thus, societal rules can be set up from a position of impartiality. For example, how would health care be constructed if a participant did not know if they were a wealthy millionaire or a homeless veteran with posttraumatic stress disorder? Rawls argues that systems created referencing the original position with the veil of ignorance would have fair policies and procedures that protect the vulnerable and provide basic liberties to all.

VIRTUE ETHICS

Both consequence-oriented decision-making and deontological decision-making differ from *virtue ethics*. In virtue ethics, the emphasis is not on consequences or rules, but on character development such that the individual inherently functions from an ethical place as a morally developed person. Inspired by Aristotle, virtues such as courage and fortitude are viewed as inherent characteristics of humans yet need nurturing. A challenge in virtue-based ethics is that it does not provide specific guidance on how to act in a particular situation. Nor are there clear directions, other than to act as a virtuous person acts. Virtue ethics relies on discernment within context referencing *the golden mean* between *excess* and *deficiency*. For example, an excess of courage is not courage at all, but recklessness. At the same time, a deficiency of this quality is cowardice. In one setting or circumstance, standing up and speaking may be courageous while in another, keeping silent is an act of great moral courage. The capacity for wise deployment of the golden mean, according to Aristotle, is projected to create *eudaimonia*, or human flourishing. Although eudaimonia is sometimes translated to mean happiness, it instead represents an evolved human condition and is the aim of this practical, applied approach to human moral development.

An Ethic of Caring

Another variant of virtue-based ethics, *an ethic of caring*, is common in professional nursing and thus deserves particular note. In many ways, it is difficult for contemporary nurses to fully appreciate the radical departure from previous ways of thinking that Gilligan's (1982) ground-breaking work offered. Aptly titled *In a Different Voice*, Gilligan challenged notions originally promulgated by Kohlberg (1958, 1984), whose description of six stages of moral development was based on samples that were disproportionately male. Kohlberg's orientation conceived laws, rights, and justice as elements of the more evolved moral reasoning. When women were included in those studies, their moral reasoning was often defined as less sophisticated and developed. Gilligan (1982) questioned the moral theory development that had been dominated by studies of men and offered an alternative perspective that demonstrated ethical decision-making based on the values of caring and responsibility rather than abstract rules. She notes that when in relationship with others, we are often on a "trampoline" of competing demands and issues and proffers that a single "best" approach is not possible. Instead, "better" choices must satisfy (see https://youtu.be/2W_9MozRoKE?si=Sx4WEk8A84w98NgH for an interview with Carol Gilligan).

USING THESE MODELS IN CLINICAL DECISION-MAKING

Nurses employ moral reasoning in *everyday ethics*. These commonplace ethical issues may not be as dramatic as end-of-life or human genome decisions, but they are real and just as important, or even more important, because they are within the authority of the nurse to address directly. In the following scenario, Lou tries out different models to deal with an issue that is creating moral anxiety for her.

> Lou is not sure what to do. She thinks that one of the providers in her practice, Dr. Sampson, is upcoding, using billing codes that are reimbursed at higher levels than what Lou sees as the correct code for the care. Lou ponders what to do and recalls her class on ethical decision-making models. She likes Dr. Sampson and thinks that a moral reasoning involving caring would mean talking to Dr. Sampson. Unfortunately, this does not go well. Dr. Sampson says that the billing code is none of Lou's concern. Moreover, Dr. Sampson says that it is appropriate to be paid more. The consequence of not upcoding, argues Dr. Sampson, would mean that the practice would not have enough money to stay afloat, and many of their staff would lose their positions. Now Lou is even more confused. Could it be okay to upcode? She recalls that in virtue-based ethics, a virtuous person should know exactly what to do. Lou does not know what to do, or even what the options are, so she does not find virtue ethics to be a helpful guide in this particular situation.
>
> Lou recalls another model, consequence-oriented ethical decision-making, but she is also conflicted about the consequences. Yes, there is the local impact on the practice, but what about the impact on the patients who are being billed at higher levels than they should be? One consequence is higher taxes and insurance premiums; in addition, patients with larger deductibles and copayments would be directly financially impacted. In other words, it is not a victimless crime. Lou now turns to rule-based ethical decision-making. "What is the rule?" Lou wonders. "Clearly, provider upcoding as a universal principle is not acceptable." Lou decides that more information might guide her. She searches the web and finds that upcoding is actually illegal and is considered a form of fraud. Lou now feels confident that she has something to help her through this situation. She checks the whistleblower protection in her health system and is pleased to find it intact and that it will support her taking action. Lou contacts the state board of nursing for assistance in navigating the reporting of this illegal practice.
>
> (See Coustasse et al., 2021, for additional information on upcoding, including findings that upcoding fraud and abuse is increasing, not decreasing. Joiner et al. [2024] found upcoding for physician services to be much greater than hospital services, $2.38 billion versus $656 million, respectively, and higher yet in Medicare Advantage at $10 to $15 billion.)

In this scenario, the ethical issue quickly turned into a legal one as well, perhaps making a rule-based ethical approach logical. Legal dimensions, however, are not always the case in ethical dilemmas. Larson (2013), for example, suggests that the top ethical issue in health care is balancing care quality and efficiency. Yet in some cases, parameters that are designed to support high-quality outcomes instead create quality and ethical conflicts

(Rambur et al., 2013). These authors detail metric-driven harm resulting from provider behavior that focuses the patient's care on achieving a metric rather than on taking the whole of the patient's preferences into consideration, a scenario that is incentivized when metrics are linked to payment of a physician or hospital. The 2014 Veterans Affairs scandal is a high-profile example. Rather than correctly reporting the inappropriately long wait times that veterans seeking service faced, a shadow set of publicly recorded reports manipulated the data to meet financially rewarding targets (Hicks, 2014). Metric-driven harm can, however, be even more subtle. Consider the example of Sam, another RN:

> *Sam is confused. As a new team leader in a large multispecialty practice affiliated with a hospital, he is puzzled to see the magnitude of routine PSA-based screening on the organizational list of quality metrics. He had assumed that the metric triggers would be irrefutable. Yet, although not an uncommon screening practice, there is longstanding evidence of overuse of such screening (Kalavacherla et al., 2023), typically driven by physicians rather than patients (Guo & He, 2015) Sam understands that the quality metrics are intended to drive behavior and will. Sam knows that the need to report on this metric will cause more providers to order PSA-based screening for prostate cancer. On the surface, this may seem like an acceptable action, but his review of the literature causes Sam to question if routine prostate specific antigen (PSA) screening is indeed a best practice or even evidence based. Sam is particularly concerned about routine screening of males over age 70, given mounting evidence of its overuse, overdiagnosis, and unnecessary treatments that may be harmful (Kensler et al., 2024). Sam uneasily wonders if this so-called quality measure may actually harm more than help. Sam is experiencing ethical tension.*
>
> *Sam needs help to sort this out, so he contacts a mentor within the organization. The mentor, speaking in confidence, states that the organization has been pushing this routine screening since hiring a new urologist and purchasing a new robot for robotic-assisted surgery. Sam ponders the potential patient outcomes, incontinence and impotence, for example, and is profoundly troubled. He decides to bring his concern about screening-induced overtreatment and downstream cascades of unnecessary care to his leadership team.*
>
> *Sam's meeting with the senior team does not go well. The consensus of the group, without reviewing the literature, is that routine PSA screening is an established practice. Sam also considers the profitable business cascade of care the screening yields but is shut out of the conversation. Sam feels both a sense of not knowing what to do, a moral dilemma between two somewhat unattractive alternatives, and also moral distress. Sam recalls the fundamental principle of nonmaleficence but feels totally stuck on how to resolve this dilemma. (See Box 9.1 for a definition of moral distress.)*

> **BOX 9.1**
>
> **WHAT IS MORAL DISTRESS?**
>
> Austin (2007) suggests that "*moral distress* distinguishes moral dilemma[s]—situations of not knowing how to act—from what is experienced when one believes one knows how to act but is thwarted by constraints. There is a sense of being morally responsible, but unable to change what is happening" (p. 84, emphasis in the original).

Note to the reader: In previous editions of this text, this scenario originally detailed routine screening mammography in an ACO. The rationale for illustration of mammography is massive evidence that details overscreening-driven harm and the commonplace nature of mammography as a payment metric. But in 2024, the US Preventive Services Task Force (2024) doubled down on their stance, recommending mammograms every other year, from age 40 to 74 rather than starting at age 50. Lown Institute has explicated the benefits and harms of this shift, noting that, without screening, 28 women of 1,000 will die of breast cancer, with only eight deaths avoided because of screening. Screening also yields 1,540 false positives, 210 unnecessary biopsies, 12 cases of overdiagnosis, and no reduction in overall mortality (Gerber, 2024) The author of this text remains concerned about this universal application of this practice and invites the reader to review the following: Gerber as well as Bleyer and Welch (2012), Keating and Pace (2018), Miller et al. (2014), Richman et al. (2023), and Welch and Frankel (2011) as well as other evidence on overscreening and its harm. The scenario in this text was switched to one in which the evidence against routine screening is unequivocal, yet continues, with an aim of illustrating the link among measurement, payment, ethics and nurse well-being.

MORAL DISTRESS

The confluence of rapid change, limitations in nurses' authority span, and providers' education and socialization to maximize treatment has created a phenomenon notable among nurses termed *moral distress*. Moral distress differs from a *moral dilemma* in which the individual does not know what to do when caught between two or more equally dubious avenues. Instead, moral distress occurs when an individual feels morally confident about a certain action but is unable to enact reconciling change due to power differentials or other organizational issues.

Contributing elements in producing moral distress include finances, power differences between disciplines, and conflicting goals and philosophies among health care providers (Corley, 2002; Sporrong et al., 2006). Hospital nurses' moral distress during COVID-19, with associated longer-term health consequences, have also been identified (Lake et al., 2022). It has also been suggested that moral tensions and strain can impel actions that modify the working environment and create moral well-being, or *moral eustress*, within a more *virtuous organization* (Rambur et al., 2010). In such a scenario, the nurse brings knowledge, skills, and experience to create organizational or systems change to better align the milieu with an informed moral compass and, in so doing, also improves the organization.

ETHICS AND CLINICAL DECISION-MAKING DURING PANDEMICS

The COVID-19 pandemic that started early in 2020 raised issues many U.S. clinicians never expected to face: Who receives lifesaving equipment and care in cases of inadequate supply? Who receives the vaccines and when? Although the mismatch between demand and services is an all-too-common experience in some developing countries, the scale and scope of shortages of ventilators, personnel, vaccines, and other lifesaving care were unprecedented in the United States. Nevertheless, the issue of distribution of ventilators was deliberated in the state of New York—the state with initially the most cases of COVID-19 and potentially at risk for other viral outbreaks due to its population density—long before the pandemic. The result was a 2015 report developed by the New York State Task Force on Life and the Law and the New York State Department of Health. The 272-page document addressed how to ethically allocate limited resources and included separate chapters on adults, children, and neonates (Zucker et al., 2015). In the height of the pandemic, additional clarification on fair allocation of resources was detailed (Emanuel et al., 2020). These authors promulgated a framework with overarching ethical guiding principles to guide allocation (i.e., rationing) of scarce resources, which can be summarized as follows:

1. *Maximize benefits*: This principle recognizes that although saving the most lives is valued, so too is saving the most "life-years." This later consideration—life-years—incorporates acknowledgment of prognosis as well as age and underlying health status. Application of this principle results in lower priority being given to those who are unlikely to benefit from treatment as well as those who are likely to recover without use of a scarce resource. Instead, the highest priority for receiving scarce equipment or treatment will go to those most likely to benefit from treatment.

2. *Treat people equally*: This principle recognizes that serving those who were sick first at the expense of those who were sick later is not the most ethical approach to allocation of scarce resources. Among patients with a similar prognosis, random selection should be used to determine who receives treatment. Principle 1, maximize benefit, would remain in place in this consideration. Moreover, pandemic patients are not inherently of higher priority for treatment. Instead, fair allocation requires that benefits of treatment must be considered across all patients. Thus, a patient with

heart failure is not inherently a lower priority for treatment with scarce resources than one afflicted with the virus. In other words, the principles are applied to all populations of patients, not just pandemic patients at the expense of others, with a similar likelihood of survival with treatment.

3. *Reward those with "instrumental value"*: Instrumental value refers to those who have made relevant contributions to the pandemic during the crisis or are likely to in the future. Application of this principle makes treatment of health care workers and research participants a high priority, given their centrality in addressing the pandemic. Emanuel et al. (2020) note that the priority placed on health care workers and pandemic research subjects is not because they are inherently more worthy than other people, but instead because more people will suffer if they are not treated. Moreover, this approach is essential to minimize absenteeism of providers who may otherwise be even more concerned about their health and the risks they are taking by being frontline providers. The principle also underscores the importance of not abusing the guidelines by giving treatment to wealthy, famous, or powerful people above first responders and health care workers. Finally, prioritizing care for research participants testing vaccines and therapeutics is only as a "tiebreaker" (Emanuel et al., 2020, p. 6) among people with similar prognoses.

4. *Give priority to those who are most sick, but only when it aligns with maximizing benefits:* Applying this principle, with all other things equal, gives priority to those who are most sick but also to the young/otherwise healthy to maximize benefits like preventing the spread of the virus.

Taken as a whole, these guidelines provide a moral compass and refuge to support decision-making in times of crises like a pandemic. Yet they are not without pain. Emanuel et al. (2020) poignantly noted:

> Because maximizing benefits is paramount in a pandemic, we believe that removing a patient from a ventilator or an ICU bed to provide t to others in need is also justifiable and that the patient should be made aware of this possibility at admission. Undoubtedly, withdrawing ventilators or ICU support from [a] patient who arrived earlier to save those with better prognoses will be extremely psychologically traumatic for clinicians—and some may refuse to do so. However, many guidelines agree that decisions to withdraw a scarce resource to save others is not an act of killing and does not require [the] patient's consent. (p. 5)

As the pandemic evolved, the focus shifted to vaccine allocation, and over time, other ethical considerations will surely arise. Understanding these principles and being prepared to apply them in any cases of scarce resources requiring rationing join the longer-standing ethical principles previously detailed. Berlinger et al. describe the central tension well. They state:

> An ethically sound framework for healthcare during public health emergencies must balance the patient-centered duty of care—the focus of clinical ethics under normal conditions—with public-focused duties to promote equality of persons and equity

in distribution of risks and benefits in society—the focus of public health ethics. Because physicians, nurses, and other clinicians are trained to care for individuals, the shift from patient-centered practice to patient care guided by public health considerations creates great tension, especially for clinicians unaccustomed to working under emergency conditions with scarce resources. (Berlinger et al., 2020, para 1)

They further illustrate the strategies used as the delivery care environment degraded (see Figure 9.1).

Consider the interactions among these domains. For example, if there are ample material supplies but too few to use them, for example, too few nurses, a scenario of scarcity exists despite ample supplies. Workforce development is a contemporary issue with both ethical and economic domains and will be detailed in Chapter 14. Although many younger readers may not have been in practice at the time of the pandemic, conditions of scarcity will surely arise again whether through natural means such as the next pandemic or declining revenues for an aging population with extensive health care needs.

Pandemics, Ethics, and Economics

The COVID-19 pandemic also highlighted the intersection of ethics and economics, with leading ethicists debating a once-unthinkable question in an article titled "Restarting America Means People Will Die. So When Do We

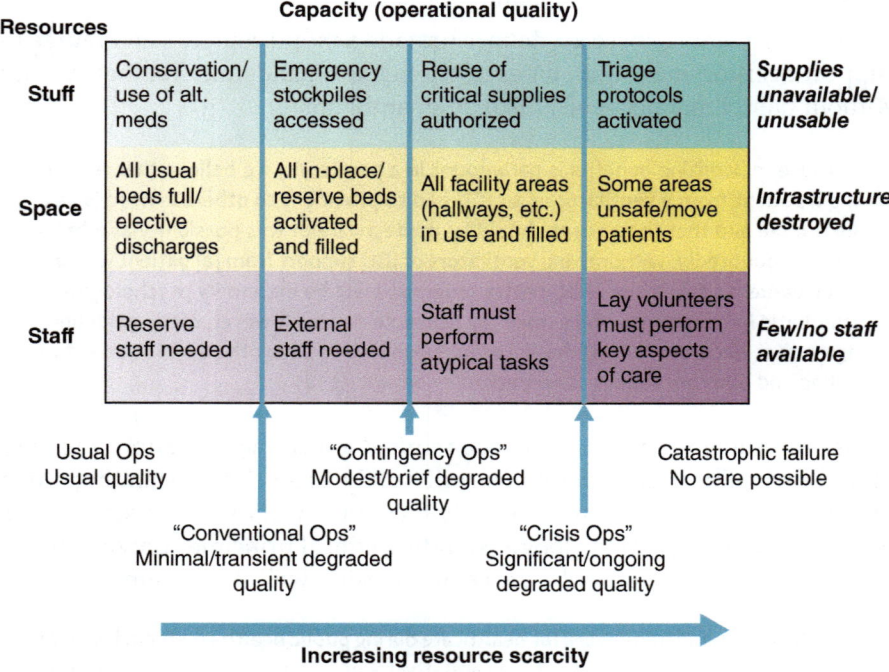

FIGURE 9.1: Resource scarcity.

Do It?" (Bazelon et al., 2020). Recognizing the differentially negative impacts of a closed economy on the poor as well as poor nations, Singer states: "Yes, people will die if we open up, but the consequences of not opening up are so severe that maybe we've got to do it anyway. If we keep it locked down, then more younger people are going to die because they're basically not going to get enough to eat or other basics" (para 12). In other words, issues of ethics and economics are always intertwined, and it is essential that nurses develop the moral muscle and economic acumen to navigate the complexities this interdigitation brings.

Finally, the pandemic educed many examples that described moral distress. One notable example is illustrated in the actions of the captain of the U.S. nuclear aircraft carrier *Theodore Roosevelt*, Captain Brett Crozier. Cozier broke rank, violating the military "chair of command" rules. He sent a desperate plea for the safety of the men aboard his ship to a higher-ranking official after he failed to obtain what he perceived as a suitable response from his own commanding officer. Arguably, it appears that he felt he knew what to do, what conduct constituted moral conduct, but was unable to execute this due to hierarchical power constraints—the very situation that breeds moral distress. Crozier was removed from his command but retained vigorous support from the hundreds of sailors on board who viewed him as "putting their safety ahead of his career" (Cooper et al., 2020, para 1). In summary, moral action is not always easy or clear-cut. Yet nurses hold an ethical obligation to develop ever more complex moral authority over the course of their career, just as other essential knowledge, skills, and abilities are developed through formal study, work with a mentor, trial and error, and application in progressively more complex situations.

ETHICS OF REFORM AND COST CONTAINMENT

The heretofore-described examples illustrate ethical issues at the intersection of clinical practice, global events, organizational culture, and market incentives. Other ethical issues are more deeply embedded in U.S. health care financing and delivery models. Saloner and Daniels (2011), for example, argue that the ethics of affordable health care coverage are rooted in "a societal obligation to protect fair *equality of opportunity*" (p. 816, emphasis added). This equality of opportunity has two major components. The first relates to the protection of health and normal functioning, so the individual has the basic opportunity to participate in society. The second aspect is financial protection, that is, ensuring that health care costs do not disproportionately erode opportunities for some, thus violating the ethical principle of fairness. Contrast, for example, the impact of an overall health care cost burden (premiums and out-of-pocket) of $10,000 for an individual who makes $30,000 per year with the impact of the same cost burden on someone making $200,000 per year.

For the low-wage worker, the impact of the cost of health care is pronounced and erodes fair opportunity. These authors conclude that the Affordable Care Act is a corrective strategy in the right direction but note that cost containment and alternative strategies that more equally distribute the cost burden, such as a more progressive tax structure, are necessary. By extension, care that is unnecessary creates cost without value and is therefore unethical. Thus, using Sam's dilemma as an example, everything we do—or do not do—matters.

Waste in the U.S. System

Unnecessary care and overtreatment are just one category of waste in the U.S. system. Berwick and Hackbarth's classic 2012 work identifies the following forms of waste as representing 18% to 37% of health care spending: failures of care delivery, failures of care coordination, administrative complexity, pricing failures, and overtreatment. When fraud and abuse are added, including such things as the upcoding example, the cost to the U.S. health system is estimated to range from 21% to a whopping 47%, with a midpoint estimate of 34%—just over one-third of U.S. health care spending (see Figure 9.2, adapted from Berwick & Hackbarth, 2012). In the ensuing years, little has changed. Shrank et al. (2019) place current estimates of waste at 25%, *excluding administrative complexities*, suggesting little improvement in eliminating waste and its associated costs (see Figure 9.3). The Lown Institute reports that over 100,000 unnecessary surgeries were performed in the first year of COVID-19 alone (Toleos, 2022) and further report the inappropriate use of stents costing

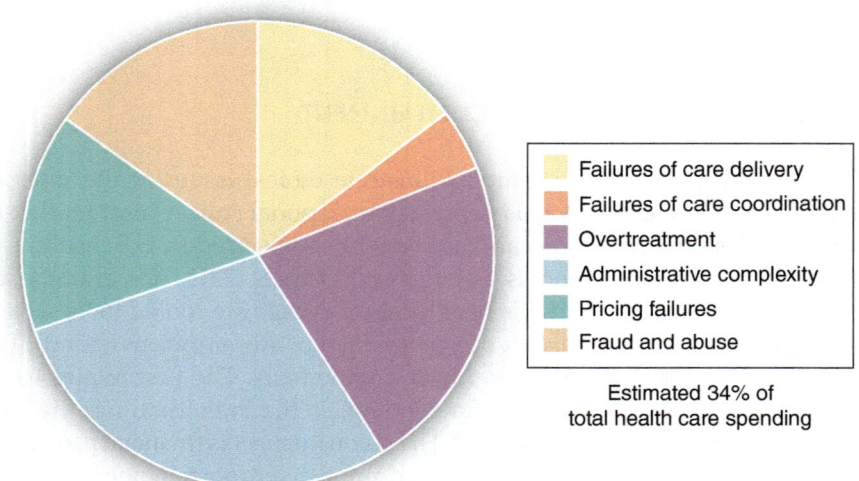

FIGURE 9.2: Waste estimate in U.S. health care spending (2011).

Source: Adapted from Berwick, D., & Hackbarth, A. (2012). Eliminating waste in U.S. health care. *Journal of the American Medical Association*, *307*(14), 1513–1516.

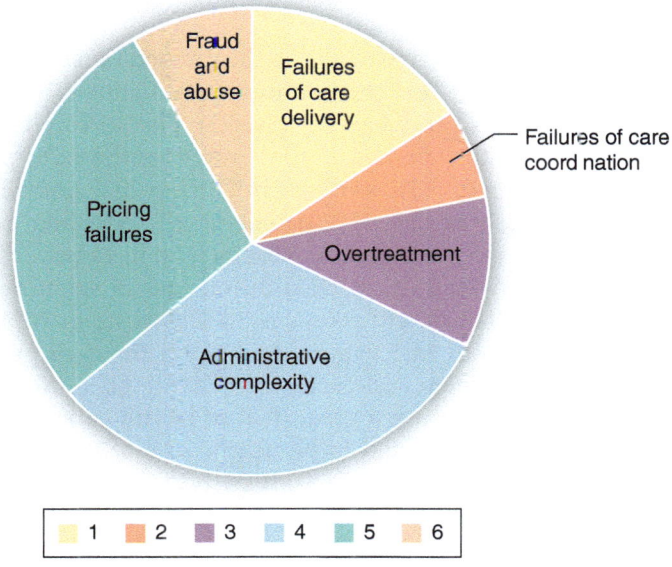

FIGURE 9.3: Waste estimate update.

Note: 1: $102.4B–$165.7B; 2: $27.2B–78.2B; 3: $75.7B–101.2B; 4: Administrative complexity $265.6B; 5: Pricing Failures 230.7–240.5B; 6: Fraud & Abuse 58.5–83.9B.

The figure represents the midpoint of the range, with the exception of administrative complexity, for which only a single data point was provided, for a total of $769 billion to $925 billion, or roughly 25% of U.S. health care costs.

Source: Adapted from Shrank, W., Rogstad, T., & Parekh, N. (2019). Waste in the U.S. health care system: Estimated cost and potential for savings. *JAMA, 322*(15), 1501–1509.

Medicare (and thus the people of this nation) $800 million per year (Toleos, 2023). These direct costs are amplified by the addition of the emotional costs to patients and their families and untold costs related to shifting resources to this procedure rather than where it clearly can make a difference.

Overdiagnosis and overtreatment impact a broad swath of conditions. McCarthy et al. (2024), for example, proffer that myocardial infarction is overdiagnosed, with resulting emotional and other negative consequences for patients. Clearly, nurses' involvement in care coordination, re-envisioned and redesigned care delivery, and focused attention to prevent overtreatment are essential elements of *role fidelity* in the current era. (See Box 9.2 to review a definition of role fidelity.)

 BOX 9.2

WHAT IS ROLE FIDELITY?

Role fidelity is an ethical principle that requires a practitioner to practice faithfully within the professional role (Edge & Groves, 1999).

SUSTAINABILITY IS AN ETHICAL ISSUE

Another area of ethical challenge relates to the financial sustainability of the current health care system. The gross domestic product (GDP) is a measure of all goods and services produced by a nation. Health care expenditures have grown faster than the average annual growth of the GDP, projected to grow at an average rate of 5.5% per year in 2018 to 2027 and reach nearly $6 trillion by 2027, nearly double the 2017 spend of $3.5 trillion, a figure that is already double that in other wealthy nations who have better health outcomes. Overall, there have been marked differences in spending per year. In 2020, for example, the growth rate was 10.3%, while in 2021, expenditures increased by 2.7% to $4.3 trillion, or $12,914 for each person in the nation (Centers for Medicare and Medicaid [CMS], 2023). Recall that this is an average; some people use a great deal of health care; others less so. Health care spending is projected to be nearly 20% of the total U.S. GDP by 2027 (CMS, n.d.). Imagine this in your own budget: 20 cents of every dollar going to health care, leaving only 80 cents for everything else. This, in turn, erodes opportunity for an array of choices that may have more personal value, particularly given the mixed outcomes of health care. And, as previously noted, it diminishes the fair equality of opportunity principle described earlier.

U.S. health care costs have long been recognized as unsustainable (Ginsburg et al., 2012; Millenson, 2018; Roy, 2023) and currently are recognized as a substantial contributor to the federal budget deficit. In response, the Federal Reserve chair, representing an organization that typically deals with financial regulation and monetary policy, noted: "…we've been on an unsustainable fiscal path for a long time . . . and there's no hiding from it" (Powell, cited in Wolff-Mann, 2018, para 2). It is thus logical to assume that what cannot be sustained will not be sustained. This raises questions about the impact of today's health care choices on future generations. Arguably, sustainability is not just important; it is actually an ethical principle that should guide health care. Fundamental flaws in the sustainability of the U.S. health care system were further revealed in the COVID-19 pandemic. This will be explicated in Chapter 13.

Ethical Principles to Augment Traditional Principles of Health Care Ethics

Taken as a whole, the examples throughout this section illustrate both the usefulness and shortcomings of traditional principles of health care ethics such as autonomy, beneficence, and nonmaleficence in the contemporary health care era, as well as the challenges in using ethical decision-making models to guide action. Accounting for decision-making not only at the individual level but also by society at large—both at the time of service and also over intergenerational time—is conceptually taxing. Nevertheless, such *full cost accounting* has been applied to fields outside of health care for decades, and several aspects of the *science of sustainability* (Costanza et al., 1997) offer parameters that translate to health care with ease. These include economic efficiency and distributional equity. The concept of distributional equity can be best understood by way of the obverse concept of distribution inequity: For example, the combined wealth of the world's 2,153 billionaires is greater than that of the bottom 4.65 billion people who constitute roughly 60% of the world's total population (Lawson et al., 2020). In the United States, 66.6% of the total wealth in the United States was owned by the top 10% of earners, and the lowest 50% of earners owned 2.6% of the total wealth (Statista, 2023).

A third element of the science of sustainability includes expanded accountability horizons. Translating this concept to health care, providers are responsible not just to the person in front of them but also for the cost of the care and the impact on unseen others, with the responsibility to maintain human well-being—individual and collective—over intergenerational time. Population health perspectives in some payment reform models have begun to nudge providers in this direction, as do organizational and policy changes toward a more just society. But how does an individual nurse begin to take action?

NURSES ON BOARDS AND IN POLITICS

One avenue for nurses to create such organizational change is through hospital and health care governance board membership. Indeed, the highly influential *The Future of Nursing* (2010) report by the Institute of Medicine (2010) (now called the National Academy of Science) called for more nurses on boards in order to better serve the public through more direct inclusion of nursing knowledge at the governance and/or policy level. In response, a Nurses on Board Collation was launched (see https://www.nursesonboardscoalition.org/). Board membership alters power dynamics and can remove the differentials that often impede nurses' full participation in needed change. Previous chapters have reviewed essential knowledge for nurses' membership on boards, such as payment models as well as ethical frameworks and rationales for these efforts. Nevertheless, nurses continue to hold only a small fraction of board seats. Many nurses may be unfamiliar with the structure and functions of boards and, importantly, how to gain access to board positions. These topics are the focus of Chapters 10 and 11, followed by a review of the political process in Chapter 12.

End-of-Chapter Resources

THOUGHT QUESTIONS

1. What tools can nurses use to ensure that the care they are involved in is necessary?
2. Imagine a scenario in which you, the RN, perceive the patient to be receiving care of little value. What do you do? What ethical principles and decision-making approaches can help guide your actions?
3. Have you experienced moral distress in a work setting? What elements of the environment contributed? What organizational, structural, or other changes could have alleviated your distress?
4. Imagine you are working in a setting that is chronically short-staffed, and you worry that patient safety is compromised. What ethical principles are in conflict? Now develop a strategy for addressing this situation, using the previously described ethical decision-making models. Which ones are most useful?

EXERCISES

1. Develop a presentation for your peers that details why cost containment, managing waste and overtreatment, and health reform are issues of ethics. Use ethics terminology.
2. Describe the process you would use to develop a plan to direct the use of scarce resources during a pandemic or other time of crisis or scarcity.

QUIZ

True or False

1. One common example of nurses using consequence-oriented ethical decision-making is triage.
2. The American Nurses Association has published a *Code of Ethics for Nurses*.
3. Another term for consequence-oriented ethical decision-making is deontology.
4. Moral eustress is another term for moral well-being following successful resolution of a situation of moral tension.
5. Gilligan's *ethic of caring* counters studies of moral reasoning that had been developed primarily using males as research subjects.

6. Rawls's approach to moral reasoning is defined as creating the greatest good for the greatest number of people.
7. Nurses use a variety of different ethical decision-making models in clinical settings.
8. One challenge with consequence-oriented ethical decision-making is that the individual may be harmed in an effort to maximize the good of the many.
9. The term deontology is derived from the Greek term for *duty*.
10. Virtue ethics focuses on consequences and rule-based decision-making.

Multiple Choice

11. Elements of Rawls's theory of justice include
    A. Decision-making from the *original position* within a *veil of ignorance*
    B. An emphasis on classic Aristotelian values such as courage
    C. Both A and B
    D. Neither A nor B
12. Moral distress
    A. Is the same as a moral dilemma
    B. Can occur when an individual feels morally confident about the most appropriate route of action but is thwarted from taking that action due to a power differential or organizational issues
    C. Both A and B
    D. Neither A nor B
13. The science of sustainability includes which of the following concepts?
    A. Distributional equity
    B. Expanded accountability horizons
    C. Both A and B
    D. Neither A nor B
14. Kohlberg's six stages of moral development suggest that the highest stages of moral development are rooted in
    A. Laws and rights
    B. Caring
    C. Both A and B
    D. Neither A nor B
15. Virtue ethics
    A. Provides clear guidelines on how to proceed in morally challenging situations
    B. Focuses on character development
    C. Both A and B
    D. Neither A nor B

NOTE

1. This situation also represents what is termed "missed care," which has been documented to create moral distress for nurses and poorer outcomes for patients and fuel nurse turnover. It will be discussed in greater detail in Chapter 14 on the workforce.

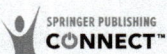 A robust set of instructor resources designed to supplement this text is located at http://connect.springerpub.com/content/book/978-0-8261-7236-5. Qualifying instructors may request access by emailing **textbook@springerpub.com**.

REFERENCES

American Nurses Association. (2015). *Code of ethics for nurses with interpretative statements*. Author.

Atomic Archive. (n.d.). *The atomic bombings of Hiroshima and Nagasaki*. Retrieved May 28, 2024, from http://www.atomicarchive.com/Docs/MED/med_chp10.shtml

Austin, W. (2007). The ethics of everyday practice: Healthcare environments as moral communities. *Advances in Nursing Science, 30*(1), 81–88. https://doi.org/10.1097/00012272-200701000-00009

Bazelon, E., Barber, W. J., Case, A., Emanuel, Z., Gupta, V., & Singer, S. (2020, April 10). *Restarting America means people will die. So when do we do it?* The New York Times Magazine. https://www.nytimes.com/2020/04/10/magazine/coronavirus-economy-debate

Berlinger, N., Wynia, M., Powell, T., Hester, M., Milliken, A., Fabi, R., Cohn, F., Guidry-Grimes, L., Carlin Watson, J., Bruce, L., Chuang, E., Oei, G., Abbott, J., & Piper Jenks, N. (2020). *Ethical Framework for Health Care Institutions & Guidelines for Institutional Ethics Services Responding to the Coronavirus Pandemic*. The Hastings Center. https://www.thehastingscenter.org/ethicalfmeworkcovid19/ra

British Broadcasting Corporation. (2012). *Fact file: Hiroshima and Nagasaki*. WW2 People's War. Retrieved August 8, 2013, from http://www.bbc.co.uk/history/ww2peopleswar/timeline/factfiles/nonflash/a6652262.shtml

Berwick, D., & Hackbarth, A. (2012). Eliminating waste in U.S. health care. *Journal of the American Medical Association, 307*(14), 1513–1516. https://doi.org/10.1001/jama.2012.362

Bleyer, A., & Welch, H. G. (2012). Effects of three decades of screening mammography on breast-cancer incidence. *New England Journal of Medicine, 367*, 1998–2005. https://doi.org/10.1056/NEJMoa1206809

Centers for Medicare and Medicaid. (2023). *National health expenditures: Historical*. https://www.cms.gov/data-research/statistics-trends-and-reports/national-health-expenditure-data/historical

Centers for Medicare and Medicaid. (n.d.). *National health expenditure projections 2018–2027*. https://www.cms.gov/Research-Statistics-Data-and-Systems/Statistics-Trends-and-Reports/NationalHealthExpendData/Downloads/ForecastSummary.pdf

Cooper, H., Schmitt, E., & Gibbons-Neff, T. (2020, April 15). *Navy may reinstate fired captain to command of Roosevelt?* New York Times.

https://www.nytimes.com/2020/04/15/us/politics/coronavirus-navy-roosevelt-crozier.html

Corley, M. (2002). Nurse moral distress: A proposed theory and research agenda. *Nursing Ethics, 9*(6), 636–650. https://doi.org/10.1191/0969733002ne557oa

Costanza, C., Cumberland, J., Daly, H., Goodland, R., & Norgaard, R. (1997). *An introduction to ecological economics.* CRC Press.

Coustasse, A., Layton, W., Nelson, L., & Walker, V. (2021). Upcoding Medicare: Is healthcare fraud and abuse increasing? *Perspectives in Health Information Management, 18*(4), 1f. https://www.ncbi.nlm.nih.gov/pmc/articles/PMC8649706/

Edge, R., & Groves, J. (1999). *Ethics of health care: A guide for clinical practice.* Delmar.

Emanuel, E. J., Persad, G., Upshur, R., Thorne, B., Parker, M., Glickman, A., Zhang, C., Boyle, C., Smith, M., & Philips, J. P. (2020). Fair allocation of scarce medical resources in the time of Covid-19. *The New England Journal of Medicine, 382*(21), 2049–2055. https://doi.org/10.1056/NEJMsb2005114

Gerber, J. (2024, May 1). *The benefits and harms of early screening for breast cancer.* Lown Institute. https://lowninstitute.org/update-the-benefits-and-harms-of-earlier-screening-for-breast-cancer/

Gilligan, C. (1982). *In a different voice: Psychological theory and women's development.* Harvard University Press.

Ginsburg, P., Hughes, M., Adler, L., Burke, S., Hoagland, G., Jennings, C., & Lieberman, S. (2012). *What is driving U.S. health care spending: America's unsustainable health care cost growth.* Robert Wood Johnson Foundation, Bipartisan Policy Center.

Guo, F., & He, D. (2015). The roles of providers and patients in the overuse of prostate-specific antigen screening in the United States. *Annals of Internal Medicine, 163*(8), 650–651. https://doi.org/10.7326/L15-5150

Hicks, J. (2014). *This memo shows that the VA knew of record manipulation in 2010.* Washington Post. Retrieved September 24, 2014, from http://www.washingtonpost.com/blogs/federal-eye/wp/2014/05/20/this-memo-shows-that-the-va-knew-of-records-manipulation-in-2010/

Institute of Medicine. (2010). *The future of nursing: Leading change, advancing health.* National Academies Press.

Joiner, K. A., Lin, J., & Pantano, J. (2024). Upcoding in Medicare: Where does it matter most? *Health Economics Review, 14*(1), 1. https://doi.org/10.1186/s13561-023-00465-4

Kalavacherla, S., Riviere, P., Javier-DesLoges, J., Banegas, M. P., McKay, R. R., Murphy, J. D., & Rose, B. S. (2023). Low-value prostate-specific antigen screening in older males. *JAMA Network Open, 6*(4), e237504. https://doi.org/10.1001/jamanetworkopen.2023.7504

Keating, N., & Pace, L. (2018). Breast cancer screening in 2018: Time for shared decision making. *JAMA Insights, 319*(10), 1814–1815. https://doi.org/10.1001/jama.2018.3388

Kensler, K. H., Mao, J., & Davuluri, M. (2024). Frequency of guideline-discordant prostate cancer screening among older males. *JAMA Network Open, 7*(4), e248487. https://doi.org/10.1001/jamanetworkopen.2024.8487

Kohlberg, L. (1958). *The development of models of thinking and choices in years 10 to 16.* PhD dissertation, University of Chicago, Chicago, IL.

Kohlberg, L. (1984). *The psychology of moral development: The nature and validity of moral stages—Essays on moral development* (Vol. 2). Harper and Row.

Lake, E. T., Narva, A. M., Holland, S., Smith, J. G., Cramer, E., Rosenbaum, K. E. F., French, R., Clark, R. R. S., & Rogowski, J. A. (2022). Hospital nurses' moral distress and mental health during COVID-19. *Journal of Advanced Nursing, 78*(3), 799–809. https://doi.org/10.1111/jan.15013

Larson, J. (2013). *Five top ethical issues in health care.* AMN Healthcare News. Retrieved September 24, 2014, from www.amnhealthcare.com/latest-healthcare-news/five-top-ethical-issues-healthcare

Lawson, M., Parvez Butt, A., Harvey, Sarosi, R., Coffey, C., Piaget, K., & / Thekkudan, J. (2020, January 20). *Time to care: Unpaid and underpaid care work and the global inequality crisis.* Oxfam International. www.oxfam.org/en/research/time-care

McCarthy, C., Wasfy, J., & Januzzi, J. (2024). Is myocardial infarction overdiagnosed? *JAMA Network Open, 331*(19), 1623–1624. https://doi.org/10.1001/jama.2024.5235

Millenson, M. (2018, September 12). *Half a century of health care crisis (and still going strong).* Health Affairs Forefront. www.healthaffairs.org/do/10.1377/hblog20180904.457305/full

Miller, A., Wall, C., Baines, C., Sun, P., To, T., & Narod, S. (2014). Twenty-five year follow-up for breast cancer incidence and mortality of the Canadian National Breast Screening Study: Randomised screening trial. *British Medical Journal, 348,* g366. https://doi.org/10.1136/bmj.g366

Rambur, B., Vallett, C., Cohen, J., & Tarule, J. (2010). The moral cascade: Distress, eustress, and the virtuous. *Journal of Organizational Moral Psychology, 1*(1), 41–54. https://www.researchgate.net/publication/230641764_The_moral_cascade_Distress_eustress_and_the_virtuous_organization

Rambur, B., Vallett, C., Cohen, J., & Tarule, J. (2013). Metric-driven harm: An exploration of unintended consequences of performance measurement. *Applied Nursing Research, 26*(4), 269–275. https://doi.org/10.1016/j.apnr.2013.09.001

Rawls, J. (1999). *A theory of justice.* Harvard University Press

Rawls, J. (2001). In E. Kelly (Ed.), *Justice as fairness: A restatement.* Belknap Press.

Roy, A. (2023). *Key findings from the 2022 World Index of Healthcare Innovation.* https://freopp.org/key-findings-from-the-2022-world-index-of-healthcare-innovation-e2a772f55b92

Richman, I. B., Long, J. B., Soulos, P. R., Wang, S. Y., & Gross, C. P. (2023). Estimating breast cancer overdiagnosis after screening mammography among older women in the United States. *Annals of Internal Medicine, 176*(9), 1172–1180. https://doi.org/10.7326/M23-0133

Saloner, B., & Daniels, N. (2011). The ethics of the affordability of health insurance. *Journal of Health Politics, Policy and Law, 36*(5), 816–827. https://doi.org/10.1215/03616878-1407631

Sporrong, S., Hoglund, A., & Arnetz, B. (2006). Measuring moral distress in pharmacy and clinical practice. *Nursing Ethics, 13*(4), 416–427. https://doi.org/10.1191/0969733006ne880oa

Shrank, W., Rogstad, T., & Parekh, N. (2019). Waste in the U.S. health care system: Estimated cost and potential for savings. *Journal of the American Medical Association, 322*(15), 1501–1509. https://doi.org/10.1001/jama.2019.13978

Statista. (2023, December 20). *US wealth distribution Q3 2023.* Author. https://www.statista.com/statistics/203961/wealth-distribution-for-the-us/

Toleos, A. (2022). *100,000 older Americans got unnecessary surgeries during dangerous first year of COVID-19*. Lown Institute. https://lowninstitute.org/press-release-100000-older-americans-got-unnecessary-surgeries-during-dangerous-first-year-of-covid-19/

Toleos, A. (2023). *Unnecessary coronary stents cost Medicare as much as 800 million/year*. Lown Institute. https://lowninstitute.org/press-release-unnecessary-coronary-stents-cost-medicare-as-much-as-800-million-per-year/

U.S. Preventive Services Task Force, Nicholson, W. K., Silverstein, M., Wong, J. B., Barry, M. J., Chelmow, D., Coker, T. R., Davis, E. M., Jaén, C. R., Krousel-Wood, M., Lee, S., Li, L., Mangione, C. M., Rao, G., Ruiz, J. M., Stevermer, J. J., Tsevat, J., Underwood, S. M., & Wiehe, S. (2024). Screening for breast cancer: US Preventive Services Task Force recommendation statement. *Journal of the American Medical Association, 331*(22), 1918–1930. https://doi.org/10.1101/jama.2024.5534

Welch, H. G., & Frankel, B. (2011). Likelihood that a woman with screen-detected breast cancer has had her "life saved" by that screening. *Archives of Internal Medicine, 17*(22), 2043–2046. https://doi.org/10.1001/archinternmed.2011.476

Wolff-Mann, E. (2018, September 26). *Powell: Our uniquely expensive healthcare system will catch up with us*. https://finance.yahoo.com/news/powell-uniquely-expensive-healthare-system-will-catch-us-212627406.html

Zucker, H., Adler, K., Berens, D., David Bleich, R. J., Brynner, R., Butler, K. A., Calderon, Y., Corcoran, C., Dubler, N., Edelson, P. J., Fins, J. J., Geer, F. H., Gorovitz, S., Henderson, C. E., Khouli, H., Koterski, J. W., Hugh Maynard-Reid, H., Murnane, J. D., Porter, K., . . . True, S. T. (2015, November). *Ventilator allocation guidelines*. New York State Department of Health Task Force on Life and the Law. https://nysba.org/app/uploads/2020/05/2015-ventilator_guidelines-NYS-Task-Force-Life-and-Law.pdf?srsltid=AfmBOor0a2bkb5eO8lvLPjd8wlfwFuIl53KpqR4cqilfLms4BKTxDQVh

SECTION IV

Pulling It All Together: Using Your Knowledge of Health Finance, Economics, and Ethics to Improve Health and Health Care

We have travelled through complex terrain together as we have navigated the twists, turns, and history of health care financing and reimbursement; plunged into deep waters of health care economics and what it means to nurses and to patients; and explored uses and limits of ethical theories to support moral reasoning and decision-making. You now have the knowledge to be an influential force not only in healthcare and in your practice, but also in the world more broadly. Nursing knowledge is necessary to shape health and healthcare beyond the borders of the bedside. But to do so, there are some additional pieces of information that are necessary.

First, understanding how institutions are organized and governed is essential for influencing change as well as maintaining things that are working well. Imagine trying to help a cardiac patient if you did not know how the heart worked. Chapter 10 discusses organizations and their governance. As noted in the preface to this text, the landmark *The Future of Nursing: Leading Change, Advancing Health* (Institute of Medicine, 2010) made important health care recommendations, including a plea for more nurses to serve on governing boards. You might wonder if this is to serve nursing. Not at all! It is to serve patients and society by bringing what nurses know to the highest level of decision-making and influence.

Nevertheless, comparatively little progress has been made in the decade since this report was released, with the proportion of hospital and health system board members who are nurses remaining constant at 5% over the last two decades (Kacik, 2022). Moreover, many nurses do not consider such roles for themselves or aspire to them. Do you? If not, Chapters 10 and 11 are dedicated to changing this. The goal is that you will consider such roles for yourself and mentor others to aspire and achieve as well. Research on nurses who serve on board has found that they perceive they "leverage expert knowledge of healthcare and caring wisdom to influence strategic thinking to meet stakeholder needs" (Sundean et al., 2022, p. 106). To do this, however, nurses need to access positions on boards.

Thus, Chapter 10 describes organizational types and differentiates between governance and management responsibilities. Because some of the readers of this text are undergraduate students seeking their first RN license, while others are more seasoned RNs seeking baccalaureate or graduate degrees, Chapter 10 laces in scenarios that describe organizational types from the perspective of a job seeker, in the hopes that the illustration will be useful to both the novice seeking a job and the seasoned professional exploring the pathways to the boardroom.

Chapter 11 describes the different routes to a board seat, reflecting different types of boards. It includes foundational information on how to run or participate in a meeting as well as a primer on financial terms you will hear in board meetings. Money is the language of power in the boardroom, so learn to speak it with authority.

But wait! Why stop with just board membership? Why not consider policy and politics? Chapter 12 provides information on ways to use all you have learned to be effectively involved in politics and influence health and health care policy.

Chapter 13 presents some lessons from COVID-19 and Chapter 14 augments this orientation with an emphasis on workforce implication and current dynamics impacting nurses. Chapter 15 concludes with some closing reflections and thoughts for your future direction and ongoing self-development in the areas of finance, economics, and politics. So, let us start by sorting out some key basics on organizations.

CHAPTER 10

Governance and Organizational Type

CHAPTER 10 describes an array of different board categories as well as their responsibilities. The intersection of governance and management is detailed, as well as common management structures nurses work within and lead from. Finally, types of organizations and their missions are described, to further the alignment between the individual nurse and selection of employment setting.

Following completion of this chapter, you will be able to

- Describe the role, responsibilities, and differences among categories of oversight boards.
- Detail the differences between governance and management.
- Illustrate common management structures.
- Describe the impact of the Sarbanes–Oxley Act on healthcare organizations.

> *Jennifer enjoys her work as a neonatal intensive care nurse. Nevertheless, she sometimes wonders if there might be an easier way to make a living. As she leaves the unit, she notices the chief executive officer (CEO) giving a tour to a group of individuals dressed in expensive suits. "Boy, that would be the life," she muses, "high salary and just walk around all day." She wonders how people access these positions.*

Jennifer likely doesn't understand the scope of responsibility of the CEO and how difficult such a position can be, despite generous compensation packages. Like much of the rest of the healthcare workforce, evidence suggests that health system CEOs turnover is increasing due to the strain of burnout (Muoio, 2023a).

Now that you know the broader dimensions of healthcare, you are ready to enact change and influence policy. Yet to do so, an understanding of organizational structure is necessary; influence cannot be leveraged without knowing what levers to push, who is responsible for what, and the manner in which an organization is "wired together." Let us start with the CEO and the governing board to which the CEO reports.

To a harried staff nurse or student, it may seem that the CEO stands far above the fray and has enormous unilateral power. Although it is true that the CEO has broad responsibilities, the CEO, too, has a boss. This "boss" is the board of trustees (BOT).

ROLE OF THE BOARD OF TRUSTEES

The role of the BOT is to ensure that the mission of the organization is met. Although healthcare organizations can be for profit or nonprofit, a definition offered by The National Council of Nonprofits is relevant for each of these categories:

> Board members are the fiduciaries who steer the organization towards a sustainable future by adopting sound, ethical, and legal governance and financial management policies, as well as by making sure the nonprofit has adequate resources to advance its mission. (National Council of Nonprofits, n.d., para 1)

They further define the role as providing "foresight, oversight, and insight" (para 3). A board member is expected to act in the best interest of the organization, with skill and due diligence. Indeed, board members may be sued for reckless or negligent behavior that harms an organization, a concept analogous to medical negligence or malpractice (see Box 10.1 for a description of *directors and operators liability insurance*, which provides protection to the board member in a manner analogous to medical malpractice insurance). Thus, when a wise nurse is a member of a governing board, they are

BOX 10.1

DIRECTORS AND OPERATORS LIABILITY INSURANCE

An individual accepting a high-level board position is well advised to ascertain if they are covered by "directors and operators liability insurance" (D and O insurance)—insurance that provides financial protection to a board member in the event that they are sued in relation to actions or inactions as a board member. In a small organization with a relatively small budget and few financial assets, it may not be necessary to have D and O insurance; at the same time, that leaves board members potentially liable. Generally, D and O insurance is not necessary when serving on an advisory board, which by its very nature does not have fiduciary responsibility for the organization. Similarly, membership on a state or federal board is again a bit different because actions are on behalf of that governmental entity, and thus there is protection for the board member through that entity. Contrast this, for example, with a hospital board in which a single board decision may mean multimillion- or even billion-dollar expenditures. Or, for example, failure to properly oversee a rogue CEO who causes harm to the institution could leave the board members liable for oversight failure. In these cases, D and O insurance would provide a form of insurance protection for financial liability, conceptually similar to medical malpractice insurance. Notably, the organization typically provides D and O insurance to board members, a likely essential approach in nonprofit boards where board members are not compensated for their time as board members.

thoughtful about board responsibilities and committed to giving the time and attention needed to be a diligent board member. At the same time, the reality of the responsibility should not be a deterrent to seeking board membership. No one board member has all the oversight skills necessary, which is why highly functioning boards are composed of individuals with diverse skills and perspectives.

Governance, Not Management

The board also hires the CEO, sets the CEO compensation package, reviews CEO performance, and—when necessary—removes the CEO. The board responsibility is *governance*, not *management*. Thus, beyond this oversight of the CEO, management is not within the purview of the BOT. Healthy organizations strike a balance whereby the board is neither overinvolved in management details that are the rightful responsibility of the management team nor merely rubber stamping governance activities for which they are responsible. Succession planning—planning to ensure continuity of leadership—is also an important but often overlooked responsibility of the board (Boardable, n.d.; Nadler et al., 2006), with PricewatershouseCooper (pwc) defining it as a core board responsibility for which *boards are often unprepared* for (PricewatershouseCooper [pwc], n.d., emphasis added). One avenue for succession planning is to build "bench strength" among the senior leadership team. However, management of the senior leadership team is a management issue, rather than a governance issue, illustrating one challenge to the succession planning responsibility of the board.

Impact of Organizational Type

Because the work of the board is to ensure that the mission of the organization is met, organizations with different missions have different board orientations. Although this is important to understand when seeking to gain influence through board membership, organizational type impacts all elements of the work of the institution. Therefore, it is valuable to consider organizational mission and type—whether seeking or accepting a board position or even when seeking employment or considering a new job—to ensure that there is a fit between individual aspirations and values and the organization.

TYPES OF HOSPITALS AND HEALTH SYSTEMS

To better understand different organizational types—a skill essential for effective board membership—it may be illustrative to first consider organizational types with a more familiar scenario, that of a new graduate seeking their first RN position.

> *Jamal is considering his first RN position after graduating with his BS in Nursing from Prestigious University. He is interested in either moving to ski country or sun country and applies to positions throughout the western United States. He receives callbacks from several institutions and narrows it down to five. In trying to make a decision, he notes that all five institutions are very different from each other. One is a large **for-profit** institution; three are **nonprofit**, with one being associated with a university **academic medical center**, the second a nonprofit **community hospital**, and the third nonprofit, a **critical** access hospital (CAH). The fifth institution falls into a still different category. It is an urban, inner-city **public hospital**. Jamal knows that he does not have the funds or emotional energy to interview at all five and needs to narrow down his job search. Perplexed, he calls his former mentor, Dr. Whitney. Dr. Whitney suggests that any of these institutions could be a great choice. "It is all a matter of fit," says Dr. Whitney. "Which mission seems like the best fit for your interests?" Jamal realizes he has no real idea what Dr. Whitney is talking about, so he thanks him and decides to do a bit more homework on organizational types and missions.*

Although healthcare is delivered by different types of organizations in the United States, as Jamal's job search revealed, they fall into three broad categories: nonprofit, for-profit, and public. Nonprofit institutions are the most common in health care and human services, with 57% of hospitals being nonprofit, 24% for profit (up from 21.3% in 2017, Murphy, 2017) and 19% being public (Taylor et al., 2023). For-profit hospitals are sometimes termed *investor owned*. Public institutions are financed through taxes. Also categorized as *governmental*, these may be state, county, city–county, city, hospital district, or federal entities.

Nonprofit and For-Profit Institutions

Let us consider the differing missions of nonprofit and for-profit institutions and how this impacts the board orientation and, by extension, the whole organization. In each case, the BOT is responsible for ensuring that the mission of the organization is met, yet there is a substantial distinction between missions of nonprofit and for-profit organizations. In for-profit organizations, the mission includes an explicit intention to return profits to owners or shareholders. Nonprofit organizations do not have owners or shareholders expecting dividends on their investments. Instead, financially healthy nonprofit organizations achieve a different sort of "profit" each year, in the form of a *budget surplus*. A budget surplus, sometimes called an *operating margin*, is intended to be garnered for an investment in the organization rather than being delivered or "paid" to owners or shareholders. A negative operating margin, a rather paradoxical term, means that a nonprofit organization spent more money than it received that year, an unsustainable situation for any organization. Thus, both these organizational types must bring in more money than they spend, with the difference being the intended use of those funds. These differing orientations create differences in organizational behavior, functioning, and even legal requirements. As one such example, nonprofit hospitals must demonstrate *community benefit* to retain nonprofit status for tax purposes, as noted in Box 3.1. See Table 10.1 for additional differences between for-profit and nonprofit hospitals.

The tax-exempt status of nonprofits, worth $28 billion/year (Goodwin et al., 2023) has been under increasing scrutiny. The data driving this scrutiny includes studies that have found that 86% of nonprofit hospitals did not provide more charity care than their tax exemption (Zare et al., 2022) and nonprofit hospitals having lower ratios of charity care to total expenses than for profit systems (Bai et al., 2021). Other evidence suggests that when profits and cash reserves at nonprofit hospitals increased, their charity care did not (Jenkins & Ho, 2023). State and federal policymakers have raised the alarm bell about this lost revenue that is not providing commiserate value to taxpayers and their communities (Miller & Hawryluk, 2023; Muoio, 2023b).

Another lens through which to understand organizations is to discern if they are private or public. For example, private hospitals can be nonprofit or for-profit organizations, but they both differ from public institutions, such as public hospitals that are funded through taxes. Service to indigent populations was the primary impetus for the growth of public hospitals, serving as a safety net for those who might not otherwise be able to access care. Such organizations may also have added services that address social determinants of health (Anderson et al., 2004). More recently, arguments have been made that all hospitals have an ethical obligation to address social determinants, given federal health reforms and expansion of medical services (Sullivan, 2019).

TABLE 10.1 DIFFERENCES BETWEEN FOR-PROFIT AND NONPROFIT HOSPITALS

For-Profit	Nonprofit
Not tax exempt—pays state and local property taxes	Does not pay state or local taxes
No community benefit requirement	Must demonstrate community benefits in accordance with state and federal guidelines (a requirement within the Affordable Care Act)
Owned by private investors or owned publicly by shareholders	Not owned
Greater cost consciousness/operational discipline[a]	

Source: [a]Cheney, C. (2019). Three strategic differences between nonprofit and profit hospitals. *HealthLeaders*. https://www.healthleadersmedia.com/clinical-care/3-strategic-differences-between-nonprofit-and-profit-hospitals.

This orientation is gaining momentum, fueled by the growing recognition that addressing social determinants improves health outcomes (Velesquez & Figueroa, 2023) and represents an important health equity strategy (Centers for Disease Control and Prevention [CDC], 2022). Nevertheless, governance of a hospital whose mission is to serve indigent or underserved populations would have very different goals and values than, for example, a private, for-profit hospital intent on returning profits to shareholders.

Mission, Hospital Type, and Reimbursement

Some hospital categories reflect unique missions and also have different reimbursement schedules. Using Jamal's job search scenario as an example, there is a range of hospital types along a continuum from very small, rural hospitals that serve as *critical access* to *community hospitals* that serve the more common and routine healthcare needs of their local community to large, *tertiary* or even *quaternary* care centers that are referral centers for a region or even a nation, providing very complex, highly unusual, specialized care. Tertiary and quaternary care centers may be affiliated with an *academic medical center*, which is a university-based teaching and research-oriented college of medicine, and possibly other health professional colleges. As with the public versus private hospitals, each of these different institutions would have very different missions and thus differing responsibilities for the governing body. For example, the mission of a tertiary care hospital with an academic medical center would include not only health care of the most critically and complexly ill but also teaching health professionals and stewarding research. Quaternary care would be even more specialized, focused on management of highly uncommon conditions and experimental treatments. Contrast this with, for example, a CAH, which—by the Centers for Medicare and Medicaid's definition—must be in a rural area without other services nearby, furnish 24-hour emergency care 7 days a week, have no more than 25 inpatient beds, and have an average length of stay of 96 hours or less. Thus, a CAH exists to provide emergency services in remote areas, stabilization services in preparation for transfer to a tertiary care center, or short-term stays for relatively uncomplicated care (Centers for Medicare and Medicaid Services [CMS], 2023). Importantly, CAHs are reimbursed at 101% of reasonable cost, as many would not be financially viable in the "marketplace" without this preferential reimbursement (review Chapter 6). Nevertheless, rural hospital closure is accelerating, with 136 closing between 2010 and 2021 and a record single year high of 19 in 2020. Reasons include low patient volumes, the shift from inpatient to outpatient, the high cost of drugs and labor (American Hospital Association, 2022), and high deductible plans in which a rural hospital—being the first stop in a patient episode that ends in a larger hospital—is more likely to serve patients who cannot pay their deductible and thus leaves the rural hospital uncompensated for care (Hawryluk, 2020). A new hospital designation, Rural Emergency Hospital, was authorized with the Consolidated Appropriations

Act of 2021. The aim was to avoid closures of essential community services. Under this designation, some rural and critical access hospitals could suspend inpatient services yet provide emergency services, observational care, and additional outpatient without needing to meet all the requirements to be a CAH (CMS, n.d.). Although a financial solution for some hospitals, there are trade-offs. Clearly, trustees must understand, or quickly become familiar with, the mission and funding streams of the institution for which they are responsible to execute their fiduciary responsibility (see Box 10.2). Again, understanding these differences in mission and scope is also useful for the novice in a job search.

> *Jamal spent a great deal of time looking at the websites of the five institutions. He finds himself attracted to two very different institutions, the inner-city public hospital and the rural CAH. He realizes that there is a commonality between these that he had not originally noticed. Both serve vulnerable, underserved populations, and he is drawn to this work. Jamal decides to interview only at these two institutions. Excitedly, he tells his best friend, Kiah, who is also a new graduate in a job search. "I don't understand you at all," says Kiah. "Don't you want to be at the academic medical center, taking part in research? It would also be so easy to pick up your master's degree because of the affiliation with a university, or maybe even a DNP or PhD."*
>
> *Jamal shares that he is very confident that, despite their differences, the inner-city public hospital or the rural hospital is the best fit for him, and he will narrow it down further after the onsite visit. He is confident that he can obtain his MS in other ways, maybe via online courses. Kiah decides instead to apply to the institutions that attract her: the tertiary care–academic medical center–university-affiliated hospital and one of the community hospitals. The community hospital is in a trendy suburb that Kia likes, and she is not sure if the degree of specialization that RNs often have at a tertiary care hospital is the best fit for her, or if a slightly more general practice in a smaller, slightly less intense setting is a better match. She is confident, however, that one of the two is the best fit for her. Both Jamal and Kia are pleased that they have chosen nursing—there are so many organizational options.*

 BOX 10.2

WHAT DOES IT MEAN TO HOLD FIDUCIARY RESPONSIBILITY?

"Fiduciary duty is a legal duty to act solely in another party's interest. Parties owing this duty are called fiduciaries. The individuals whom they owe a duty are called principals. Fiduciaries may not profit from their relationship with their principals unless they have the principals' express informed consent. They also have a duty to avoid any conflict of interest between themselves or their principals or between their principals and the fiduciaries' other clients. *A fiduciary duty is the strictest duty of care recognized by the U.S. legal system.*"

Source: Legal Information Institute. (n.d.). *Fiduciary duty.* www.law.cornell.edu/wex/fiduciary_duty.

Note that as job seekers, Jamal and Kia have choices as to which hospital type they are interested in and can determine which one feels like the best fit. This is typically not the case for nurses seeking board membership. As nurses access board positions (as discussed in Chapter 11), the process typically is facilitated through proximity, connections, and knowledge base relative to the organization's needs, so knowledge of all organizational types is helpful for a nurse seeking a board position. Finally, this example illustrated hospitals, which are among the most diverse category of organizational type. Home health agencies tend to be either for-profit or nonprofit and operate under a similar board structure. Other organizations, like accountable care organizations, are in evolution but may be affiliated with several of these organizational types. Increasingly, mergers and acquisitions have created systems along a care continuum that may have integrated many organizations and organizational types under one overall service entity. Hospitals, home healthcare agencies, skilled nursing facilities, physician offices, and other services, for example, may have vertically integrated to become one legal entity. This overarching entity typically will have its own board and may have sub-boards at the level of the individual organizations. These consolidations in the form of mergers and acquisitions accelerated in response to changes in the Affordable Care Act as well as to prepare for value-based payments across the care continuum, but later slowed as their value has come into question (Kacik, 2019) only to rise again in response to financial pressure (Kacik, 2023) Nevertheless, these system-level boards wield substantial power; serving at the institutional board level is excellent training for service on the system board. Recall also that role of the Federal Trade Commission in overseeing potential mergers or acquisitions. Finally, a nurse should not expect to serve on a board in an organization in which they are employed unless they are there in a designated position such as a staff liaison. Few boards have such a position for nurses as the employed person has an inherent conflict of interest (although employed physicians often serve on the board of their employing entity), so it is important to look outside for these opportunities.

NAVIGATING GOVERNANCE–MANAGEMENT BOUNDARIES

Luciana is fuming! Newly elected as the president of the hospital nurses' union, she cannot understand why the board is so unresponsive to the union's demands. They have negotiated in good faith with the administrative bargaining team led by the vice president (VP) of human relations, but—in frustration—Luciana presented a passionate plea at the open session of the BOT meetings at both of the last two sessions. Both times the board members listened politely, but nothing seemed to come of it. "Why doesn't the board do something?" she laments.

Clara is dismayed. As the newly elected chair of the BOT, she hopes to foster a climate of inclusion and respect. Yet, the union's spectacles at the board meetings

> are accelerating. Clara admires the fiery Luciana, sees much of her own young self in Luciana, and appreciates her zeal and passion for the work of the institution they both so clearly love. "But why does Luciana continue to bring management issues to the board?" wonders Clara. "Does she understand that union negotiations are management issues, and not under the purview of governance?" She considers telling Luciana directly, yet is concerned that Luciana would misperceive the intention. She decides that if the union contract is still unsettled next month and Luciana and her troops present again to the board, then she, Clara, will again politely thank her, but directly ask if she and the other union leaders understand that union negotiations are a management issue, not a governance issue, and thus not within the board's scope of responsibility and authority.

Perhaps one of the areas of greatest blurring for the nurse new to board work is to understand the difference between management and governance. Yet to appropriately apply influence, it is fundamental to understand the governance role of boards and differentiate it from management. With the exception of the CEO, who reports to the BOT, all senior management, sometimes called the *senior leadership team*, reports to the CEO, not the board.

The Senior Leadership Team

Different organizations divide the responsibility of senior management differently; however, a very common structure is the CEO—who may also hold the title of president—in the lead yet reporting to the board, with a chief financial officer (alternately titled VP for finance) and chief operating officer (COO; alternate titles include VP for operations) reporting to the CEO. In some organizations, the COO and chief nursing officer (CNO) are combined, with a title reflective of that role, such as VP for patient care services. In other organizations, the CNO reports to the COO, while in still other settings, the reporting line is to the CEO or chief medical officer (CMO). CMOs typically report to the CEO. See Figure 10.1 for examples of different senior-level management structures commonly found within healthcare.

Why Do Reporting Lines Matter?

Reporting lines are important, as the further the position is from the CEO, the less likely the individual is to interact with and influence the CEO on a daily basis, and the less likely they are to have board contact. An organization in which the CNO and CMO have similar authority and an equally broad *span of control* creates a very different sort of organization from one in which the CNO reports to the CMO, as just one example. The term *span of control* means the number of services, people, or functions for which an individual

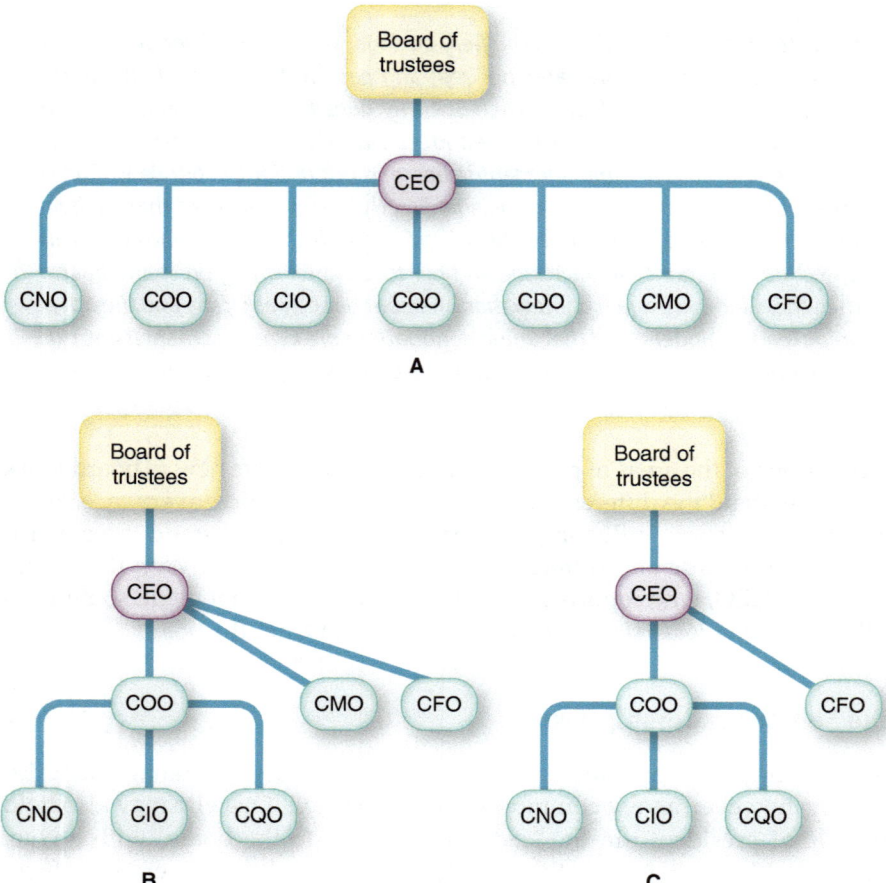

FIGURE 10.1: Examples of different organizational senior leadership reporting lines.
CEO, chief executive officer/president; CFO, chief financial officer/vice president of finance; CIO, chief information officer/vice president of information management; CMO, chief medical officer/vice president of medical affairs; CNO, chief nursing officer/vice president of nursing; COO, chief operating officer/vice president of operations; CQO, chief quality officer/vice president of quality.

is responsible. Inherent in the definition is the notion that the individual has both the *responsibility* and the corresponding *authority* to execute that responsibility. Nurses remain underrepresented in health care organizations, filling less than 25% of leadership roles (Rappleye, 2018). Bean et al. note that accurately identifying the proportion of CEOs who are nurses is unclear due to a lack of data, but they recognize the role of gender, with women representing just 15% of health care CEOs (Bean et al., 2022). This is recognized as a global phenomenon. Note, for example, the prescient nature of World Health Organization document titled *Delivered by Women, Led by Men: A Gender and Equity Analysis of the Global Health and Social Workforce* (World Health Organization, 2019). Take a moment to review the organizational structure of some of the hospitals and agencies you have practiced in. Where is the most senior nurse leader located in the organizational structure? How many nurses are there in senior leadership positions? How many organizations are led by CEOs who have a nursing background?

Senior Leadership Positions Reflect Health Care Change: Who Is on the Team in Your Organization?

Early in the 21st century, two new high-level roles have emerged: chief quality officer (CQO), who may also or instead be the VP for performance improvement, and chief information officer (CIO). These may be stand-alone roles reporting to the president/CEO or—with a different title, reporting line, and level of influence—reporting only indirectly to the CEO/president, with the direct report being through a VP. Health care is also highly regulated and accountable to the public. Moreover, given that over 50% of health care is publicly funded through taxes, state and federal relations are an important interface for any contemporary organization. Thus, VPs for government relations and community relations are also common and typically report directly to the president/CEO. Depending on the size of the organization, this may be a conjoined position or two different posts occupied by two different individuals. COO–CNO roles held by a single person are increasing, with an aim of aligning services (Bean, 2023) and giving nursing the opportunity to oversee all operations, not just nursing services. Finally, some institutions have a chief diversity officer/VP for multicultural affairs among their senior leadership team.

The postpandemic landscape gave rise to additional C-suite roles, including elevated roles for leaders in infection control. As Kayser notes: "Unprecedented times call for unprecedented C-suite titles" (Kayser, 2023, para 1). These titles reflect the changing health care landscape. Other emerging roles are chief artificial intelligence officer and chief innovation officer. Kayser further notes that these new titles may not have longevity; for example, chief diversity officer was the fasting-growing role in 2022, but people are "now vacating the position. It is unclear if a chief AI officer will be a necessity in 10 years" (para 8). Roles merge—and disappear—as institutions seek, and often struggle, to redefine themselves in a rapidly changing, resource-limited health care environment. Understanding the roles and responsibilities of these individuals is very important for any nurse wanting to be influential in the corollary areas.

What About Fundraising?

The goal of raising external funds through philanthropy is an extraordinarily important realm in today's health care milieu. This arm of an institution is commonly structured in one of two ways. There may be a separate foundation with a separate board that is responsible for fundraising or, instead, there may be a VP for development who reports to the CEO/president. In this latter configuration, the role may also include community outreach and public relationships, as well as marketing and press relation functions. This sort of position is often termed VP of advancement. All board members are expected to provide at least some level of philanthropic support; it can be difficult to ask others for money if board members don't ante up.

What Does It Mean to Be an Ex Officio Board Member?

In for-profit organizations, the CEO is sometimes also chair of the board. The CEO is typically an *ex officio* board member. Ex officio members are board members by virtue of being in a particular job role, and depending on the organization, ex officio members may be voting or nonvoting as prescribed in organizational bylaws. In academic medical centers, the dean of medicine is routinely an ex officio board member, yet inclusion of the dean of nursing in board membership is less common. This, in turn, creates a very different span of influence for the educational and research opportunities for the students represented by the dean. Moreover, aside from these potential ex officio board posts, nurses are markedly underrepresented on boards of health organizations. In 2008, for example, Myers noted that in a study of community health system governance, only 2.4% of board seats were held by nurses, in stark contrast to physicians, who held 22% of board seats. Since that time, and catalyzed by *The Future of Nursing* report, there has been a concerted effort to facilitate the inclusion of more nurses on boards. The Nurses on Boards Coalition, for example, set a goal of 10,000 nurses on boards by 2020 but fell short of that goal as the year opened, with roughly 7,000 nurses on boards, but numbers rose to over 10,000 in 2021. Note that not all of these are hospital or health care governance boards but include a wide array of board types, including advisory boards. Clearly, the effort continues, and your time and talents are needed to ensure that nursing wisdom is present on every health-related board.

THE RELATIONSHIP BETWEEN ORGANIZATIONAL STRUCTURE AND ORGANIZATIONAL VALUES

Why are the structure and makeup of this senior leadership team and boards so important? Organizational structure reflects organizational values. It is illustrative to examine where in the hierarchy the most senior nurse is situated. To whom does the chief nurse report? This has implications not only for influence but also for span of control. A CNO who is also the COO and reports to the president/CEO has a very different span of control than one who, for example, reports to a COO or CMO.

The role of all of these individuals is senior management. The various VPs, or "chiefs," report to the CEO/president, who in turn reports to the board. Sullivan (2013) elegantly describes the problems that can arise when new nurse leaders do not understand the senior management lines—for example, a new CNO preparing her first budget but going to the board chair for help, rather than to her immediate supervisor, the CEO. In the scenario detailed, the board chair—appropriately—chastises her. First, budget preparation is a management issue, and boards later approve the overall budget. In other words, the board has fiduciary responsibility that includes budget approval as a form of governance oversight over the work of the management team that prepared the budget. Second, the new CNO could be perceived as insubordinate and attempting to circumvent her supervisor. In any case, no matter where they are positioned in an organization, the savvy nurse understands the reporting lines and roles.

THE ROLE OF BOARD COMMITTEES

Boards commonly divide their governance oversight into different working committees, termed *standing committees*. Although each board member has a legal, fiduciary responsibility to the overall mission of the organization, committees allow members with different expertise to bring those skills to board work in a more focused way. These various committees typically have a lead staff member from among the VPs—for example, the CQO would be a logical lead staff for the quality/performance improvement committee of the board. Common standing committees in health care organizations are listed in Box 10.3. Note, however, that the exact committee name varies by organization. Typically, all work of the standing committees goes to the full board for approval. So, for example, the executive compensation committee will do foundational work to develop the CEO's compensation package, but implementation would require approval of the full board.

Committee Charters, Bylaws, and Ad Hoc Committees

Board committees typically have *charters* that delineate the role and responsibility of the committee. The rules for modifying the charter of a committee can be found in the *organizational* or *board bylaws*. Although organizational bylaws may seem arcane and cumbersome to read, bylaws codify organizational rules and are therefore an important item for thoughtful review by any new board member. Finally, boards may also form *ad hoc committees* and

BOX 10.3

COMMON STANDING BOARD COMMITTEES

Audit committee
Finance committee
Performance improvement/quality committee
Development committee (unless there is a separate foundation responsible for fundraising)
Facilities and planning committee
Nominating committee (generating names of qualified individuals for board membership)
Mission and ethics committee (in nonprofit organizations, particularly religiously affiliated)
Compensation committee (typically reviews and approves the benefit packages and wage plan for staff, physician incentive compensation plan, overview of senior leadership team incentive compensation plan)
Executive compensation committee (designs and reviews CEO's compensation package and incentive compensation)
Executive committee (may consist of all committee chairs or just officers of the board; it is a powerful committee that often meets between board meetings to conduct business and deal with emergencies)

advisory committees. An ad hoc committee is a short-term, temporary committee that is formed to study and address a particular issue, report back to the full board, and then dissolve, whereas an advisory committee invites nonboard members with complementary areas of expertise to provide advice on key areas. A home health agency, for example, may have an end-of-life advisory board composed of palliative care experts, ethicists, social workers, and religious advisors/clergy. Such advisory boards do not have fiduciary responsibility (see Box 10.2) for the organization and offer advice without authority for governance or oversight of the CEO or president. They are a valuable way for an organization to connect community leaders and interested parties, ensuring that stakeholders and potential benefactors remain engaged in the work of the organization.

Governance boards have additional responsibility since the passage of the Sarbanes–Oxley Act of 2002, which is outlined in the next section.

THE SARBANES–OXLEY ACT

"How could it have happened?" Fred and Regina lost all the investments that they had carefully made over the course of a lifetime. A retired former employee of Enron, Fred had felt well prepared for retirement. Now, 2 years into retirement, Enron's swift collapse—from an organization ranked as the world's

> seventh largest energy company in April 2001 to bankruptcy filing in December 2001—has wiped out all but Social Security payments for Fred and Regina. "You know what sticks most in my craw?" Fred asks Regina. "That as the stock value was falling, we couldn't sell our stocks but the brass—all the bosses—could. Someone needs to be sure this never happens to anyone else again."[1]

That "someone" was Congress, with the passage of the Sarbanes–Oxley Act of 2002.

Traditionally, the central role of a governing board has been to "act as a watch dog" (Nadler et al., 2006, p. 6) and to oversee the overall functioning of the organization as well as the CEO. A series of corporate scandals—Enron was just one example—rocked the United States and resulted in passage of the Sarbanes–Oxley legislation, sometimes called SOX, in 2002. This legislation was designed to minimize the opportunity for fraud, financial mismanagement, and conflicts of interest among corporations and their leaders. Although SOX is directed at for-profit organizations, there has been substantial spillover to nonprofit organizations, including hospitals and health care organizations. Although only two provisions of SOX pertain directly to nonprofit organizations—whistleblower protection and stipulations related to document destruction—many nonprofit organizations have voluntarily adopted SOX provisions (Worth, 2024). Many of these adoptions seem inherently logical and ethical, such as the provision that prohibits organizational loans to board members or executives. A more complex and nuanced SOX provision relates to audit committee responsibilities.

The Board Audit Committee

Prior to SOX, the typical role of the audit committee detailed in most audit committee charters was responsibility for the selection of external auditors, recommendations for payment of external auditors, review of the performance of external auditors, and assessment of the accounting report. The SOX Act dramatically changes the role and responsibility of audit committees, requiring more independent conversations between the audit committee of the board and the independent auditor, exclusive of an intermediary function by the CEO and senior leadership. Logically, it makes sense for the board, which has a fiduciary responsibility to the organization and for CEO performance, to have the opportunity to assess the financial operations of the organization independent of the CEO and senior management involvement. Yet, as Rossiter (2004) notes, this requirement constituted a substantial change in the manner in which business had been conducted, given that this board committee–auditor communication is "without management functioning as a filter or even providing context" (p. 2).

Rossiter further notes that the audit committee may be required to make many more difficult judgments than in the pre-SOX era, potentially diminishing the pool of those willing, or prepared, to serve on the audit committee. Finally, each member of the committee must be an audit expert or explain why such expertise is not necessary. In health care organizations, midsized and large hospitals typically have a similar overall audit committee orientation, with the audit committee having direct interaction with auditors and at least one member of the committee holding a firm background in finance (Bader, 2010). Although SOX is not currently drawing much public attention, it continues to be relevant. As Peregrine noted on the 15th anniversary of the law in 2017, SOX "has had an enormous impact on the governance, operations, financial reporting, and legal/compliance functions of healthcare companies [and has] perhaps irrevocably altered the relationship of the board and senior management to its internal and external legal, financial and accounting advisors" (Peregrine, 2017, para 1).

The Board Performance Improvement and Quality Committee

Some authors also suggest that a greater understanding of quality of care on the part of board members is essential. Bader (2010) proposes that there should be "quality audits," a concept conceptually analogous to financial audits. Warden (cited in Myers, 2008) highlights the important contribution nurses bring to boards in this area, stating:

> *The nurse brings the ability to translate and demonstrate evidence-based kinds of safety and quality improvements to the board and brings an in-depth understanding of the patient care process. The nurse can make or break an institution in terms of quality and safety. (p. 12)*

As discussed in previous chapters, reimbursement is increasingly linked to quality outcomes and safety measures. Thus, the nurse on a board is well positioned to cross-pollinate finance and quality committees with key information. Value-based purchasing (discussed in Chapters 4 and 6), for example, includes metrics nurses are familiar with that are now linked to payment, for example, surgical site infections. The clinical "knowledge gap" board members have (Castellucci, 2020, para 7) can be addressed with nurses' firsthand knowledge. Moreover, the nurse can provide mentorship to other board members as they begin to learn the safely and quality issues plaguing the U.S. health care system. Kaplan states: "I think it is interesting that many boards don't fully appreciate that they are ultimately responsibility for the safety and quality of the care within the institution they govern" (cited in Castellucci, 2020, para 5). Sundean, interviewed in 2020 about her career that facilitates and expands nurses' roles on boards, offers the following advice to nurses: ". . . be confident about the strengths [you] bring to the table, whatever table it is! . . . pay it forward . . . help others . . . and encourage them to pursue a wide range of leadership" (cited in Reid Ponte, 2020, p. 62). In summary, nurses are well positioned to play pivotal roles on boards, provided they can access board membership. This latter issue, accessing board membership, is the focus of the next chapter.

End-of-Chapter Resources

THOUGHT QUESTIONS

1. A colleague reports frustration at the number of vice presidents in her organization. What thoughts can you share about the roles of these vice presidents?
2. What organizational structure do you see as optimal for nursing practice and why?
3. Define the following key terms:
   Academic medical center
   Ad hoc committees
   Advisory board or committee
   Budget surplus
   Charter
   Community benefit
   Community hospital
   Critical access hospital
   Directors and operators insurance
   Ex officio committee member
   For-profit organization
   Fiduciary responsibility
   Governance
   Investor-owned institution
   Management
   Nonprofit organization
   Operating margin
   Organizational bylaws
   Public hospital
   Quaternary care center
   Senior leadership team

Span of control
Standing committee
Tertiary care center

EXERCISE

1. Develop a presentation to share with your peers that describes the various types of hospitals in the United States. What are the strengths and limitations of each type in terms of mission? Employment? Defend your answer. What type of organization would you prefer to be employed in? Why? Serve on a board of? Why?

QUIZ

True or False

1. Most hospital governing boards include equal numbers of physicians and nurses.
2. Governance and management are different terms for the same set of responsibilities.
3. Directors and operators liability insurance offers financial protection to board members who are named in a lawsuit as a result of their board activities.
4. Nonprofit organizations are termed nonprofit because they return financial profits to stockholders.
5. In addition to hospital care, the mission of academic medical centers includes university-based teaching and research-oriented colleges of medicine.
6. The term *span of control* refers to the number of services, people, or functions a leader is responsible for.
7. Ad hoc board committees are ongoing, permanent board structures.
8. The COO typically reports directly to the board.
9. Advisory boards hold fiduciary responsibility.
10. All health care organizations are governed by the same board structure.

Multiple Choice

11. Critical access hospitals
    A. Must provide 24-hour emergency care 7 days a week
    B. Are reimbursed differently than hospitals that are not designated critical access hospitals
    C. Both A and B
    D. Neither A nor B

12. Ex officio board members
    A. Are board members by virtue of holding a particular job role or title
    B. Are always voting members of the board
    C. Both A and B
    D. Neither A nor B
13. The Sarbanes–Oxley Act
    A. Is an extension of Sherman antitrust legislation
    B. Dramatically changed the role of governing-board quality committees
    C. Both A and B
    D. Neither A nor B
14. Board committees
    A. Typically have charters to define the role of the committee
    B. May include focus areas such as quality and finance
    C. Both A and B
    D. Neither A nor B
15. A governing board
    A. Typically sets the compensation level for the chief executive officer of an organization
    B. Is responsible for the hiring and, when necessary, firing of the chief executive officer
    C. Both A and B
    D. Neither A nor B

NOTE

1. This scenario is adapted from the overview of Enron authored by Sridharan et al. (2002).

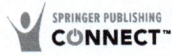

A robust set of instructor resources designed to supplement this text is located at http://connect.springerpub.com/content/book/978-0-8261-7236-5. Qualifying instructors may request access by emailing textbook@springerpub.com.

REFERENCES

American Hospital Association. (2022). *Rural hospital services.* https://www.aha.org/advocacy/rural-health-services

Anderson, R., Boumbulian, P., & Pickens, S. (2004). The role of U.S. public hospitals in urban health. *Academic Medicine, 79*(12), 1162–1168. https://doi.org/10.1097/00001888-200412000-00008

Bader, B. (2010). *Applying Sarbanes–Oxley to healthcare quality: Great Boards* (Vol. 10). Bader and Associates Governance Consultants.

Bai, G., Zare, H., Eisenberg, M. D., Polsky, D., & Anderson, G. F. (2021). Analysis suggests government and nonprofit hospitals' charity care is not aligned with their favorable tax treatment. *Health Affairs, 40*(4), 629–636. https://doi.org/10.1377/hlthaff.2020.01627

Bean, M., Carbajal, E., & Gleeson, C. (2022, March 31). *Is it time for more nurse CEOs? Becker's hospital review.* https://www.beckershospitalreview.com/nursing/is-it-time-for-more-nurse-ceos.html?oly_enc_id=9085F7288456J5N

Bean, M. (2023, June 6). *The rise of the hybrid CNO–COO.* Modern Healthcare. https://www.beckershospitalreview.com/hospital-management-administration/the-rise-of-the-hybrid-cno-coo

Boardable (n.d.). *A nonprofit's checklist for better board succession planning.* Author. https://boardable.com/resources/board-succession-planning

Castellucci, M. (2020, February 8). *Quality often an oversight for system, hospital boards.* Modern Healthcare. https://www.modernhealthcare.com/governance/quality-often-oversight-system-hospital-boards

Centers for Disease Control and Prevention. (2022). *Why is addressing social determinants of health important for CDC and public health?* Author. https://www.cdc.gov/about/sdoh/addressing-sdoh.html

Centers for Medicare and Medicaid Services. (2023). *Critical access hospitals.* Author. https://www.cms.gov/medicare/health-safety-standards/certification-compliance/critical-access-hospitals

Centers for Medicare and Medicaid Serivces. (n.d.). *Rural Emergency Hospital.* https://www.cms.gov/medicare/health-safety-standards/quality-safety-oversight-guidance-laws-regulations/hospitals/rural-emergency-hospitals

Goodwin, J., Levinson, Z., & Hulver, S. (2023, March 14). *The estimated value of tax expemption for nonprofit hospitals was about 28 billion in 2020.* Kaiser Family Foundation. https://www.kff.org/health-costs/issue-brief/the-estimated-value-of-tax-exemption-for-nonprofit-hospitals-was-about-28-billion-in-2020/

Institute of Medicine. (2010). *The future of nursing: Leading change, advancing health.* National Academy of Sciences.

Hawryluk, M. (2020, January 10). *Rural hospital closures leave communities reeling—and high deductibles contribute.* USA Today. https://www.usatoday.com/story/news/health/2020/01/10/rural-hospitals-high-deductibles-give-financial-hit-communities/4422129002/

Jenkins, D., & Ho, V. (2023). Nonprofit hospitals: Profits and cash reserves grow, charity care does not. *Health Affairs (Project Hope), 42*(6), 866–869. https://doi.org/10.1377/hlthaff.2022.01542

Kacik, A. (2019, December 14). *Year in review: M&A slows down as the benefits called into question.* Modern Healthcare. https://www.modernhealthcare.com/hospitals/healthcare-mergers-and-acquisitions-slow-down-benefits-called-question

Kacik, A. (2022). *How nurses are making inroad in hospital boardrooms.* https://www.modernhealthcare.com/esg/nurses-on-boards-hospital-governance-palo-pinto-aha

Kacik, A. (2023, December 26). *Hospital merger activity to increase in 2024.* Modern Healthcare. https://modernhealthcare.com/mergers-acquisitions/hospital-merger-activity-continue-rise-2024

Kayser, A. (2023, August 28). *Healthcare's newest C-suite roles.* Becker's Hospital Review. https://www.beckershospitalreview.com/hospital-management-administration/healthcares-newest-c-suite-roles.html

Miller, A., & Hawryluk, M. (2023, July 10). *Nonprofit hospitals under growing scrutiny over how they justify billions in tax breaks.* CNN. https://www.cnn.com/2023/07/10/health/nonprofit-hospitals-community-benefits-kff-health-news/index.html

Muoio, D. (2023a, January 23). *Health system CEO turnover rose in 2022 as more executives feel the strain of burnout.* Fierce Healthcare. https://www.fiercehealthcare.com/providers/health-system-ceo-turnover-rose-2022-more-executives-say-theyre-feeling-burnt-out

Muoio, D. (2023b, August 8). *Citing lax enforcement, senators ramp up scrutiny of nonprofit hospital tax exempt status.* Fierce Healthcare. https://www.fiercehealthcare.com/providers/citing-lax-enforcement-senators-ramp-scrutiny-nonprofit-hospitals-tax-exemptions

Murphy, B. (2017). *50 Things to know about the hospital industry.* Becker's Hospital Review. www.beckershospitalreview.com/hospital-management-administration/50-things-to-know-about-the-hospital-industry-2017.html

Myers, S. (2008). A different voice: Nurses on the board. *Trustee, 6*(6), 10–14. https://pubmed.ncbi.nlm.nih.gov/18590097/

Nadler, D., Behan, B., & Nadler, M. (2006). *Building better boards: A blueprint for effective governance.* Wiley.

National Council of Nonprofits. (nd). *Board roles and responsiblities.* https://www.councilofnonprofits.org/running-nonprofit/governance-leadership/board-roles-and-responsibilities

Peregrine, M. (2017). *The continuing relevance of Sarbanes–Oxley to the health care sector.* American Health Lawyers Association. https://www.mwe.com/insights/the-continuing-relevance-of-sarbanes-oxley-to-the/

PricewatershouseCooper. (n.d.). *How the best boards approach CEP succession planning.* Author. https://www.pwc.com/us/en/services/governance-insights-center/library/ceo-succession-planning.html

Rappleye, E. (2018, December 10). *Nurses fill less than 25% of leadership roles in most healthcare organizations.* Becker's Hospital Review. https://www.beckershospitalreview.com/hospital-management-administration/nurses-fill-less-than-25-of-leadership-roles-at-most-healthcare-organizations.html

Reid Ponte, P. (2020). Nurses on boards: An interview with Lisa J. Sundean, PhD, MHA, RN. *The Journal of Nursing Administration, 50*(2), 61–62. https://doi.org/10.1097/NNA.0000000000000842

Rossiter, P. (2004). Supporting the audit committee after Sarbanes–Oxley: A practical guide. *Bank Accountingand Finance, 17*(5), 1–9. https://link.gale.com/apps/doc/A121572001/AONE?u=tel_oweb&sid=googleScholar&xid=48dc0ef0

Sridharan, U., Dickes, L., & Royce Caines, W. (2002). The social impact of business failure: Enron. *American Journal of Business, 17*(2), 11–22. https://doi.org/10.1108/19355181200200006

Sullivan, E. (2013). *Becoming influential: A guide for nurses* (2nd ed.). Pearson.

Sullivan, H. (2019). Hospitals' obligation to address social determinants of health. *AMA Journal of Ethics, 21*(3), E248–E258. https://doi.org/10.1001/amajethics.2019.248

Sundean, L. J., O'Lynn, C. E., Christopher, R., & Cherry, B. (2022). Nurses' perspectives of their impact while serving on boards. *The Journal of*

Nursing Administration, 52(2), 106–111. https://doi.org/10.1097/NNA.0000000000001110

Taylor, L., Franz, B., Zink, A., Fair, A., & Cronin, C. (2023). Public perceptions of US for-profit, nonprofit, and public hospitals. *Health Affairs Scholar, 1*(4), qxad046. https://doi.org/10.1093/haschl/qxad046

Velasquez, D., & Figueroa, J. (2023). Learning from Massachusetts hospitals on programs to address Social Determinants of Health. *NEJM Catalyst, 4*(4). https://doi.org/10.1056/CAT.22.0344

World Health Organization. (2019). *Delivered by women, led by men: A gender and equity analysis of the global health and social workforce.* Human Resources for Health Observer Series, No. 24. https://www.who.int/publications/i/item/9789241515467

Worth, M. (2024). *Nonprofit management: Principles and practices* (7th ed.). Sage.

Zare, H., Eisenberg, M. D., & Anderson, G. (2022). Comparing the value of community benefit and tax-exemption in non-profit hospitals. *Health Services Research, 57*(2), 270–284. https://doi.org/10.1111/1475-6773.13668

CHAPTER 11

Building Skills for Board Membership

CHAPTER 10 described a range of organizational categories as well as types of boards. Chapter 11 expands on this foundation to prepare the reader to access a board position or to effectively report to one in a senior leadership position.

Following completion of this chapter, you will be able to:

- Identify personal skills and growth areas for board membership.
- Describe board selection processes.
- Determine board types of greatest personal interest and develop a plan toward board appointment.
- Describe basic elements of organizational financial statements.

> Abby's twin sister, Emma, has just secured a position on the board of the regional home health agency. Abby states, "It is great you are there to represent nurses on the board!" Emma, who understands the governance responsibility to the mission, shakes her head, responding, "I don't represent nursing on the board. This is not a constituency board. Instead, I hope to exemplify what nurses can bring to a board."

ZEAL, ORGANIZATIONAL FIT, AND PHILANTHROPY

Securing a position on a board is not about what the board can contribute to the board member's career, but instead is about what the individual can contribute to the board. At the same time, board membership builds important skills and connections and widens the board member's sphere of influence. It is also time-consuming. Thus, there are key dimensions to consider regarding becoming a board member. First, is the mission of the organization of interest? Zeal for the cause is a great mobilizer of both time and energy. This is important, as a committed board member will need both. Second, a commitment to a nonprofit board typically means not only time and energy but also at least some level of financial commitment to the organization on a yearly basis. Philanthropy, fundraising for the institution, is an important responsibility of a board, and it is difficult to ask others to give to an organization if there is no commitment to philanthropy from 100% of the board members, demonstrated by giving personal funds to the organization. In other words, if the organization is not valuable enough for board members—who are the stewards and living logo for an organization—to give to, why would anyone else? For-profit boards generally do not involve fundraising and members may be financially compensated for their time. In that case, it is important to assess any potential conflicts of interest or influence that could undermine your credibility. In general, it is easier to start with small, local, nonprofit boards, who often are looking to expand their membership.

Board Skill Mix

A second domain of exploration is an assessment of strengths and areas of potential impact and contribution. Every board needs members with complementary skills, and nurses offer valuable understanding of the delivery of health care. More important, however, the role of a governing board member is not to represent a constituency (e.g., nurses) on the board. Instead, each board member brings their knowledge, skills, and experience to serve the overall mission of the organization. Moreover, although nurses often know their own particular unit, specialty, or service delivery area, a board member is responsible to the whole organization, including finances. Lundean states:

> Considering the state of healthcare outcomes in the US today, it is incumbent on hospital boards of directors to convene the most broadly diverse board composition with the right expertise to guide board deliberations and decision making. Boundary spanning leaders, nurses on boards make the critical connections between the care, outcomes, and health of patients/populations with the mission, vision, and growth of the organization. Nurses understand and articulate well the healthcare needs and determinants of health for community stakeholders who must be centered in boardroom discussions. While we are seeing an uptick in the engagement of nurses on boards across sectors, intentional focus on engaging more nurses on healthcare delivery organization boards is imperative to the business proposition of these organizations and their mission for high quality care and outcomes. (personal communication, February 15, 2024)

Most boards hold an orientation to acquaint members with the range of efforts and activities of the board. Expanded understanding of the domains of governance responsibility will not only enhance effectiveness of the board member but also increase the likelihood of an appointment in the first place.

TYPES OF BOARD APPOINTMENTS—HOW POSITIONS ARE ACCESSED

Self-Perpetuating Boards

Board membership occurs in three main ways: self-perpetuating, appointed, and elected. Many boards are *self-perpetuating boards.* In this model, existing board members identify potential new board members. This scenario creates obverse strengths and weaknesses. On the positive side, the board can shape itself to meet the demands of its responsibility, adding new skill sets to complement those of existing board members and address gaps or weaknesses in collective expertise. In contrast, underrepresented groups will often continue to be underrepresented, as members naturally look among those they know or those with whom they share business or social interests, which can limit identifying a new population from which to draw potential board members (Worth, 2024).

Nurses have traditionally been dramatically underrepresented in hospital boards, which tend to be self-perpetuating boards. Stephen Shortell, founder of the University of California, Berkeley Center for Healthcare Organizational and Innovation Research, notes, "It is a function of the perceived hierarchy within medicine and also gender issues. . . . The process for recruiting board members has historically relied on board members reaching out to their own networks, so it is self-perpetuating" (cited in Kacik, 2022, paras. 14 and 15). One study of 15 top ranked medical centers found only 0.9% of board members to be nurses (Kacik, 2022). Clearly, there is much work to do.

Appointed Boards

Other boards are *appointed boards*, with membership accessed through appointment by an official or authority who is not a direct part of the organization. This may involve a political dimension, as the appointing authority may be composed of elected officials themselves. Many public universities, for example, are governed by boards that are appointed by the governor or through some other state-level political process. Regulatory boards fall into this category and will be discussed shortly.

Elected Boards

A still different governance structure is that of *elected boards*. In the case of elected boards, as the name implies, the board members are elected by those being governed—the members of the organization. In this case, a level of visibility and perceived competency is necessary to be elected as a board member. Such visibility can be difficult for frontline staff, such as staff nurses, to obtain. Therefore, involvement in organizational committees and working groups is a valuable first step, both in skill building and network formation.

WHAT A GOVERNING BOARD IS NOT

Advisory Boards

It is important to reiterate that not all boards are governing boards, even if they hold the title of "board." Governing boards hold legal and fiduciary responsibility for the organization. *Advisory boards* serve important functions, providing insight, connections, and even philanthropic support, but do not hold legal, fiduciary responsibility. Moreover, they offer recommendations that are nonbinding. The leader in the organization does not report to such a board, but rather to someone else. As an example, a dean of a college of nursing may have an advisory board, but that dean reports to the provost/vice president for academic affairs, who in turn reports to the president of the university. The president, a role parallel to a chief executive officer (CEO), reports to a governing board.

Nevertheless, a role on an advisory board for an organization is also an important way to contribute and build board skills. Similar to governing boards, there may be a committee structure. Those committees would reflect the needs of the individual or organization that created the advisory board. Such a board is not responsible for quality and financial status of the organization, and, correspondingly, these committees are not a typical part of the advisory board structure, but again—depending on the organization—either or both may exist on some advisory boards. Friend raising and fundraising is one role of many advisory boards, as is expanding the sphere of influence of the organization. Another may be to give programmatic advice. Take a look at your college or program website. Do you see an advisory board? Note the types of people who are on it. Now look at the website of a hospital, health system, or university. Note the trustees, who are sometimes called *directors*, and the group termed board of directors. These terms are telling; members of governing boards *direct*, advisory boards *advise*.

OTHER TYPES OF BOARDS

Constituency Boards

A still different variation of board type with a different route to board seat acquisition is a *constituency board*. In a constituency board, individuals represent a single agency, entity, or even a nation. In such a model, the board member has the responsibility to promulgate the views of the entity that they represent, rather than putting that identity aside to address the collective mission, as would be expected in a governing board. The role of constituency board members must include a mechanism by which the representative can garner the views of the constituency group as well as report back to them. Therefore, unlike a typical nonprofit fiduciary board role where the individual board member uses their own best judgment in the organization's overall best interest, constituency board membership involves substantial, ongoing communication with constituency members. An example of a constituency board would be one in which the board members represent the nurses' association, medical association, physical therapy association, small businesses, and so on. Board members representing such different entities may have conflicting agendas, as often the representative board member is also a lobbyist for that organization and has the responsibility to work for the best interests of its members, including their financial well-being. This is unlike the previously detailed nonprofit governing boards, in which the responsibility includes putting personal interests aside.

Regulatory Boards

A regulatory board is not a governing board, constituency board, or advisory board. Instead, a regulatory board has the responsibility for the enforcement of a particular *statute* or law to ensure compliance with that law, typically via *administrative rules*, in which the administrative rule is the more detailed policies and procedures. The regulatory board, sometimes called *regulatory authority* or *regulatory body*, is a governmental entity that has the responsibility for oversight in the best interest of the public. An example would be a state *board of nursing*. Such a body's responsibility is to protect the public, not to represent nurses or nursing. State regulatory boards are typically appointed by the state governor in a process that varies by state and by the particular regulatory body. Health care is a highly regulated function in society, and regulatory bodies may oversee Certificates of Need and hospital budgets, as just two examples, while a board of nursing oversees nursing practice and education to ensure that the public is protected. Importantly, the board of nursing is not accountable to nursing per se, nor does it represent nurses in the same way as a nursing association, but instead is accountable to the public for safe nursing practice.

In many regulatory boards, the *executive director* of the board is a staff person who is hired by and reports to the board, similar to the CEO in a governing board. Again, to underscore, unlike a governing board, there is no direct fiduciary responsibility for board members. Instead, there is a responsibility to ensure the execution of the state law. Take a moment to review the process for appointment to the board of nursing in your state by viewing the board website. This will give you a sense of how nurses are appointed to one regulatory body in your state.

BUILDING THE SKILL SET FOR BOARD MEMBERSHIP

There is no clear-cut set of strategies or experiences that lead to board membership, but there are skills and competencies that you can foster to be ready to comfortably seek or be ready to accept a board position. Test your skill set for board membership and determine your strengths and growth areas using the following skills checklist.

Skill 1: I Understand How Meetings Are Run and the Protocols Around Rules of Order, Such as Robert's Rules of Order or the Modern Rules of Order

In some boards, the culture is such that meetings are run loosely or at least more loosely than a full formal protocol or set of rules would demand. Other boards maintain strict attention to protocol. Although the best way to have a sense of the culture in a particular group is to participate in different meetings as an active member, here are a few guidelines.

Typically there is a *chair* and *members* of the board. The chair, often with input from management or other board members, develops the *meeting agenda*. This agenda, inclusive of date, location, times, and items for discussion and vote, is distributed prior to the meeting, typically via email (see Exhibit 11.1 for an example of an agenda). The details of how to access the meeting—time, location, weblink—are critical. Notably, since the beginning of the COVID-19 pandemic, virtual board meetings are becoming more common. Different organizations have different bylaws on the length of time before the meeting that the agenda must be distributed, but a common time frame is 1 to 2 weeks. Certain critical voting elements may have to be *warned* at least a month prior to the meeting, warned meaning informing the board of the upcoming vote on a particular issue. This sort of structure would also be common in a body like a university senate, in which many members need to be assembled and, thus, must have sufficient notice, not only to be sure that they can attend but also to obtain input from the constituencies they represent about an issue under consideration.

CALL TO ORDER

The chair calls the meeting to order and "runs the meeting." A *permanent chair* differs from a *convening chair*, whose role is simply to pull the group together and thus has a different level of power and influence and, indeed, a different role.

ESTABLISHMENT OF A QUORUM

Most boards and other groups such as a university senate require that there be a predefined *quorum*, a proportion or percentage of the membership that must be present if a vote is to occur. The proportion of the group needed to constitute a quorum is typically established in the organizational *bylaws*. You can think of bylaws as a set of organizational rules.

EXHIBIT 11.1

Sample Agenda

Pleasant Valley Hospital and Health System Board of Trustee Meeting
Date: April 15, 20XX
Time: 1:00 p.m.
Location: Pleasant Valley Hospital Board Room A, 10th Floor, West Corridor, 1353 Fictitious Lane, Anytown, USA or via weblink

1. Call to order—Tierra Jackson, Board Chair	1:00 p.m.
2. Review of previous minutes—Tierra Jackson, Board Chair	1:01 p.m.
3. Chair's report—Tierra Jackson, Board Chair	1:05 p.m.
4. CEO's report—David Hernandez, CEO, Pleasant Valley Hospital	1:15 p.m.
5. Standing committee reports	
A. Audit Committee: Peter Smith, Audit Committee Chair	1:25 p.m.
B. Finance Committee: Aki Chang, Finance Committee Chair	1:35 p.m.
C. Planning Committee: Jada Kennedy, Planning Committee Chair	1:45 p.m.
D. Quality Committee: Xavier Gonzalez, Quality Committee Chair	1:55 p.m.
6. Old business	
A. Union negotiations: Lamar Jones, Vice President for Human Resources	2:05 p.m.
B. Quality Institute planning: Lakshmi Chada, Chief Quality Officer	2:30 p.m.
7. New business	
A. ACO acquisition: David Hernandez, CEO, & Jada Kennedy, Planning Committee Chair	3:00 p.m.
8. Adjournment: Tierra Jackson, Board Chair	4:00 p.m.

Note: All names represent fictitious characters.
ACO, accountable care organization; CEO, chief executive officer.

Thus, the first order of business is to establish if there is a quorum of members in attendance. The absence of a quorum is unlikely in major boards, but some small, new, or struggling boards may suffer from attendance issues among board members. If there is no quorum in attendance, those attending can decide to hold the meeting for the purpose of discussion, but no voting can occur. Or the group may decide to reschedule. The quorum criterion is also a necessary aspect of committee meetings, and small committees are more likely to be plagued by quorum issues because the absence of one or two members may mean a majority of members are not in attendance.

APPROVAL OF MINUTES FROM THE PREVIOUS MEETING

Once the quorum is established, the next line of business is approval of previous minutes. Although this may seem like a perfunctory issue, these minutes become the permanent record of board action. In the event of a legal challenge to board action or an inquiry of any type, the minutes are a key reference. As a board member, it is wise to read minutes carefully, be sure they are complete and correct, and if not, to offer *corrections and additions.* A motion and second to accept the corrected minutes will likely follow. Also, a member who was not at the meeting should abstain from this vote, as it is not possible for them to assess the accuracy of minutes for a meeting they did not attend.

OPEN MEETING LAWS

Some public bodies function under an *open meeting law,* meaning all business except personnel or contract issues must be open to the public, including the minutes being open and individuals being free to choose to *attend* a meeting as a spectator. Such meetings may be video recorded, creating a permanent public record. The written minutes are then often terse, as the full record is available on video.

CHAIR'S REPORT AND CHIEF EXECUTIVE OFFICER'S REPORT

At this point, the protocol in different boards varies. A common approach is for a *chair's report*, updating the board, followed by a *CEO's report*. Alternatively, these may be previously provided in written form and this time used simply for questions about the written materials.

COMMITTEE REPORTS

Committee reports, provided by the committee chairs, are next. If there are recommendations that come from the committee, they are vetted by the full board at that time. Recommendations coming from a committee do not require a seconded motion for discussion leading to a vote. This, of course, makes sense: The recommendation has already been, in essence, supported by at least two people, which is what is needed for a motion and a second. The full board then discusses committee recommendations, and a vote is taken. Prior to a vote, several actions can take place.

VOTING PROCESS

A *friendly amendment* is a recommended change to a motion or recommendation that is in keeping with the original motion but offers some refinement or small change. The original maker of the motion or recommendation must agree to the friendly amendment, as must the individual who offered the second to the original *motion*. If so, the vote is on the new language. A more formal means to alter a motion or recommendation is with a motion for an amendment. This, if moved and seconded, is then discussed and voted on. If it is approved, the discussion then returns to the *main motion as amended*. If it is not approved, the discussion returns to the original motion. In either case, at the conclusion of discussion, there is a vote. If there is a great number of unanswered questions or a conflict, a member may make a motion to *table* the item, which means to put the issue aside and not vote on it at that time. If seconded, there would be a vote on tabling the item. If the motion to table is supported, the item is not discussed further at that time, although a plan for further information gathering or to revisit it at some point in the future is common. A timetable or set date to return to the item may also be required. If the motion to table the item is not supported, the conversation returns to the motion under discussion.

A still different action prior to the vote is to *call the question*. This typically happens if there is protracted conversation about a motion. If the question is called, a mistake typically made is for the chair to immediately cease all conversation and go to the vote on the main motion (or main motion as amended, if that is the motion under discussion). Instead, the correct protocol is that when the question is called, and if it is seconded, there must be a vote on calling the question, that is, a vote on whether or not discussion should cease. If the motion and second to call the question are supported by majority vote, discussion does cease and a vote is taken on the main motion, or the main motion as amended, depending on what previously ensued. If the vote to call the question does not pass, discussion continues.

STANDING REPORTS, OLD BUSINESS, AND NEW BUSINESS

As noted in Exhibit 11.1, standing committee reports are typically followed by a discussion of old and new business, which may also present items requiring a vote. State regulatory boards may have a mandatory period for public *comment* and a process by which the public can comment before a board can act on an item, meaning that no item can be introduced and voted on in the same meeting.

CONSENT AGENDAS

This meeting pattern would be altered if a consent agenda is used. A consent agenda, termed a consent calendar in Robert's Rules of Order, is a meeting practice that bundles routine, noncontroversial business, reports, or votes into a single item. The aim is to conserve meeting time for complex issues needing discussion or educational sessions. A person who is part of a board that uses consent agendas should carefully review all the materials in the consent agenda and, if uncomfortable with any element in it, ask for that item to be removed from the consent agenda for open discussion. Some board chairs ask members if they want any item removed from the consent agenda before proceeding with a vote. BoardSource cautions: "Board members need to be vigilant so that debatable issues do not accidentally pass through without appropriate deliberation" (2023, para 11).

ACTION ITEM OR EDUCATIONAL SESSION?

In addition to meetings including *action items*, those needing a vote, many boards hold educational sessions. These may be a part of full board meetings or the board may alternate *action meetings* with *educational meetings*. Clearly, board membership requires a level of communication between and among group members as well as the public. This will be the next item on the skill set checklist.

Skill 2: I Can Speak in a Clear and Direct Way in Public, and My Appearance Creates Confidence in My Message and Abilities

This skill may come naturally to you. If not, it is a skill that can be practiced. Many colleges and universities require graduates to demonstrate some level of an oral proficiency competency and offer courses to enhance the student's "public speaking," as it is often called. Such courses offer an ideal time to hone skills with guided feedback. A more independent way to augment your public speaking skills is to video record yourself on either a phone or a medium like YouTube. If you are practicing on YouTube and do not want this publicly disseminated, be sure to select the setting as "private." Self-recording provides an unparalleled way to identify strengths and growth areas. Self-query questions as you review the presentation include the following:

- Is my manner direct? Confident? Trustworthy? Do I have any mannerisms that distract from these important qualities, such as eye shifting or eye rolling? Do the "uhs" or "likes" get in the way of the message?
- Does my visual appearance inspire confidence in the audience I am trying to connect with? Remember that your physical appearance can help forge a form of overlap between yourself and the group. Thus, your clothing, accessories, and makeup presence/absence are extremely important. There is an almost instantaneous impression based on appearance, which is closely followed and informed by language, tone, and grammar: Who are you saying you are with your visual messages? Generational issues are also at play in this arena, as many tech start-up millionaires and even billionaires are young and casually dressed. Know that these issues are critical when presenting virtually as well; be sure to check the backdrop

that your viewers will be seeing; ensure proper lighting; raise the camera so that viewers see your eyes, not a neck or "nose shot"; and have pets and other distractions cloistered.

Finally, while it is important to be yourself, recall that there are different elements of your skills and abilities that you can bring to the forefront in different settings that may either be more or less readily accepted, based on appearance. If, for example, you are meeting with a group of homeless adolescents, bonding would likely be facilitated if you *did not* arrive in the sort of polished business attire that would be the norm for the corporate boardroom. Conversely, wearing jeans, shirts without ties, and other casual wear may not inspire the desired impression in a group of business and political leaders. The local culture also makes a difference in what constitutes *appropriate professional attire*. In a meeting at a small nonprofit in a very rural remote area, casual rainboots may be appropriate footwear in bad weather, but out of place—marking you as an outsider—if that meeting were in Washington, DC. Nurses sometimes attend meetings in scrubs, as do physicians. Although this can reinforce the image of the practicing clinician, it may be inappropriate or at the least not optimal for a board-level meeting. Gordon's (2005) observation remains relevant over two decades later: Nurses undermine their own authority by "showing up in what looks like pajamas," particularly when these scrubs have images on them such as animals. A trusted mentor can help you navigate these various issues. Also be sure to observe board politics and power dynamics for clues on how to best present your message so that you will be heard and taken seriously. This is particularly important for women, given their persistent challenges with being ignored, interrupted, or challenged at meetings (Kramer, 2023).

Skill 3: I Understand Financial Operations and Financial Reports

This is a particularly important competency for governing board members because one of the key responsibilities of the board is to provide and oversee the organization's budget, revenue and expenditures, and fiscal benchmarks needed for credit ratings. It is critical to understand, however, that this approval and oversight occur at a high level; the board members do not determine specific budget line expenses. Instead, a strategic vision is developed by leadership in collaboration with other members of the organization, typically with performance targets. These may be approved by the board, but the institutional budget represents the living strategic plan. It details the organization's priorities by illustrating where and how financial resources are allocated. Moreover, many financial allocations translate to human resources, for example, the salaries of individuals doing the work of the organization, including nurses. Therefore, attention to the distribution of resources between human and material resources illustrated on the financial report is warranted.

WHAT ABOUT FINANCIAL STATEMENTS?

The organization's financial statements will first be vetted by the finance committee and only then reviewed by the full board. They are organized in a standard manner, with assets listed first and liabilities second. The *budget to actual* is typically included, as is a comparison to a previous year-to-date budget, to be discussed in greater detail later in this chapter. Negative numbers are shown in parentheses or may literally be illustrated in red ink, hence the colloquialism of being *in the red*.

SALARIES AND FRINGE BENEFITS

As a human resource–intensive industry, health care organizations typically employ a large number of individuals. This is reflected in budget sheets as salaries. Note also, however, that fringe benefits such as health insurance and retirement contributions are a notable portion of a budget. Using a hypothetical employee with a salary of $100,000/year, for example, an organization whose fringe rate is 38% would need to have budgeted—and have available—$138,000/year for compensation for that employee. The largest portion of fringe benefits is typically health insurance.

WHAT DOES THE TERM "DAYS CASH ON HAND" MEAN AND WHY IS IT IMPORTANT?

A second key background concept important to all organizational types is *days cash on hand*. This concept is similar to a personal checking account for meeting regular, ongoing expenses, and a cushion is needed to ensure that the organization can meet ongoing obligations—paying its nurses, for example.

WHAT ARE BOND RATING AND BOND COVENANTS?

Not only is days cash on hand important in *making payroll*, that is, having the financial resources to pay employees and other regular expenses, it is one element that determines an organization's *bond rating* and impacts *bond covenants*. The term bond rating refers to an organization's *credit worthiness*, while the term bond covenant refers to a set of rules or parameters around a borrowing arrangement. Bond rating will impact how much an organization can borrow and how much borrowing costs the organization in terms of interest rating. An organization may need funds to expand the physical plant (buildings) of a hospital, for example, and a higher credit rating enables the organization to borrow money at a lower interest rate and thus creates less long-term debt. In the United States, there are three common raters,

Moody's Investors Services, Standard and Poor's, and Fitch, and the rating for an organization may differ slightly among them. An organization that has obtained bonds for some sort of project must abide by the previously noted bond covenants or rules of the borrowing arrangement. Days cash on hand is a key financial "vital sign" in an organization, as is the amount of *long-term debt* and the ratio of *debt to total capital* (see Exhibit 11.2 for analogous simple, everyday examples of these concepts). This latter concept is sometimes termed *debt-to-cap* or *D/C ratio*. This ratio is simply an index of the amount of debt compared to other assets; you can think about this as the loans-to-assets ratio.

WHAT DOES "BUDGET TO ACTUAL" MEAN?

When attending a board meeting or a meeting of the finance committee, organizations also provide a written report of *budget to actual revenues* and *budget to actual liabilities*. Although these may seem like very foreign terms, these concepts are actually familiar to you in your everyday life. You can consider these terms parallel to the following statements in your own household. Budget to actual revenue: "I thought I was going to have *x* amount of money coming in (budgeted revenue), but I actually have *y* amount of money coming in (actual revenue)." Budget to actual liabilities: "I thought I was going to have *z* amount of money I would need to pay out (budgeted liability), but I actually have *q* amount of money I need to pay out (actual liabilities)." The difference between *x* and *y* is called a *variance*, as is the difference between *z* and *q*.

EXHIBIT 11.2

Defining Common Financial Terms

Long-term debt can be differentiated from short-term debt in the following manner. Imagine you decide to buy a new dining room set, and you are able to obtain a 12-month loan from the furniture company. This is short-term debt, in contrast to, for example, a home mortgage in which the loan for your home will be paid with a monthly amount over 30 consecutive years. The mortgage constitutes long-term debt.

Debt-to-capitalization ratios can be conceptualized in the following contrasting situations, the first with a low debt-to-capitalization ratio and the second with a high debt-to-capitalization ratio. Imagine you owe $10,000 on a new car valued at $30,000 and you own a fully paid-off $300,000 home. In this case, you have very little debt in relationship to assets. Contrast this with a situation in which you owe $10,000 on your car, which is worth only $12,000, but also have $100,000 in student loans and no other assets.

It is a bit more complicated in health care, of course, but these scenarios illustrate the basic ideas. Which of the two preceding individuals would you rather be? If you were a bank, which one would you rather give a loan to? Similarly, organizations with lower long-term debt and a low debt-to-capitalization ratio are in better financial health and considered more creditworthy.

Obviously, an organization that consistently has more actual liabilities than actual revenue is not in sound financial health. Remember also that budgeted revenues are *predictions* of what an organization believes it will receive, and these estimates may never be perfectly on target with the actual numbers, no matter how skillful the organization. Some variance is expected, just not dramatic, consistent, or growing negative variance.

WHAT SORTS OF CIRCUMSTANCES CREATE BUDGET VARIANCES?

Revenue in a health care organization includes payment from Medicare, Medicaid, and commercial insurance reimbursement, among others. When an organization sets its budget based on an expected rate of Medicaid reimbursement, for example, and that state later responds to budget shortfall by cutting Medicaid reimbursement rates midyear, that actual revenue will be lower than initially budgeted. (The term for this sort of change is *rescission*, which means cutting out or repealing something that was previously approved.) Variance can also be related to how many health services people are using. *Lower-than-expected volumes*—that is, the amount of services given to patients in an organization—will result in a lower actual revenue than budgeted in an organization receiving fee-for-service reimbursement. A variance can also be created following expenditures or costs that are higher or lower than expected. If, for example, there is an extremely harsh winter, actual heating costs (noted in the budget sheet under the term *utilities* and inclusive of other utilities such as electricity) may be much higher than budgeted. Conversely, an unexpectedly mild winter may result in lower-than-budgeted utility expenses. The important concept to take away here is that, unlike how the term budget is used more commonly, the "budget" of an organization is a *plan*, whereas "actuals" *are what actually happens*. Finally, liabilities in a health care organization will include things like salaries for staff and payment on debts. Take a moment to locate and review these financial reports on your institution's website.

WHAT ABOUT PAYER MIX?

The items just discussed are common to all organizations, but there are financial elements (discussed in earlier chapters) that are unique to health care and merit reconsideration as you review financial reports. Key among these are *payer mix*, the proportion of revenue from commercial insurers, Medicare, and Medicaid, as well the proportion of *bad debt* and *charity care*, which represents charges that are not collected (see Exhibit 11.3). As detailed in previous chapters, cost, charges, and reimbursement are not the same. Therefore, organizations may look similar in terms of cost and charges but be compensated at very different levels based on payer mix. Again, take a moment to search the website of a local health care organization and see if you can locate and read a financial statement to further acquaint yourself with these aspects of financial operations and reports.

NEXT STEPS

In summary, three major areas of strength that complement your clinical and nursing practice knowledge will help you access a board position. These are being meeting savvy, effective presentation of self, and financial acumen. Create a list of your strengths and gaps. Then, if possible, review it with a colleague who will give you an honest critique. Then, develop a plan to fill those gaps.

EXHIBIT 11.3

What Is the Difference Between Bad Debt and Charity Care?

Bad debt and **charity care** are both ways in which hospitals report care given to those who are uninsured or underinsured. Hospitals typically have a policy about how this care is charged; for example, they may set the charge at the Medicare rate rather than the much higher commercial insurance rate. They may also work with uninsured individuals to see if they are indeed eligible for some sort of coverage such as Medicaid. Even so, some individuals will not have coverage, meaning that the facility is providing uncompensated care. This **charity care** is known upon admission, and the magnitude of **charity care** is carefully monitored because some states provide reimbursement to hospitals for some portion of the **charity care**, and **charity care** is part of a financial formula that reimburses hospitals that serve a high proportion of uninsured individuals and Medicaid patients. This is called a disproportionate share hospital (DSH) payment, commonly voiced as "dish" payment. There is also a DSH formula for Medicare (see https://www.cms.gov/medicare/payment/prospective-payment-systems/acute-inpatient-pps/disproportionate-share-hospital-dsh). Charity care is also a component of the community benefit requirement for nonprofit tax-exempt status, a situation under scrutiny, as previously discussed.

Bad debt refers to a different phenomenon and basically refers to individuals who do not pay their bill after receiving services. Unlike **charity care**, where the situation is known up-front, **bad debt** is discovered after the treatment. These persons may be insured but have a high deductible, for example, and be unable or unwilling to pay what insurance did not cover.

End-of-Chapter Resources

THOUGHT QUESTIONS

1. How do board member roles vary on different kinds of boards? Why are there these differences?
2. What strengths would you bring to a governing board? Regulatory board? Advisory board?
3. What is appropriate professional attire for participation in a hospital board meeting? Defend your answer.
4. Define the following key terms:
   Action item
   Action meeting
   Administrative rules
   Appointed board
   Appropriate professional attire
   CEO's report
   Chair's report
   Consent agenda
   Constituency board
   Convening chair
   Corrections and additions to minutes
   Days cash on hand
   Education meeting
   Elected boards
   Main motion
   Main motion as amended
   Open meeting law
   Quorum
   Self-perpetuating board
   Warned vote

EXERCISES

1. Role-play a governing board meeting. Assign peers and yourself to different governing board roles and hold a mock board meeting. Be sure to have the chair prepare the agenda in advance and have voting items.
2. Attend an open meeting of the state board of nursing or other state regulatory board.

3. Does your nursing program have an advisory board? Are there students on it? Or is there a student advisory board in which students provide insight to the dean? If so, who are these students, and how did they get appointed, selected, or elected?
4. Obtain the bylaws of your college or university or local hospital (try the institution's website). What do they say about a quorum? What other rules are identified?
5. Many hospital board meetings include a session for the public. Attend and report back to peers on what you observed. What financial terms did you understand? Which ones were confusing to you? Develop a learning agenda to address that gap.

QUIZ

True or False

1. In self-perpetuating boards, existing board members identify potential new members.
2. One strength of a self-perpetuating board is the capacity to easily expand board membership to underrepresented groups.
3. Typically, a quorum of board members is needed for board action items that require a vote.
4. Another term for statute is administrative rule.
5. Another term for statute is law.
6. Similar to a chief executive officer, the executive director is hired by and reports to the board.
7. Charity care differs from bad debt in that care that will be charity is known by the institution at the time of admission, whereas bad debt will not be known by the institution until the individual fails to pay whatever remains on the bill.
8. The financial term debt-to-cap ratio is synonymous with the term days cash on hand.
9. The term bond covenant refers to rules that are part of an organization's borrowing agreement.
10. An organization's deemed credit worthiness is identified by its bond rating.

Multiple Choice

11. Different types of boards secure new members using different approaches. These include
    A. Election
    B. Appointment
    C. Both A and B
    D. Neither A nor B

12. Regulatory boards
    A. Represent the interests of shareholders
    B. Hold fiduciary responsibility
    C. Both A and B
    D. Neither A nor B
13. Which is a type of board in which members are typically appointed by a political entity such as the state governor?
    A. Governing board
    B. Regulatory board
    C. Advisory board
    D. All of the above
14. The type of board that is most likely to be responsible for enforcement of a statute is a:
    A. Governing board
    B. Regulatory board
    C. Advisory board
    D. All of the above
15. What constitutes appropriate professional attire?
    A. May vary depending on the audience, venue, or group
    B. May be discerned with the help of a trusted mentor
    C. Both A and B
    D. Neither A nor B

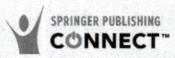

A robust set of instructor resources designed to supplement this text is located at http://connect.springerpub.com/content/book/978-0-8261-7236-5. Qualifying instructors may request access by emailing **textbook@springerpub.com**.

REFERENCES

BoardSource. (2023, October 20). *Consent agendas*. Author. https://boardsource.org/resources/consent-agendas/

Gordon, S. (2005). *Nursing against the odds: How health care cost cutting, media stereotypes, and medical hubris undermine nurses and patient care*. Cornell University Press.

Kacik, A. (2022). *How nurses are making inroads in hospital boardrooms*. Modern Healthcare. https://www.modernhealthcare.com/esg/nurses-on-boards-hospital-governance-palo-pinto-aha#

Kramer, A. (2023, December 11). *Why women face a sound barrier in their fight to be heard*. Forbes. https://www.forbes.com/sites/andiekramer/2023/12/11/why-women-face-a-sound-barrier-in-their-fight-to-be-heard/

Worth, M. (2024). *Nonprofit management: Principles and practices* (7th ed.). Sage.

CHAPTER 12

Applying Health Economics to Improve Health Care Through Federal and State Policy Formation

Following completion of this chapter, you will be able to:
- Describe U.S. governmental structures.
- Describe the policy process.
- Detail points of influence in policy formation.
- Explore the unique contribution of nurses in policy formation.
- Develop a learning agenda for enhancing personal political influence.

> *I see clinicians and other people who work in healthcare as incredibly committed, really trying to do the right thing. They are advocating for people's health on a daily basis. Yet they are not always adept about policy because it is not a world they travel in. So I would like to see more clinicians integrated into the policy process—in part because they have such a rich voice.*
> —Julie Sochalski, in an interview by Pulcini (2014, p. 19)
>
> *Too little has changed since this interview over a decade ago.* Joyce Pulcini (personal communication, May 30, 2024)

Two hundred years ago, women did not have the right to vote. Neither did people of color. Today, all citizens, including nurses, have the opportunity to influence policy in meaningful ways. Nurses have held positions in Congress, state legislatures, and other prominent positions. However, a nurse does not need to run for political office to be influential. Numbering 5.2 million (Smiley et al., 2023), nurses have a collective opportunity to be a substantial force in health care policy, health policy, and economic and social policy writ large. Too few nurses, however, seize this opportunity. Hajizadeh et al. (2021) note that although nurses constitute the majority of the health care workforce, few are involved in policy making at any level, including within their own clinical setting. They further note that nurses' lack of involvement in policy is so significant that it is a concern of not only the International Council of Nurses but also the World Health Organization.

Arguably, nurses may subconsciously view their role as a private relationship between patients and their families and themselves, the individual nurse. In the same vein, nurses studied nursing in college, not political science or law, alternative pathways that might have indicated an intention to become active in politics. Yet even one small policy change may impact thousands or even millions of lives and offers a profound means of beneficence. What follows, therefore, is a dissection of the political process, with suggestions for active involvement at various scales and levels of intensity. After all, *politics* means, literally, *the work of the people*, given that the Latin origin of the word "poli" means "many." Nothing could be more compatible with nursing than policy formation, offering broad solutions to societal problems through policy and politics.

First, a short review of the basics of U.S. governance. Although this may seem like basic knowledge, a 2022 Annenberg Public Policy survey reported that less than half of respondents were able to name all three branches of government and one in four could not name any branches of government. In the same vein, less than half could correctly identify the role of the Supreme Court (Annenberg Public Policy Center, 2022). Yet understanding the responsibilities the U.S. Constitution gives each branch of government is essential to influencing health policy and, arguably, even participate in voting and public life as an informed citizen. Understanding the roles of each branch of government is also critically important in understanding the fate of key pieces of legislation, such as the Affordable Care Act (ACA) and the Supreme Court challenges to its constitutionality, as well as other health care–related laws, executive orders, and Supreme Court decisions.

BRANCHES OF GOVERNMENT

The three branches of government exist to provide a system of checks and balances, whereby each branch has both influence and limitations. For example, the legislative branch, Congress, makes the laws; the executive branch, the president, executes the law; and the judicial branch, the Supreme Court, adjudicates when there is a question of constitutionality or there are conflicting decisions from the "lower courts." The lower federal courts include district courts and circuit courts. At the federal level, the circuit courts form the first level of appeal of decisions made in the district court and thus serve as an intermediary review step before the U.S. Supreme Court (see Figure 12.1). The term "circuit" court refers to the original concept of this intermediary court in which judges from different legal jurisdictions "rode the circuit" to hear cases.

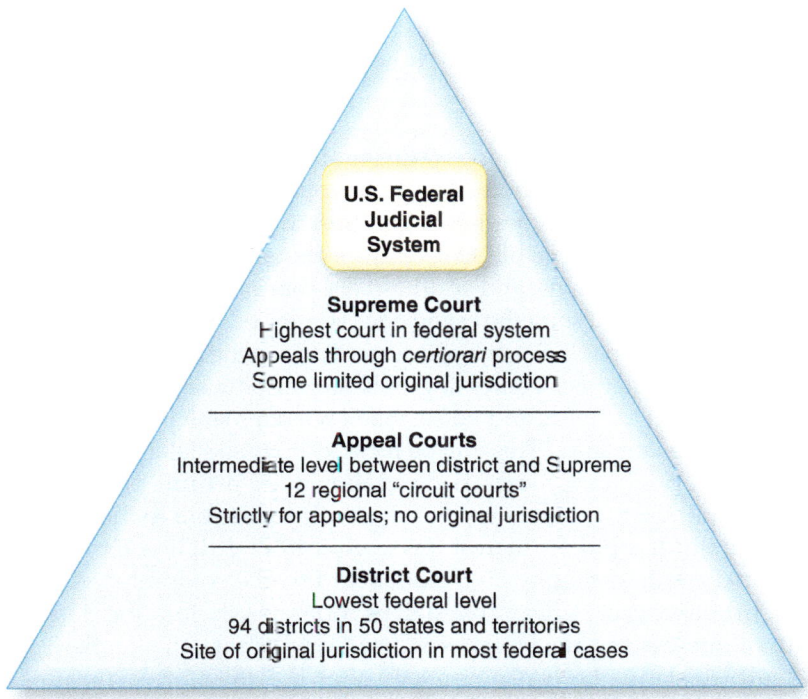

FIGURE 12.1: The federal judicial appeals process.

These three branches of government also exist at the state level, wherein the legislative branch is the state legislature, the executive branch the governor, and the judicial branch the state Supreme Court.

How Are Laws Made?

The U.S. Constitution vests the power to make laws in the legislative branch of government. The very first part of the Constitution, Article 1, Section 1, states: "All legislative Powers herein granted shall be vested in a Congress of the United States, which shall consist of a Senate and House of Representatives." Again, in a similar pattern to the federal chambers, each U.S. state has a state Senate and state House of Representatives who hold the power to make state law. The state of Nebraska is the exception to this structure, with only one chamber, which is termed unicameral from the Latin "one chamber." Although uncommon in the United States, of the 240 nations with legislative bodies, nearly two-thirds are unicameral (Central Intelligence Agency [CIA], n.d.; Kenton, 2024).

Legislative Committees

> *Laws are like sausages—it is best not to see them being made. (Attributed to Otto Von Bismarck)*[1]

Senators and representatives serve on committees, and much of the "hammering out" work is done there. As the famous Bismarck quote illustrates, like sausage, what initially goes into a bill draft may look very different from the final product, that is, the bill that receives enough votes to be passed into law. Amendments, deletions, and additions are common. A bill may change so much in the process that something you once supported, you may now oppose. Thus, it is important to follow a bill of interest through the entire legislative process. Moreover, sometimes competing bills are introduced, again illustrating why fully engaged lobbyists and government relations staff can be so valuable to an organization or cause. This will be further discussed later in this chapter.

The first step in the process is development of a draft of the bill (see Box 12.1). A bill sponsor or sponsors will introduce the bill to the House, the Senate, or both. If a bill of interest has been introduced, it is first reviewed in committee, with testimony on the bill heard by the committee. A committee is a sort of working group that delves more deeply into the details of a domain of interest and develops expertise by which it can shepherd issues to the full legislative body. Committees offer a form of specialization, for example, in areas such as health, environment, and education, to name just a few. Other committees deal with the actual funding of bills, for example, the appropriations committee or—at the national level—the House Ways and Means Committee. Take a moment to review the website for your state governance structure as well as the parallel information at the national level (www.house.gov and www.senate.gov).

 BOX 12.1

WHAT IS A BILL DRAFT?

Long before something becomes a law, it exists in earlier forms. First, there needs to be an idea, and this idea is then drafted into a bill or a preliminary version of what the law might look like.

Many bills *die in committee*, meaning the bill does not return to the Senate or House for a vote. In the 117th Congress, only 4% of the bills introduced were voted on by the full assembly and only 2% of the bills introduced were enacted into law (Govtrack, n.d.). Each Congress has two 1-year sessions; for example, the 117th Congress met from January 3, 2021, to January 3, 2023. The 118th Congress convened January 3, 2023, and concluded on January 3, 2025. If a bill is not enacted during this time, it is not carried over and must be reintroduced to be considered. Thus, involvement at the committee level is an essential skill for politically active nurses.

INFLUENCING AT THE COMMITTEE LEVEL

Whom should you contact? If the chair of the committee is in your legislative district, contacting the chair of the committee with your input is a particularly effective strategy; committee chairs set agendas and tones, an explicit and implicit form of influence, respectively. Understandably, they want to have and keep your vote. The committee chair is not the only avenue. Committee members are also key influencers during the committee review process. Look to see if any of your representatives or senators serve on key committees.

TIMING MATTERS

Timing matters! If the bill is still in committee, contacting committee members is most effective. If it has gone to the floor for a vote, then it is very effective to contact whomever represents you. Indicate your position clearly and succinctly. Also know that in small states, state representatives and senators are largely without full staff support. Thus, if there is an area in which you are an expert, a short list of *talking points* may aid the policy maker if they wish to articulate that position on the floor of the House or the Senate. At the federal level, companion bills may go through the House and the Senate at the same time and, if passed in both, differences reconciled in a conference committee, as noted in the "How a Bill Becomes a Law" diagram (see Figure 12.2). Bills may be introduced by any member of either chamber, House or Senate, with the exception of bills imposing taxes; the Constitution states: "All bills for raising Revenue shall originate in the House of Representatives." Instead of companion bills, 24 states include a *bill crossover deadline* approach, with the crossover deadline being the last day a bill in one chamber can be passed to the other for consideration (Statescape, 2020). In this model, committee hearings and votes happen on one side, say the House, and then *cross over* mid-session, that is, switch to the Senate. There, in the Senate, the process starts anew as a bill to be considered by that body. Take a moment to review how a bill becomes a law in your state, noting when legislators are in session (annually, biannually, selected months), legislators' employment status (full time/part time), their salaries, and key dates such as crossover.

A bill that has survived this process then goes to the executive branch—the president or governor—to sign into law or veto. This step offers one last chance to advocate for or against a bill by contacting the president on a federal bill or the governor for a state bill (see USA.gov, n.d. for an additional illustration of the federal process).

The president may sign the bill into law or *veto* the bill and return it with objections to Congress. Congress may override the veto if there is two-thirds support in both chambers. Finally, in a *pocket veto* a bill dies due to lack of

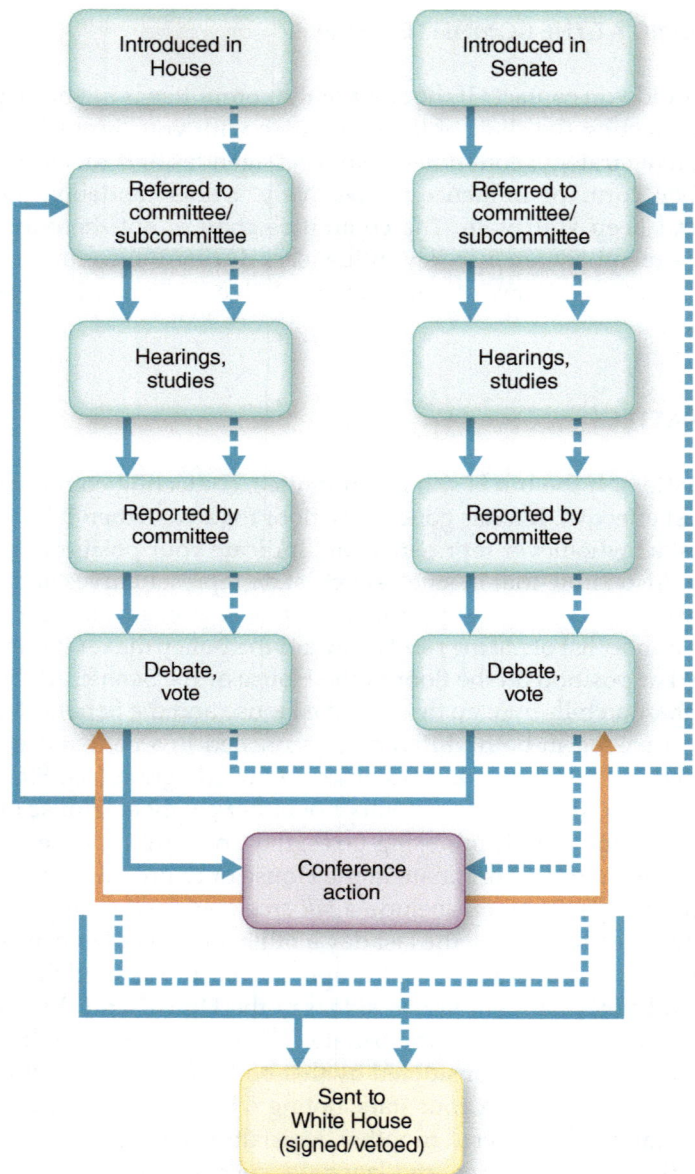

FIGURE 12.2: How a bill becomes a law.

executive signature and is not returned to Congress within the required 10 days. A total of 38 of the 45 presidents have vetoed 2,576 bills, and only 4.3% of these had sufficient congressional support to override the veto and become law (Stuessy, 2019). At the time of this writing, 44 U.S. states allow *line-item* veto, in which the governor cancels or nullifies specific provisions of a bill without vetoing the whole bill. The presence or absence of the potential for line-item vetoes dramatically changes political strategies and gives a governor substantially more power to shape nuances of a bill. Again, take a moment to look at your state laws on this issue. The practice was deemed unconstitutional at the federal level because the president would be, in essence, acting in a legislative capacity—a role that the Constitution assigns to Congress (Cornell Law School, n.d.).

MAINTAINING A CONNECTION WITH POLICY MAKERS TO INFLUENCE HEALTH AND HEALTH CARE

A sustained connection with a policy maker or policy makers can result in the nurse and nursing agendas having considerable influence throughout the legislative process, from bill drafting and committee hearings to full chamber review. Nursing interests may be forgotten not out of malice but simply because nurses are not visible in the process. In many states, the absence of a constant nursing presence at the statehouse results in comparative invisibility. In such cases, identification of additional stakeholders and subsequent coalition building are valuable ways to foster a nursing presence. Finally, nursing involvement in health policy may be focused on health care, but activities directed toward the broader social determinants of health are a worthy contribution as well. Nurses are credible to the public, and advocating for policies that do not directly benefit nurses adds additional credibility to the cause under review. Similarly, engaging stakeholders who are not directly affiliated with nurses, for example, the chamber of commerce, strengthens nurses' influence.

Beyond the Legislative Process

Despite its prominent place in the U.S. Constitution, the legislative process is not the only way societal laws are determined. Twenty-four states allow *direct democracy* in the form of initiatives or referendums whereby voters directly determine law (see Box 12.2). Other means that occur at both the state and federal levels include administrative rulemaking (sometimes called administrative law), executive order, and judicial review. These will now each be reviewed in turn.

Administrative Rule Making

When a law is passed, the approved bill is now called an act, but that is just the first step toward implementing the new law. Most laws lack the specificity necessary to execute the law and—as the name implies—this responsibility

BOX 12.2

DIRECT DEMOCRACY

The 24 states that allow direct democracy differ in their approach, but in general include the option for (a) an *initiative* whereby, following the attainment of a required number of citizens' signatures, a law is decided directly by the voters or (b) a *referendum* in which voters demand a popular vote on a new law passed by the legislature. Examples include the state of Maine's referendum that expanded Medicaid following the vote of nearly 60% of residents and Massachusetts's initiative to mandate nurse staffing ratios, the latter of which did not carry the popular vote and thus did not become law. Since the *Dobbs* decision overturning *Roe v Wade*, citizen-initiated efforts to place abortion access as a constitutional amendment has emerged as a "powerful tool that is being utilized to allow voters to garner signatures to place abortion on the ballot without directly involving the legislature or the governor" (Felix et al., 2024, para 3). Learn more about your state at www.ncsl.org/research/elections-and-campaigns/chart-of-the-initiative-states.aspx.

to develop the details goes to the executive branch of government. Take a moment to review the statute (law) in your state that gives registered nurses the authority to practice. Then review the administrative rules that provide the details governing nursing in your state. These rules are promulgated by an agency of state government. Similarly, on the national level, a health care law—even a detailed one—does not provide sufficient particulars for execution, and these are typically developed and promulgated by the U.S. Department of Health and Human Services or one of its branches such as the Centers for Medicare & Medicaid Services.

How significant is the role of administrative rules? Recall that these rules have the force of law, and they provide an enormous amount of detail guiding how the law will be carried out. The ACA, for example, is over 900 pages long (roughly 380,000 words), and its administrative rules are 30 times as long as the law. The administrative rules also can reflect the views of a particular president's administration more so than the statute itself. Why is this so?

The president nominates and then appoints the heads of executive agencies following confirmation in the Senate. The heads of these agencies serve as the president's cabinet. These agencies develop the administrative rules and—although public comment is accepted and the planned rule can be modified—the agency has broad discretion to promulgate and enforce the rule. Thus, the president, through selections of agency heads, shapes the execution of federal law. A similar process occurs at the state level, with the governor appointing heads of state agencies and these individuals serving as the governor's cabinet. This is an indirect manner by which the executive branch can shape the execution of a law. In addition, the executive branch can directly shape law through executive orders.

On June 28, 2024, the Supreme Court made a major ruling that will impact the authority of federal agencies, the implications of which are not fully clear as this text goes to press. In a 6–3 ruling, the justices overturned a 1984 ruling that gave rise to what is known as the Chevron doctrine or Chevron deference. The Chevron doctrine gave power to the agencies' interpretations of the law if it was reasonable, with the courts required to uphold the agency interpretation. The 2024 decision cuts this power and instead ruled that courts should interpret ambiguous laws, not the agencies, with far-reaching implications for health care (Howe, 2024).

Executive Orders

An executive order is a dictate by the chief executive, that is, the president at the national level and the governor at the state level. These orders have the power of law, yet they are determined by the decree of one person, the chief executive officer, rather than through the legislative process. An executive order may also be used to create organizations and committees. The Peace Corps, for example, was created by John F. Kennedy through an executive order. Presidents may also issue a proclamation that has the force of law; for example, the Emancipation Proclamation issued by Abraham Lincoln changed the status of more than 3.5 million people from slave to free. More recently, President Trump issued a proclamation to suspend the entry of immigrants who have the potential to financially burden the U.S. health care system (White House, 2019), and in 2023 President Biden issued a proclamation that grants pardon for the offenses of possession of marijuana or use of marijuana (see a list of all proclamations since 1994 here: https://www.federalregister.gov/presidential-documents/proclamations). Each U.S. president, except for James A. Garfield who only served as president for 6 months, has issued at least one proclamation. Proclamations are typically largely ceremonial and affect private individuals, a scope usually and not otherwise within presidential power (Ballotpedia, n.d.). President Biden, however, issued substantive proclamations and letters immediately after becoming president. A proclamation ending Trump-era travel restrictions for citizens from seven Muslim-majority and African countries was signed on the day of the inauguration, for example, as were letters returning the United States to membership in the World Health Organization and the Paris Climate Accord.

Executive orders have been used by presidents since George Washington, who issued eight. The record to date is President Franklin Delano Roosevelt, who issued 3,721. More recently, there has been concern among some that important policy debates are bypassing the legislative process and the debate and compromise typically required to pass a bill. But are executive orders really increasing?

George W. Bush issued 291 executive orders in his two terms as president, and, similarly, Barack Obama issued 296. Donald Trump issued 220 executive orders during the 4 years of his first administration (see www.federalregister.gov/presidential-documents/executive-orders/donald-trump/2020). President Biden signed almost as many executive orders in his first 2 weeks of office as FDR (the previous record holder) signed in his first month. The number per year decreased over time with 142 signed between 2021 and October, 2024.

Despite far fewer executive orders in the Bush and Obama years than in the years surrounding FDR's presidency and the COVID-19 era of the Trump and Biden administrations, high-profile Obama and George W. Bush executive orders have created echoing controversy. One such example is President Obama's Deferred Action for Childhood Arrivals (DACA), which allowed people who are in school, who have graduated, or who have been honorably discharged from the military to stay in the United States without fear of deportations. This action was largely supported by liberals and many moderates, deplored by many conservatives, and was subject to a Supreme Court review and decision in 2020 (see Downey & Garnick, 2020, for explication of this complex ruling). On the other side of the aisle, a controversial, initially secret order by George W. Bush authorized the National Security Agency to eavesdrop on U.S. phone calls without a warrant. Mayer (cited in Rothman, 2017) noted that "[a] person's attitude about executive action depends almost entirely on whether the President is of your party," but the debates about the extent or limits of presidential power have been present since the beginning of our nation. "Hamilton and Madison fought over it. Those debates have not been tempered in the centuries since" (para 5).

What do executive orders have to do with nursing and health care? Presidents can issue an array of health care–related executive orders, some of which directly impact nurses. An October 2019 executive order, for example, was directed toward impeding Medicare for All. It also included provisions to reduce the price and payment discrepancies between physicians and "nonphysician" providers, including nurse practitioners, to ensure that "clinicians, including physicians, physician assistants, and nurse practitioners, are appropriately reimbursed in accordance with the work performed rather than the clinician's occupation" (White House, 2019, para 18). A 2023 executive order was directed toward increasing access to care and supporting caregivers and included language directed toward long-term care staffing and turnover (White House, 2023). These represent just two executive orders with implications for nurses. Details on recent executive orders, listed by U.S. president, can be found on the U.S. Federal Register webpage at https://www.federalregister.gov/presidential-documents/executive-orders.

Why do presidents and governors use executive orders to create law? An executive order has the advantage of great speed compared with the relative slow speed and uncertainty of the legislative process. President Bill Clinton's administration described the lure of an executive order as "Stroke of a pen, law of the land. Kind of cool." (cited in Bennet, 1998, para 5). Nevertheless, laws created in this way may not have staying power. With the same stroke of a pen that created the law, the next president can undo a previous executive order. Moreover, Congress can overturn an executive order by passing a bill that modifies or eliminates it. Although the president can veto that law, Congress would need a two-thirds vote to override the veto and remove the provisions of the executive order. Finally, the Supreme Court can determine that an executive order is unconstitutional. This resulting decision creates a new law and is the highest, final determination of what constitutes U.S. law. (Similar processes occur at the state level, with the result being state law rather than federal law.) Notably, all three of the mechanisms of creating law detailed herein—congressional action, administrative rules, and executive order—can face Supreme Court challenges and be reaffirmed, modified, or eliminated. The Supreme Court is the final arbiter, and its decisions become the definitive law. For example, during the COVID-19 intense spring of 2020, the governor of the state of Wisconsin issued a "stay at home" executive order. In a 4–3 decision, the Wisconsin state Supreme Court ruled this as "unlawful" and "unenforceable," and the order was thus struck down. Note, this was a decision by a state Supreme Court related to a governor's executive order. The federal Supreme Court has similar powers at a national level, for example, striking down President Biden's plan to cancel more than $400 billion in student loan debt through the authority of the U.S. Secretary of Education (PBS News Hour, 2023). Finally, the Supreme Court also has overruled itself in subsequent decisions, including the highly controversial *Dobbs v. Jackson Women's Health Organization* that overturned *Roe v. Wade*. A comprehensive list of Supreme Court decisions overruled by subsequent decisions can be found at https://constitution.congress.gov/resources/decisions-overruled/.

Judicial Review and Case Law

The U.S. Constitution limits the Supreme Court to "cases" and "controversies" and does not allow for the Supreme Court to provide advisory opinions. At least five of nine judges must vote in the same manner for a particular decision to become law. In this manner, acts, administrative rules, and executive orders may be reinforced, modified, or eliminated.

When does the Supreme Court step in? Conflicting judicial decisions between a state Supreme Court and federal circuit courts or between or among federal circuit courts may cause the Supreme Court to step in. Or the Supreme Court may step in when there are issues that are deemed to be a highly important social issue, for example, *Roe v. Wade* that made abortion legal in all 50 states and was subsequently overruled in 2022. They may also step in to review unusual circumstances that are deemed critical to the nation. Examples in this category include *U.S. v. Nixon* regarding the Watergate tapes or *Bush v. Gore* to determine the outcome of an extremely close presidential election in

2000 that hinged on voter counts and recounts in the state of Florida. Other routes to a Supreme Court hearing may occur if a lower court disregards a past Supreme Court decision. In this circumstance, the Supreme Court may hear that case or simply correct the lower court without a hearing. Finally, some cases are reviewed because of an interest or a particular judge (FindLaw, n.d.). Of the 7,000 to 8,000 requests received each year, the court accepts only about 100-150 cases for review (U.S. Courts.gov n.d.-a).

How does the process work? Parties who are not satisfied with a decision of a lower court must first petition the Supreme Court to hear their case. Four of the nine judges must vote to accept a case (U.S. Courts.gov, n.d.-b). The agreement to hear the case is termed granting a *writ of certiorari*. To come to this decision, the Supreme Court is aided by their own set of attorneys, led by the solicitor general. Wermiel suggests that the solicitor general must "strike a sometimes delicate balance between serving the legal interests of his [*sic*] superiors (the president and attorney general), the long-term interests of the United States (as opposed to the present Administration), and his responsibility as a special officer of the Court itself" (Wermiel, 2012, para 2). In regard to the latter, the solicitor general has been called "the 10th Chief Justice of the Supreme Court," an important role that is largely invisible to the American public. You can learn more about this powerful role at https://www.justice.gov/osg/about-office.

Taken as a whole, the president and political party in the majority have not only the visible impact of who occupies the executive branch but also shape agency appointees and the potential for Senate confirmation for that presidential nomination, committee membership and leadership, and who is appointed to lifetime positions on the Supreme Court. Next we discuss ways you can influence who occupies these roles and other ways to impact health policy.

WAYS OF INFLUENCE

Voting

A foundational and basic way to have influence is at the ballot box: Vote! As simple as it seems, many Americans do not vote. As previously noted, a mere 100 years ago, slightly more than five generations ago, women did not have the right to vote—they did not win the right to vote until 1920—whereas "race, color, or previous condition of servitude" were addressed 50 years earlier, in 1870, with the passage of the 15th Amendment. These victories were hard won. As a first step toward influence, register to vote . . . and vote!

Political Campaigns

A next level is to become involved with a political campaign. Offering time for a worthy candidate or a cause is an excellent way to demystify the political process. Activities can range from preparing social media to stuffing envelopes, dropping flyers off door to door, fundraising, or working on the *get-out-the-vote effort*—activities designed to ensure that supporters actually arrive at the ballot box. No activity is so small as to be insignificant. What if time is short? Do not underestimate the power of even a small contribution to a campaign. In the world of politics, money matters. Money materializes in the world as human and material resources. Contributing time, money, or both is a valuable way to further a cause.

Political Action Committees

Financial resources go further when they are merged with those of like-minded others. *Political action committees*, or *PACs*, offer a way of pooling funds with others. Political action group funds may support particular candidates or causes, so it is important to carefully consider which groups to join. Key questions to ask before providing financial support include the following:

1. What are the views or platform of the group?
2. Do you agree with these views and resulting strategies, or are you—through your dues or additional PAC contributions—supporting something that is not aligned with your interests and ideals?

Lobbyists

Many organizations fund a *lobbyist*. A lobbyist is an individual who actively works to influence policy makers to take a particular view or vote a particular way. At a state level, nursing organizations may not be sufficiently financed to support a lobbyist at the statehouse full-time, whereas better-resourced organizations such as hospital and medical associations employ lobbyists who become part of the trusted—or at least influential—fabric of state politics. This creates an unfortunate power differential in political influence that can be difficult for nursing to overcome. The many different nursing groups, sometimes with conflicting views and messages, may also be confusing to policy makers. A unified message or set of messages from the various groups representing nurses and nursing is warranted whenever possible.

Is All Advocacy Lobbying?

What is the difference between being a lobbyist versus simply advocating for an issue? Although there are some similarities, there are important distinctions. *Lobbying* is activity to influence legislators or federal policy makers to vote a particular way on a piece of legislation. *Direct lobbying* is done by a registered lobbyist who is officially representing the views of a particular group, frequently having been hired to do so. The process by which to register as a lobbyist varies by state, but an individual cannot lobby without taking the appropriate actions that include a process, forms, and fees. Typically, there are also strict ethical guidelines regarding gifts from lobbyists to policy makers. Professional lobbyists may also analyze regulatory proposals or drafts of proposed bills to inform the organization of the potential impact of proposed legislative action. Take a moment to review lobbying guidelines on your state government's website.

LOBBYING AS OFFICIAL AUTHORITY TO REPRESENT A GROUP VIEW

In summary, active lobbying signifies *official authority* to represent the group. A responsibility of a lobbyist for a state nurses' association is to represent the interests and views of that group, which are not necessarily the lobbyist's own. In some controversial areas—patient-directed dying, for example—the organization may poll members to determine what stance they want officially represented. Alternatively, based on stated values or following polling of a group, the official organizational stance may be to take no position. Individual members of groups can always be in contact with policy makers representing their own views, but they cannot simply hold themselves up as representatives of the group's collective position.

GRASSROOTS LOBBYING

Conversely, *grassroots lobbying* is the mobilization of individuals within a group to influence legislation. Such groups may promulgate a *call to action* suggesting that individuals contact their state or federal policy makers to support, oppose, or amend a particular bill. As a citizen, of course, you can contact policy makers at any time, with or without such an action prompt. Nevertheless, alignment with a group that continually monitors federal and/or state legislation and promulgates calls to action is a helpful way to keep track of the myriad of constantly shifting details that characterize the political process without having to navigate it alone.

HOW TO CONTACT POLICY MAKERS

Gabriella is amazed at how easy it was to influence legislation to increase the student loan repayment program in her state. The nursing student association forwarded an action alert, and Gabriella took a deep breath and called her state representative who, incidentally, is on the committee that reviewed the bill draft. Gabriella initially left a phone message to detail her perspective. Representative Smith then asked Gabriella to testify to the committee on the issue of student debt load and the value of loan repayment as a state workforce retention strategy.

Obviously, to take a step like Gabriella did, it is critical to know who to call. Do you know who represents you in the House and Senate? Please take a moment to identify your district, representatives, and senators at both the state and national levels. This is essential, basic knowledge for political influence.

Is It Just a Good Idea or a Good Idea That Should Become a Law?

With this knowledge, you can now influence policy in a number of ways. If there is an issue you would like to see become a law, first ponder if it is just a good idea or a good idea that should become a law. This is an important distinction. Not every good idea should be a law, as laws have enforcement requirements as well as other costs. If you decide on the latter, it is helpful to first explore if a bill on this issue had previously been introduced and trace what happened to that bill. This creates an "in the know" starting platform. If you continue to believe state legislation should be proposed, you can contact your state senator or representative and ask them to sponsor a bill. Recall that these individuals are elected to represent you. That is the whole idea of a representative form of government. Alternatively, you may bond with like-minded others and create a collective strategy for approaching legislative action. Coalitions of interested parties can bring issues to the attention of policy makers. Unusual alliances are particularly powerful. Ponder, for example, the difference between students and universities promoting loan repayment and these groups' stance reinforced by the hospital association and statewide chamber of commerce. The broader nature of the latter creates political momentum. Similarly, nursing and consumer groups that together advocate for a policy change are in a much more powerful political position than when either group is advocating in isolation.

Phone Calls and Emails to Policy Makers

If instead there is a current bill or item of a bill that you strongly support or oppose, a phone call or email is effective. Federal legislators typically have a comment portal to aid easy transmission of your views. Letters are also effective but know that at the federal level this is less inefficient; there may be a long delay between when you send the letter and when it is received. This is because land mail is extensively screened following the 2001 anthrax bioterrorism scare; a phone call or e-message is better. Also, arrange to visit the federal staff in person, either in your congress member's state office or when you are in Washington, DC. Unless you are officially representing an organization, be sure to use your personal email address, not that of your organization.

Health Staff to Federal Policy Makers

Do you know who is staffing your federal representatives and senators in the area of health and health-related issues? Do you know where the state offices of these Congress members are located? Organized meetings with staff members can be a powerful tool, provided the message is clear and well organized. These individuals work for your representatives and senators, and again, these representatives of the people cannot represent you if they do not know your thoughts. They depend on all of their constituents for re-election, so do not conclude that they are powerful and you are not; you have the power of your own voice—your vote—and your connection with coalitions of similar-minded individuals and groups. Careful use of social media also offers an effective tool for promulgating your positions and becoming a thought leader (Shattell & Darmoc, 2017; Shattell et al., 2022). Yet there are mixed views on the impact of social media in democracy. When compared to other nations, more Americans view social media as a divisive force with negative impacts on democracy (Wike et al., 2022). Nevertheless, for the foreseeable future, social media will continue to intersect with policy and politics. Nurses can, and should, learn how to responsibly harness its power.

OVERCOMING IMPEDIMENTS TO INVOLVEMENT

Tensions With Powerful Others

Des Jardin (2001a) suggests that nurses' involvement in the political process is hampered by more than just a lack of knowledge about the process. Nurses may feel an inconsistency between the goals of professional nursing and those of the institutional and physician sector of health care. A contemporary illustration is the continuing tensions between organized medicine and authority roles for nurses; for example, the American Medical Association chastising The Joint Commission for not mandating that physicians must be the heads of medical homes, in contrast to the stance promulgated by the American Association of Nurse Practitioners, which stated: "A patient's needs should determine who leads a team and leadership should not be 'defined by a profession'" (Robeznieks, 2014, para 15). A second example is the potential tension between an employing hospital that does not support legislated limits on nurse–patient ratios and a nurse who does support staffing ratios. It is important to recall that an organization such as the American Medical Association or American Hospital Association exists to support the interests of physicians and hospitals, respectively, which may or may not be aligned with the interests of nurses or society at large. As the nurse in these crosshairs, these potential schisms are easily reconciled from an ethical perspective: Any and all potential or real conflicts of interest must be resolved in the best interest of the patient.

Stereotypical Images of Nurses and Policy: Do Nurses Internalize Politically Powerless Self-Images?

Stereotypical images of nurses have long been a focus of study and critique. Des Jardin (2001b) also suggests that stereotypical images of nurse as mother, servant, religious symbol, and military angel such as Florence Nightingale may not only be held by society but also internalized by nurses. Gordon (2005) has argued that the "virtue script" and complex adaptation of nurses to ensure deference to physicians artfully conceals the genuine mastery of health care by nurses. Moreover, these emotional and societal stances do not encourage the acquisition of voice and comfort with controversy, yet controversy is inherent in the political process. Similarly, Summers and Summers (2010) suggest that media images of nurses as backdrops, gurney pushers, and agents in romantic plots devalue and dismiss nurses. Again, the extent to which nurses internalize these images is difficult to estimate. Nevertheless, such images matter and impact the policy process because "what nursing is said to be constitutes what nursing is" (Kelly et al., 2011, p. 1804). Negative, demeaning, or powerless images of nurses have another negative impact, that of nurse invisibility in the marketing materials or web presence of many medical facilities (Carty et al., 2000). Such invisibility does not socialize nurses to consider roles of *public ambassador* for a political cause. Nurses were more visually present in media outlets during the COVID-19 pandemic, and, arguably, this can create momentum for greater impact in the future. There remains much work to do in this area. The Woodhull study revisited the issue of nurses' public visibility and found that nurses were only cited as sources for 2% of health-related news stories and never cited in policy news stories (Mason et al., 2018). A systematic review of research exploring nurses' involvement in policy noted an array of internally perceived barriers, including feeling powerless, fear of facing new challenges, and a perceived lack of the skills needed to engage in the health policy process and in public relations (Hajizaden et al., 2021). Finally, Teresa-Morales et al.'s (2022) integrative review of stereotypes found marked differences by gender, with men perceived as more capable of managerial roles. Such stereotypes have consequences. The pay gap persists, with female RNs paid 91 cents for every dollar paid to RNs who are male (Nursing Journal Staff, 2023). These dynamics will be discussed in greater detail in Chapter 14 on workforce.

Strategies Toward Becoming a Confident Public Ambassador for Nursing

Fortunately, there are effective strategies to create a core of confidence that supports the role of nurse as an effective political agent. A sound starting place is the identification of powerful examples or models of effective political force in action.

LEARNING FROM DISTANT OTHERS

Although there are many examples of politically powerful men to consider as potential role models—and behaviors and styles you wish to avoid—politically powerful women represent a smaller proportion of the politically powerful. Regardless of alignment with your personal politics, individuals like Angela Merkel, Germany's first female prime minister; former ambassador and Republican presidential candidate, Nikki Haley; Janet Yellen, first female U.S. Federal Reserve chief and secretary of the Treasury; former U.S. Vice President and presidential candidate, Kamala Harris; Christine Legarde, managing director of the International Monetary Fund; Jacinda Ardern, former prime minister of New Zealand; Nancy Pelosi, 52nd Speaker of the U.S. House of Representatives; Condoleezza Rice, 66th U.S. Secretary of State, Mary Barra, CEO of General Motors; Sandy Ran Xu, COO for Chinese e-commerce giant JD; and even Taylor Swift, to name but a few, offer examples of women in power, worthy of study (see Forbes' most powerful women list https://www.forbes.com/power-women/list/; Taylor Swift was #5 in 2023). Moreover, it is useful to identify individuals who mirror your race, ethnicity, gender, and—if possible—age and then study strengths you admire as models to emulate. What qualities make them effective in the public arena? How did they become who they are? What skills did they develop, and what experiences fostered that skill development? Did they layer in parenting and partnering? If so, how and when? What lessons about the navigation of personal and professional life can be gleaned? Biographies, autobiographies, and documentaries can offer useful illustrations.

LEARNING FROM AT-HAND MENTORS

Useful as it is to study the biographies, history, and style of influential people, a more immediate role model may be found in a mentor or collection of mentors, all of whom have different backgrounds and skill sets from which you can identify examples you wish to follow to become your best self. Although the professional and popular literature frequently touts the mentor route, an effective mentor–mentee relationship is not automatic or easy and must meet the needs of both the mentor and protégée. Box 12.3 outlines essential elements of effective mentoring, based on a qualitative study of 117 dyads.

BOX 12.3

ELEMENTS OF AN EFFECTIVE MENTORING RELATIONSHIP

Open communication and accessibility
Goals and challenges
Passion and inspiration
Caring personal relationship
Mutual respect and trust
Exchange of knowledge
Independence and collaboration
Role modeling

Source: Sanzero Eller, L., Lev, E., & Feurer, A. (2013). Key components of an effective mentoring relationship: A qualitative study. *Nurse Education Today, 34*, 815–820.

These classic characteristics have evolved over time, yet Mullen and Klimaitis (2019) note that although there are varied definitions of and forms of mentoring, there is broad agreement on core characteristics. Drawing from Kram, they offer that mentoring is relational and developmental, has career and psychosocial functions, and includes the phases of initiation, cultivation, and separation inclusive of a redefinition of the relationship. They note that although traditional mentoring was largely career focused, their review of contemporary literature suggests much broader functions (see Table 12.1).

Unlike the exploration and potential applications of skills viewed at a distance in leaders, the mentor–mentee dynamic is an actual relationship and, like any relationship, takes work and compatibility. In addition,

TABLE 12.1 EXAMPLES OF CONTEMPORARY MENTORING RELATIONSHIPS DESCRIBED IN THE LITERATURE

Formal mentoring	Planned and programmatic, typically led by the organization
Informal mentoring	Spontaneous interactions between mentor and mentee
Diverse mentoring	Cross-gender and/or cross-race mentoring between or among those who differ
Electronic mentoring	A significant culture change enabled by technology; may include group mentoring
Group mentoring	Although relatively new to contemporary research investigations, it represents an "age old practice" (p. 27); increasingly aided by virtual group meetings both formal (planned) and informal (spontaneous)
Comentoring, also known as collaborative mentoring	A dynamic partnership in a mutually beneficial relationship; may be an evolution of a previous mentee–mentor relationship or the evolution of two peers who share goals and values, for example, two nurses with an interest in developing a business
Peer mentoring	A formal or informal process in which someone who has recently lived through a phase supports one going through it, for example, senior nursing students serving as mentors for sophomore nursing students
Multilevel mentoring	Intention and programmatic to achieve specific ends, for example, retention of new graduates, with mentors spanning all levels of the organization (e.g., frontline nurses with an array of experience levels, supervisors, chief nursing officer)
Cultural mentoring	Typically attracting people who are excluded from other networks or exposed to discrimination, this form of mentoring unites diverse cultures toward a common goal

Adapted from: Mullen, C. A., & Klimaitis, C. C. (2019). Defining mentoring: A literature review of issues, types, and applications. *Annals of the New York Academy of Sciences*, 1483(1), 19–35. https://doi.org/10.1111/nyas.14176.

although the mentor's role is to help the mentee create a larger vision of what is possible and then fulfill the promise of that extended self, some mentors become caught in their own needs, for example, the need to be the rescuer and thus foster a codependent relationship (Kets de Vries, 2013). Conversely, the mentee may have unreasonable expectations of the mentor's time and talents. Eby (2007) further notes that relational problems such as personality clashes, jealousy, and unwillingness to learn may mar the mentoring and undermine growth potential. Similarly, if goals are not met, interaction costs may leave the mentor or mentee feeling the outcomes are not worth the effort. Seek out those with admirable political skills and become an apprentice. If mentors are easily identified, this approach can augment what can be learned from world and historical figures.

End-of-Chapter Resources

THOUGHT QUESTIONS

1. What qualities make an individual an effective ambassador for a cause? How can essential skills be practiced?
2. What bills of interest to nurses are under consideration in the current or last state legislative session in your state?
3. How would you advise nurses who are interested in creating a political learning agenda for themselves? What sources of information and connection can you advise them to explore? What else would you need to know to help them?
4. Define the following key terms:
   Administrative rule
   Advocate
   Call to action
   Crossover
   Direct lobbying
   Executive order
   Get-out-the-vote efforts
   Grassroots lobbying
   How a bill becomes a law
   Lobbyist
   Political action committee
   Talking points

EXERCISES

1. Create a presentation for your peers that details the political process in your state. Include tangible suggestions for how to become involved.
2. Consider exemplary political role models. What skills do you share with them? What are your growth edges?

QUIZ

True or False

1. All advocacy is lobbying.
2. Grassroots lobbying can only be done by registered lobbyists.
3. Unusual alliances among groups to advocate on behalf of a particular bill or issue usually are looked on with suspicion by policy makers and should therefore be avoided.
4. Once introduced into the legislature, a bill draft rarely changes.
5. A foundational strategy to influence policy is to vote.
6. Political action committees have been deemed illegal in the United States since 1992.
7. Ethical guidelines generally prohibit lobbyists from giving gifts to policy makers.
8. Bill drafts are debated by the full Senate or House of Representatives before being reviewed by the appropriate committee.
9. Political action is inconsistent with the roles and responsibilities of the professional nurse.
10. Personality clashes, jealousy, and unwillingness to learn can mar the mentor–mentee relationship.

Multiple Choice

11. One strategy to support political campaigns is
    A. Fundraising for worthy candidates
    B. Working on get-out-the-vote efforts
    C. Both A and B
    D. Neither A nor B
12. Lobbyists
    A. Have the moral responsibility to present their personal view on an issue
    B. Do not need to be registered in the state
    C. Both A and B
    D. Neither A nor B

13. Ways to influence policy makers include
    A. Phone calls to the policy maker's office or staff
    B. Emails to the policy maker's office or staff
    C. Both A and B
    D. Neither A nor B
14. An effective mentor–mentee relationship requires
    A. Collaboration
    B. Independence
    C. Both A and B
    D. Neither A nor B

NOTE

1. Shapiro (2008) offers that although associated with Bismarck starting in the 1930s, the original quote was coined in 1869 by lawyer-poet John Godfrey Saxe, who was cited in *The Daily Cleveland Herald* on March 29, 1869, as stating, "Laws, like sausage, cease to inspire respect in proportion as we know how they are made."

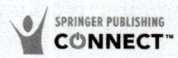

A robust set of instructor resources designed to supplement this text is located at http://connect.springerpub.com/content/book/978-0-8261-7236-5. Qualifying instructors may request access by emailing **textbook@springerpub.com**.

REFERENCES

Annenberg Public Policy Center. (2022). *Americans' civics knowledge drops on first amendment and branches of government*. https://www.asc.upenn.edu/news-events/news/americans-civics-knowledge-drops-first-amendment-and-branches-government

Ballotpedia. (n.d.). *Presidential proclamation*. https://ballotpedia.org/Presidential_proclamation

Bennet, J. (1998, July 5). *True to form, Clinton shifts energies back to U.S. focus*. The New York Times. https://www.nytimes.com/1998/07/05/us/true-to-form-clinton-shifts-energies-back-to-us-focus.html

Carty, B., Coughlin, C., Kasoff, J., & Sullivan, B. (2000). Where is the nursing presence on the medical center's website? *The Journal of Nursing Administration*, *30*(12), 569–570. https://doi.org/10.1097/00005110-200012000-00004

Central Intelligence Agency. (n.d.). *The world fact book: Field listing-legislative branch*. Author. https://www.cia.gov/the-world-factbook/field/legislative-branch/

Cornell Law School. (n.d.). *The line item veto*. www.law.cornell.edu/constitution-conan/article-1/section-7/clause-1-3/the-line-item-veto

Des Jardin, K. E. (2001a). Political involvement in nursing—Politics, ethics, and strategic action. *Association of Operating Room Nurses Journal*, *74*(5), 614–618, 621–622. https://doi.org/10.1016/S0001-2092(06)61760-2

Des Jardin, K. E. (2001b). Political involvement in nursing—Education and empowerment. *Association of Operating Room Nurses Journal, 74*(4), 468–475. https://doi.org/10.1016/s0001-2092(06)61679-7

Downey, M., & Garnick, A. (2020, July 7). Explaining the Supreme Court's DACA decision. The Regulatory Review. https://www.theregreview.org/2020/0707/downey-garnick-explaining-supreme-court-daca-decision/

Eby, L. (2007). Understanding relational problems in mentoring: A review and proposed investment model. In B. Ragins & L. Kran (Eds.), *The handbook of mentoring at work: Theory, research, and practice* (pp. 323–344). Sage.

Felix, M., Sobel, L., & Salganicoff, A. (2024, February 9). *Addressing abortion access through state ballot initiatives*. Kaiser Family Foundation. https://www.kff.org/womens-health-policy/issue-brief/addressing-abortion-access-through-state-ballot-initiatives/

FindLaw. (n.d.). *How does the U.S. Supreme Court decide whether to hear a case?* https://www.findlaw.com/litigation/legal-system/how-does-the-u-s-supreme-court-decide-whether-to-hear-a-case.html

Gordon, S. (2005). *Nursing against the odds: How health care cost-cutting, medical stereotypes, and medical hubris undermine nursing and patient care*. Cornell University Press.

Govtrack. (n.d.). *Congress bills: Statistics and historical comparison*. www.govtrack.us/congress/bills/statistics

Hajizadeh, A., Zamanzadeh, V., Kakemam, E., Bahreini, R., & Khodayari-Zarnaq, R. (2021). Factors influencing nurses participation in the health policy-making process: A systematic review. *BMC Nursing, 20*(1), 128. https://doi.org/10.1186/s12912-021-00648-6

Howe, A. (2024, June 28). Supreme Court strikes down Chevron, curtailing power of federal agencies. Scotusblog. https://www.scotusblog.com/2024/06/supreme-court-strikes-down-chevron-curtailing-power-of-federal-agencies/

Kelly, J., Fealy, G., & Watson, R. (2011). The image of you: Constructing nursing identities in YouTube. *Journal of Advanced Nursing, 68*(8), 1804–1813. https://doi.org/10.1111/j.1365-2648.2011.05872.x

Kenton, W. (2024). What is a *unicameral system*: How legislature works and examples. Investopedia. https://www.investopedia.com/terms/u/unicameral-system.asp

Kets de Vries, M. F. R. (2013). *The dangers of codependent mentoring* [Blog post]. Harvard Business Review. http://blogs.hbr.org/2013/12/the-dangers-of-codependent-mentoring/

Mason, D., Nixon, L., Glickstein, B., Han, S., Westphaln, K., & Carter, L. (2018). The Woodhull study revisited: Nurses' representation in health news media 20 years later. *Journal of Nursing Scholarship, 50*(6), 695–704. https://doi.org/10.1111/jnu.12429

Mullen, C. A., & Klimaitis, C. C. (2019). Defining mentoring: A literature review of issues, types, and applications. *Annals of the New York Academy of Sciences, 1483*(1), 19–35. https://doi.org/10.1111/nyas.14176

Nurse Journal Staff. (2023, March 23). The gender pay gap in nursing. Nurse Journal. https://nursejournal.org/resources/the-gender-pay-gap-in-nursing/

PBS News Hour. (2023, June 30). *Biden pledges alternative plan after Supreme Court strikes down student debt relief*. Author. https://www.pbs.org/newshour/show/biden-pledges-alternative-plan-after-supreme-court-strikes-down-student-debt-relief

Pulcini, J. (2014). Interview with a nursing policy leader: A hopeful look at a changing profession. *American Journal of Nursing, 114*(1), 19–22. https://doi.org/10.1097/01.NAJ.0000441785.39914.ea

Robeznieks, A. (2014). *AMA to Joint Commission: We're the head of the medical household*. Modern Healthcare. Retrieved June 10, 2014, from www.modern healthcare.com/article/20140610/NEWS/306109947

Rothman, L. (2017, February 5). *9 Executive orders that changed American history*. Time. https://time.com/4655131/executibe-orders-history/

Shattell, M., & Darmoc, R. (2017). Becoming a public thought leader in 140 characters or less: How nurses can use social media as a platform. *Journal of Psychosocial Nursing and Mental Health*, 55(6), 3–4. https://doi.org/10.3928/02793695-20170519-06

Shattell, M., Batchelor, M., & Darmoc, R. (2022). *Social media in health care: A guide to creating your professional digital presence*. Slack Incorporated.

Shapiro, F. (2008). *Quote . . . misquote*. The New York Times. http://www.nytimes.com/2008/07/21/magazine/27wwwl-guestsafire-t.html?_r=0

Smiley, R., Allgeyer, R., Shobo, Y., Lyons, K., Letourneau, R., Zhong, E., Kaminski-Ozturk, N., & Alexander, M. (2023). The 2022 National Nursing Workforce survey. *Journal of Nursing Regulation*, 14(1), S1–S90. https://doi.org/10.1016/S2155-8256(23)00047-9

Statescape. (2020). *Bill crossover deadlines: When a bill must cross a chamber*. www.statescape.com/resources/legislative/bill-crossover-deadlines/

Stuessy, M. (2019, June 18). *Regular vetoes and pocket vetoes: In brief*. Congressional Research Service. https://sgp.fas.org/crs/misc/RS22188.pdf

Summers, S., & Summers, H. J. (2010). *Saving lives: Why the media's portrayal of nurses puts us all at risk*. Kaplin.

Teresa-Morales, C., Rodríguez-Pérez, M., Araujo-Hernández, M., & Feria-Ramírez, C. (2022). Current stereotypes associated with nursing and nursing professionals: An integrative review. *International Journal of Environmental Research and Public Health*, 19(13), 7640. https://doi.org/10.3390/ijerph19137640

U.S. Courts.gov. (n.d.-a) *About the Supreme Court*. https://www.uscourts.gov/about-federal-courts/educational-resources/about-educational-outreach/activity-resources/about

U.S. Courts.gov. (n.d.-b). *Supreme Court procedures*. https://www.uscourts.gov/about-federal-courts/educational-resources/about-educational-outreach/activity-resources/supreme-1

USA.gov. (n.d.) How laws are made. https://www.usa.gov/how-laws-are-made

Wermiel, S. (2012, May 2). *SCOTUS for law students: What does the Solicitor General do?* (sponsored by Bloomberg Law), SCOTUSblog. https://www.scotusblog.com/2012/05/scotus-for-law-students-what-does-the-solicitor-general-do-sponsored-by-bloomberg-law/

White House. (2019, October 4). *Presidential proclamation on the suspension of entry of immigrants who will financially burden the United States Healthcare system*. https://trumpwhitehouse.archives.gov/presidential-actions/presidential-proclamation-suspension-entry-immigrants-will-financially-burden-united-states-healthcare-system/

White House. (2023). *Executive order on increasing access to high quality care and supporting caregivers*. https://www.whitehouse.gov/briefing-room/presidential-actions/2023/04/18/executive-order-on-increasing-access-to-high-quality-care-and-supporting-caregivers/

Wike, R., Silver, L., Fetterolf, J., Huang, C., Austin, S., Clanc, L., & Gubbala, S. (2022, December 6). *Social media seen as mostly good for democracy across many nations, but U.S. is a major outlier*. Pew Research Center. https://www.pewresearch.org/global/2022/12/06/social-media-seen-as-mostly-good-for-democracy-across-many-nations-but-u-s-is-a-major-outlier/

CHAPTER 13

Lessons From the COVID-19 Pandemic and a Look to the Future

Earlier chapters detailed preliminary lessons from COVID-19 that intersect with the focus of the chapter. Inclusive of and yet beyond these, the impact of COVID-19 is sweeping and profound. This historic pandemic illuminated foundational cracks in the U.S. education, health care, and justice systems. The trajectory of the pandemic and its long-term echo are still in play as this text goes to press. What follows, therefore, are early, critical perspectives for nurses to consider as we live and lead in a forever changed world.

But first, how did the United States, a wealthy nation by any standard, arrive to the world of the pandemic so unprepared? First, the nation has been underinvesting in the public health infrastructure and public health surveillance for decades. Arguably, perhaps the nation felt it immune from the catastrophes that have recently plagued other nations, for example, Western Africa's challenges with Ebola—an extraordinarily deadly disease—and severe acute respiratory syndrome of 2003 and Middle Eastern respiratory syndrome of 2012 primarily impacted Asia and the Middle East, respectively. COVID-19 has been a deadly reminder that today's world is interconnected, and each nation's public health preparedness is only as strong as the weakest link.

Next, the known fragility of the *supply chain* was not addressed to ensure adequate personal protective equipment (PPE) for our nation's health care and other frontline workers (Box 13.1).

BOX 13.1

WHAT IS A SUPPLY CHAIN?

A supply chain is a set of interconnections among people, products, resources, and companies that may span nations to produce a final product. *Supply chain management* is a process to maximize the efficiency of that process and reduce the cost of the final product. Disruptions in the supply chain can—and likely will—result in reduced availability of the final product. During the pandemic, supply chain disruptions resulted in shortages of PPE, bicycles, and toilet paper, among other products, although some of the shortages were due to increased demand and—in the case of toilet paper—consumer hoarding.

The U.S. health care system has experienced previous supply chain impacts following natural disasters. After Hurricane Maria's devastation of Puerto Rico,

(coninued)

BOX 13.1

WHAT IS A SUPPLY CHAIN? (*CONTINUED*)

for example, saline solution was in critical shortage in the United States because Puerto Rico was a key provider of saline solution; manufacturing delays were rampant as Puerto Rico struggled to recover from the hurricane (Mazer-Amirshahi & Fox, 2018). Gibson and Prasad Singh (2018) have detailed the substantial risks the United States has taken because of its dependence on medicines from China. Beyond an individual product such as saline or a single category such as medications, health care's supply chains infuse the health care system, with multifaceted dimensions below the awareness of many nurses—except in time of shortages. Michandandi (2020), for example, noted that the U.S. health care supply chain is not one chain, but instead includes five distinct chains: PPE, medical devices, medical supplies, pharmaceuticals, and blood. Disruption in any one of these creates havoc. This author further notes that "urgent action must be taken to ensure that our supply chain supports our healthcare providers at this critical time and in the future" (para 8). Another high-profile supply chain issue was the infant formula shortage in 2022. Although the acute stage of the pandemic has abated, supply chain disruptions continue, with 93% of health care executives experiencing product shortages (Health Industry Distributers Association, 2023) that can delay surgeries and other needed care (Kaufman Hall, cited in Hagland, 2023). Compounding these challenges are ongoing natural disaster. Damage from Hurricane Helene, for example, halted production in the largest U.S. manufacturer of intravenious solutions and peritoneal dialysis (Johnson, 2024).

The counterproductive competition among states for the same supplies, and between states and the federal government, illustrates the fundamental tensions between issues of "states' rights" perspectives that support autonomous state action and, instead, centralized federal oversight and control for a more systematic, nationwide, uniform response across states. This directly impacts nurses at all levels of preparation. Dai et al. (2021) note that "nurses have been on the frontline of the failures of supply chain[s] without essential tools to protect themselves and the patients they care for" (para 1). As nurses work to become *upstreamists* who address social determinants of health before people become patients, they should also strive to understand and influence the supply chain stream in their work setting. This is essential to not only nurses' well-being and safety but also to ensure that patients and coworkers are served and protected. St. Pierre calls on organizations to more directly involve nurses in supply chain improvement initiatives, noting: "As a critical end [user], nurses have unique visibility into supply chain inefficiencies and problems. . . . Nurses can reveal key supply chain vulnerabilities and weakness that other staff members don't see" (St. Pierre, 2021, para 1). Technology-enhanced strategies such as artificial intelligence (discussed in Chapter 6) are key tools toward this end (Dai et al., 2021). What supply chain improvement initiatives are underway in the health care settings you are working in or have clinical assignments?

Reliance on Elective Procedures and Fee-for-Service Reimbursement

The challenges inherent in fee-for-service reimbursement, including its potential for overuse of health care, have been detailed in previous chapters and will not be recounted here. COVID-19 revealed additional foundational weaknesses that have had a dramatic impact on nurses' employment. Specifically, most health care organizations in fee-for-service arrangements depend on *elective* procedures for the financial revenue to maintain base operations and personnel, including nurses. *High-margin procedures* can account for up to 80% of the revenue in an organization. Examples of such high-margin procedures include orthopedics and heart procedures (Respaut & Spaulding, 2020), and many organizations have *chased revenue* by overbuilding high-margin service lines and investing less in others, such as mental health. Recall supplier-induced demand discussed in an earlier chapter, that is, "build it and they will come." Yet many elective procedures (see Box 13.2) were delayed by hospitals and health care providers to ensure their services would be available for an expected surge of COVID-19 patients.

Finally, there are key lessons at the intersection of the limitations of a predominantly volume-based fee-for-service reimbursement and employer-based insurance. These will now be detailed in turn.

BOX 13.2

WHAT IS AN ELECTIVE PROCEDURE IN HEALTH CARE?

Elective procedures are those health care interventions that are not immediately medically essential but instead can happen at the time and discretion of the patient and availability of the provider. Some, such as orthopedic joint replacement or opening of a clogged tear duct, are primarily done to improve the quality of life of the patient and reduce discomfort. Others, such as cosmetic surgery, aim to improve the patient's appearance and are not medical in any way. Wolfson (2020) notes the pandemic's impact on "the joint replacement *goldmine*," a "cash cow" before the pandemic (para 18, emphasis added).

Other procedures and health care visits were cancelled, postponed, or eliminated because people were fearful of contagion and avoided the medical system. ED visits were also down, as people who typically would have visited the ED with symptoms or concerns chose not to seek treatment. Hospitals estimated losses of $1.4 billion *per day* (with the American Hospital Association estimating 2020 losses at $323 billion) (LaPointe, 2020). Nevertheless, in some health care settings, upticks in telehealth and COVID-19 relief funds addressed that financial loss. COVID-19 funds were released by *traunch* (see Box 13.3), with some health systems eventually returning funds. Bryant (2020), for example, suggests that "public shaming" and audit concerns caused one financially flush post–acute care health system to return $237 million of relief funds to the federal government.

> ### BOX 13.3
> **WHAT IS A TRAUNCH?**
> A traunch is one in a series of payments. The payments are typically over a pre-defined period and subject to achievement of performance metrics. Derived from the French word for "slice" ("tranche"), this approach is commonly used in startup efforts by venture capitalists to reduce investor risk (Fernando, 2020): COVID-19 relief funds, for example, much of the Coronavirus Aid, Relief, and Economic Security (CARES) Act funds, were released by the federal government in traunches.

During the pandemic, many nurses, once essential health care workers, were furloughed as their role, or at least the revenue for their role, evaporated. Jarman (2020) notes: "The coronavirus means doctors, nurses and PAs are essential workers—until they get laid off." Indeed, a record number of nurses and other health care workers were furloughed or laid off during the pandemic. In 1 month alone, April 2020, a record 1.4 million health care workers lost their jobs (Gooch, 2020). Across payers, there were strong rebounds in health care use late in spring 2020, with care use largely rebounding to prepandemic levels in 2022; however, missed care due to costs continues (McGough et al., 2023). Finally, Shen et al. (2024) note persistently higher rates of turnover in health care workers post–COVID-19 and posit that this will continue. Contemporary workforce issues are detailed in Chapter 14.

VALUE-BASED CARE

As the limitations of volume-based fee-for-service were amplified, perspectives on value-based payments also shifted. Livingston (2020) notes:

> The COVID pandemic . . . has highlighted like never before the pitfalls of paying for healthcare based on the number of patients seen and services rendered. It simultaneously reinforced the benefits of financing healthcare in a way that's not tied to volume, but to value with perspectives that COVID-19 may "end up boosting value based payments." (para 6)

Others suggest a particular form of value-based payments, global budgets, as a strategy to secure the financial health of rural hospitals (Fried et al., 2020), many of whom were already in deep financial struggles before the pandemic (Diaz et al., 2020); the shift from patient coverage by traditional Medicare to the lower-reimbursing Medicare Advantage is also deemed a threat to rural hospital survival (McCauliff, 2024). Still others have argued that the situation demands *value-informed nursing practice*—nurses who can articulate the value of care inclusive of cost and quality and direct practice accordingly (Yakusheva et al., 2020). These skills will be essential to the professional nurse of the future working in value-based settings and potentially others such as hospital at home (HaH), to be described later in this chapter.

Challenges With Employer-Based Insurance

The majority of Americans who have private commercial insurance obtain it through their employer. Representing roughly 160 million people, or half of the U.S. population, job loss can result in loss of health insurance. Indeed, two out of five people or their partners who were furloughed or lost their job because of the pandemic had health coverage through their job, with one-fifth then uninsured (Collins et al., 2020). Moreover, COVID-19–related job loss disproportionately impacted women, likely because they are more likely to be or have been employed in jobs deeply impacted by COVID-19, raising concerns about women's access to reproductive health services (Sonfield et al., 2020) even before the *Dobbs* decision of 2022.

Recall also that commercial insurance reimburses providers at a much higher rate than Medicaid. Thus, health care providers giving the exact same services to the exact same person will be reimbursed less if the person transitions from commercial insurance to Medicaid. Note, however, that even this lower rate is still higher than the zero reimbursement received if the person is uninsured. Cross-Call and Broaddus (2020) note that states that have expanded Medicaid were in a stronger position to address not only COVID-19 but also the pandemic-related economic downturn. For example, they note that 650,000 uninsured frontline or essential workers would have become eligible for Medicaid if the states who have not expanded Medicaid do so. Beyond this pandemic, what about the health care system of the future?

Telehealth and Virtual Care

Just as the pandemic uncorked virtual and e-connected learning for students at all levels of the educational system, it also unshackled virtual care. Prior to the pandemic, payment for virtual care was limited to those in rural areas or in payment arrangements such as Medicare Advantage or next-generation accountable care organizations. These arrangements hold payers at risk for cost of care or providers at risk for cost of care, accordingly. As such, they do not have a financial incentive to decant virtual care to enhance revenue, but instead to enhance value and access and contain costs. Telehealth reimbursement in traditional fee-for-service Medicare was limited because of concerns about explosive cost, given that providers have a financial incentive to maximize the use of services. Also, there is the risk of greater reach of "unscrupulous providers" (Cohen, cited in Schulte, 2020, para 4). Indeed, one of the largest illegal Medicare schemes was a telehealth scheme, in which 35 people fraudulently obtained over $2.1 *billion* from Medicare. Mehrota et al. (2020) thus suggest that telehealth expansion occur when services substitute for face-to-face or in alternative payment models where providers do not have the incentive to increase telehealth service volume to enhance finances. As this text goes to press, the U.S. Ways and Means Committee passed an additional 2-year extension (until December 2026) of the temporary Medicare telehealth waivers enacted during the pandemic, with virtual and televisits inclusive of audio only for mental health already a permanent Medicare payment change. This latter change may be particularly useful, given the prevalence of "diseases of despair" in the United States (alcohol dependency, substance misuse, and suicidal thoughts and behavior; Brignone et al., 2020) and elevated concerns about mental health and substance use post–COVID-19 (Panchal et al., 2023).

Hospital at Home

The pandemic also spurred the growth of the acute care HaH movement. Unlike traditional home care, in this model, hospital-level acute care is provided in the home for selected acutely ill people. This, in turn, minimizes the person's risk for hospital-acquired airborne infections and potentially other conditions as it simultaneously debulks hospitals, thus enabling them to serve others whose condition requires care within a brick-and-mortar facility. This model has been successfully used in other nations, resulting in decreased costs of care and better outcomes, and Johns Hopkins has operated such a program since 1994 (Klein, n.d.). Adoption accelerated when the pandemic prompted the Centers for Medicare and Medicaid Services to allow some Medicare-certified hospitals to provide this level of acute care in the home and be reimbursed as if a brick-and-mortar hospitalization; criteria are strict because the same level of care must be offered regardless of the setting of the care. Leff and Milstein (2022) note the strong empirical base for HaH's capacity to deliver safe, high-quality, equitable, and effective care, yet some groups, including some nurses' unions, have voiced opposition. Nevertheless, HaH continues to grow despite a somewhat uncertain regulatory and payment history, and there has been bipartisan support for the potential of HaH to improve care in rural and underserved areas (Eastabrook, 2024). In the view of the author of this text, HaH will continue to grow as virtual technologies and remote monitoring capacities become increasingly refined. There is also greater potential to address social determinants of health, as the nurse is in the home with the patient and their supports and thus can discern realistic discharge planning and foster effective implementation. This attribute of HaH—contextual discharge planning—may be the force behind the ongoing findings that HaHs have lower readmission rates than similar, traditionally hospitalized patients. As Leff et al. state: HaH "puts the patient at the center of care at home, where they have more agency and power to affect their care. HaH is the keystone of this future home-based care ecosystem. It is time to claim the future" (Leff et al., 2024, para 13). Nurses can and should be the key to the success of this model, provided we are willing to challenge traditional notions and expand beyond walled care. Let's not let this opportunity pass nursing by; if nurses are not willing and able to provide such care, someone else will.

Other Trends

Emerging trends prior to COVID-19 are likely to continue or even accelerate, with weighty implications for nursing practice. Reese's (2020) interviews of 10 health care thought leaders underscored the following: ongoing transitions from fee-for-service to value-based care; telehealth; efforts to better understand the total cost of care; heightened attention to upstream determinants of health; care in the least restrictive environment; emerging technology, precision medicine, and artificial intelligence; and heightened attention to cybersecurity, among others (Reese, 2020). As a result of virtual health implementation, "health systems in the United States have been reorganizing their care delivery process with unprecedented speed" (Stahl et al., 2022, para 1). All of these have a great impact on you, regardless of your career phase and interest—or lack of interest—in innovation. Greater accountability for cost as well as outcomes is laced throughout these projections, as is the movement toward care delivery that is person-centric, focusing on serving the population, not the health care system. Impacting costs through value-informed practice is essential; so, too, is progressive adoption of new forms of care delivery. If the nursing role is to be upskilled, with corollary enhancement of career opportunities and compensation, nurses must be prepared to contribute in new ways. This will be particularly important as the outcomes and cost of an individual nurse's work become more traceable through universal adoption of national provider identifiers (such NPIs are required for nurses who bill but are optional for those who do not) and/or unique nurse identifiers (see Chan et al., 2023, for additional explication of these two routes to greater transparency in nursing care delivery). As Blumenthal et al. (2020) note: "One thing is certain: The healthcare system that emerges from the pandemic will not be the same" (para 1). Thoughtful nurses have the opportunity, perhaps even the responsibility, to shape a just, equitable, affordable health care system.

End-of-Chapter Resources

THOUGHT QUESTIONS

1. What are the pros of HaH? Cons? What skills do you have that prepare you for such work? What skills would you need to further develop?
2. Some nurses' unions have voiced concerns about the safety of HaH and its potential impact on availability of nursing positions. What do you think? Defend your position.
3. What are the pros of virtual care? Cons? What skills do you have that prepare you for such work? What skills would you need to further develop?
4. Define the following key terms:
   Acute care hospital at home
   Disease of despair
   Elective procedure
   Supply chain
   Telehealth fraud
   Traunch

EXERCISES

1. Select any product in your work setting or home. Describe the supply chain, including all subcomponents and processes, from its origin to your hands.
2. Consider a recent experience in clinical practice. How could care be delivered more efficiently and cost-effectively? What steps could you, as an individual nurse, take to make this happen?
3. Consider leading a supply chain improvement strategy for a clinical setting. What information would you need to get started? Who would be in the strategy team, and how would you recruit them?

QUIZ

True or False

1. Financial resources provided to health care during the COVID-19 pandemic were carefully calibrated to meet societal need.
2. Human resources were carefully deployed during COVID-19 to ensure capacity to meet societal need.
3. Telehealth has the potential to expand care to underserved populations.

4. Telehealth has been associated with fraud.
5. Some providers previously deemed "essential" were furloughed during the COVID-19 pandemic.
6. The U.S. health care supply chain depends heavily on other nations.

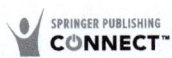

A robust set of instructor resources designed to supplement this text is located at http://connect.springerpub.com/content/book/978-0-8261-7236-5. Qualifying instructors may request access by emailing textbook@springerpub.com.

REFERENCES

Blumenthal, D., Schneider, E., Seerval, S., & Shah, A. (2020, July 24). *Three scenarios for how the pandemic could change U.S. health care*. Harvard Business Review. https://hbr.org/2020/07/3-scenarios-for-how-the-pandemic-could-change-u-s-health-care

Brignone, E., George, D. R., Sinoway, L., Katz, C., Sauder, C., Murray, A., Gladden, R., & Kraschnewski, J. L. (2020). Trends in the diagnosis of diseases of despair in the United States, 2009–2018 A retrospective cohort study. *BMJ Open, 10*(10), e037679. https://doi.org/10.1136/bmjopen-2020-037679

Bryant, B. (2020, May 19). *"Public shaming," audit concerns prompt Encompass Health to return $237M in CARES Act funding*. https://homehealthcarenews.com/2020/05/public-shaming-audit-concerns-prompt-encompass-health-to-return-237m-in-cares-act-funding

Chan, G. K., Cummins, M. R., Taylor, C. S., Rambur, B., Auerbach, D. I., Meadows-Oliver, M., Cooke, C., Turek, E. A., & Pittman, P. P. (2023). An overview and policy implications of national nurse identifier systems: A call for unity and integration. *Nursing Outlook, 71*(2), 101892. https://doi.org/10.1016/j.outlook.2022.10.005

Collins, S., Gunja, M., Aboulafia, G., Czynewicz, E., Kline, C., Rapoport, R., & Glancy, S. (2020, June 23). *An early look at the potential implications of the COVID-19 pandemic for health insurance coverage*. The Commonwealth Foundation. https://www.commonwealthfund.org/publications/issue-briefs/2020/jun/implications-covid-19-pandemic-health-insurance-survey

Cross-Call, J., & Broaddus, M. (2020, July 14). *States that have expanded Medicaid are better positioned to address COVID-19 and recession*. Center on Budget and Policy Priorities. https://www.cbpp.org/research/health/states-that-have-expanded-medicaid-are-better-positioned-to-address-covid-19-and

Dai, T., Zaman, M. H., Padula, W. V., & Davidson, P. M. (2021). Supply chain failures amid COVID-19 signal a new pillar for global health preparedness. *Journal of Clinical Nursing, 30*(1–2), e1–e3. https://doi.org/10.1111/jocn.15400

Diaz, A., Chhabra, K., & Scott, J. (2020, May 3). *The COVID-19 pandemic and rural hospitals—Adding insult to injury*. Health Affairs Forefront. https://www.healthaffairs.org/do/10.1377/hblog2020429.583513/full/

Eastabrook, D. (2024, May 17). *Hospital-at-home grows despite regulatory uncertainty*. Modern Healthcare. https://www.modernhealthcare.com/providers/hospital-at-home-congress-regulation

Fernando, J. (2020, January 11). *Traunch.* Investopedia. www.investopedia.com/terms/t/traunch.asp

Fried, J., Liebers, D., & Roberts, E. (2020). Sustaining rural hospitals after COVID-19: The case for global budgets. *Journal of the American Medical Association, 324*(2), 137–138. https://doi.org/10.1001/jama.2020.9744

Gibson, R., & Prasad Singh, J. (2018). *China Rx: Explaining the risks of America's dependence on China for Medicine.* Prometheus Books.

Gooch, K. (2020, June 5). *Record number of healthcare workers laid off, furloughed during pandemic.* Becker's Hospital Review. https://www.beckershospitalreview.com/workforce/record-number-of-healthcare-workers-laid-off-furloughed-during-pandemic.html

Hagland, M. (2023, October 24). *Kaufman Hall: Workforce issues remain key challenges for hospital performance.* Healthcare Innovation. https://www.hcinnovationgroup.com/finance-revenue-cycle/news/53076228/kaufman-hall-workforce-issues-remain-key-challenges-for-hospital-performance

Health Industry Distributers Association. (2023). *Supply chain. A look ahead.* https://www.hida.org/distribution/news/healthcare-distribution-supply-chain-magazine/2023/Supply_Chain__A_Look_Ahead

Jarman, R. (2020). *The corona virus means doctors, nurses and PAs are essential workers—Until they get laid off.* https://www.nbcnews.com/think/opinion/coronavirus-means-doctors-nurses-pas-are-essential-workders-until-they-ncna1234289

Johnson, SR. (2024, October 17). *Hurricane Helene leaves IV fluid shortage in its wake.* U.S News and World Report. https://www.usnews.com/news/national-news/articles/2024-10-17/hurricane-helene-leaves-iv-fluid-shortage-in-its-wake

Klein, S. (n.d.). *"Hospital at home" programs improves outcomes, lowers costs but face resistance from providers and payers.* The Commonwealth Foundation. https://www.commonwealthfund.org/publications/newsletter-article/hospital-home-programs-improve-outcomes-lower-costs-face-resistance

LaPointe, J. (2020). *Hospital revenue falling $1.4B a day as patient volume drops.* Revcycle Intelligence Practice Management News. https://revcycleintelligence.com/news/hospital-revenue-falling-1.4b-a-day-as-patient-volume-drops

Leff, B., Levine, D., & Siu, A. (2024, May 3). *The acute hospital care at home waiver and the future of hospital at home in the US.* Health Affairs Forefront. https://www.healthaffairs.org/content/forefront/acute-hospital-care-home-waiver-and-future-hospital-home-us

Leff, B., & Milstein, A. (2022, June 27). *What we learned from the acute hospital care at home waiver—and what we still don't know.* Health Affairs Forefront. https://www.healthaffairs.org/content/forefront/we-learned-acute-hospital-care-home-waiver-and-we-still-don-t-know

Livingston, S. (2020, June 13). *COVID-19 may end up boosting value-based payments.* Modern Healthcare. https://www.modernhealthcare.com/insurance/covid-19-may-end-up-boosting-value-based-payment

Mazer-Amirshahi, M., & Fox, E. (2018). Saline shortages—Many causes, no simple solution. *New England Journal of Medicine, 378,* 1472–1474. https://doi.org/10.1056/NEJMp1800347

McCauliff, M. (2024, May 14). *Medicare advantage will 'sink' hospitals, experts warn.* Modern Healthcare. https://www.modernhealthcare.com/politics-policy/rural-hospitals-medicare-advantage-pay-closing

McGough, M., Amin, K., & Cox, C. (2023, January 24). *How has healthcare utilization changed since the pandemic*. Peterson Kaiser Family Foundation Health System Tracker. https://www.healthsystemtracker.org/chart-collection/how-has-healthcare-utilization-changed-since-the-pandemic

Mehrota, A., Wang, B., & Snyder, G. (2020, August). *Telemedicine: What should the post pandemic regulatory and payment landscape look like?* The Commonwealth Fund. https://www.commonwealthfund.org/publications/issue-briefs/2020/aug/telemedicine-post-pandemic-regulation

Michandandi, P. (2020, May 5) Health care supply chains: COVID-19 challenges and pressing actions. *Annals of Internal Medicine, 173*, 300–301. https://doi.org/10.7326/M20-1326

Panchal, N., Saunders, H., Rudcwitz, R., & Cox, C. (2023, March 20). The implications of COVID-19 for mental health and substance use. Kaiser Family Foundation. https://www.kff.org/mental-health/issue-brief/the-implications-of-covid-19-for-mental-health-and-substance-use/

Reese, E. (2020, January 1). *2020 Vision: What to expect in healthcare finance over the next decade*. Healthcare Financial Management Association. https://www.hfma.org/topics/hfm/2020/january/healthcare-2020s-views-on-healthcares-changing-landscape-from-thought-leaders.html

Respaut, R., & Spaulding, R. (2020, March 31). *U.S. hospitals halt lucrative procedures amid coronavirus crisis; jobs cuts follow*. Reuters. https://www.reuters.com/article/us-health-ccronavirus-usa-hospitals-idUSKBN21I388

Schulte, F. (2020). *Coronavirus fuels explosive growth in telehealth—And concern about fraud*. Kaiser Family Foundation. https://khn.org/news/coronavirus-fuels-explosive-growth-in-telehealth—and-concern-about-fraud/

Shen, K., Eddelbuettel, J. C, & Eisenberg, M. D. (2024). Job flows into and out of health care before and after the COVID-19 pandemic. *JAMA Health Forum, 5*(1), e234964. https://doi.org/10.1001/jamahealthforum.2023.4964

Sonfield, A., Frost, J., Dawson, R., & Lindberg, L. (2020). *COVID-19 job losses threaten insurance coverage and access to reproductive health care for millions*. Health Affairs Blog. https://www.healthaffairs.org/do/10.1377/hblog20200728.779022/full/

Stahl, M., Cheung, J., Post, K., Valin, J. P., & Jacobs, I. (2022). Accelerating virtual health implementation following the COVID-19 pandemic: Questionnaire study. *JMIR Formative Research, 6*(5), e32819. https://doi.org/10.2196/32819

St. Pierre, W. (2021, July 26). *Four ways to engage nurses in supply chain optimization initiatives*. GHX Healthcare Hub. https://www.ghx.com/the-healthcare-hub/four-ways-to-engage-nurses-in-supply-chain-optimization-initiatives/

Wolfson, B. (2020, August 10). *Pandemic hampers reopening joint replacement gold mine*. Modern Healthcare. https://www.modernhealthcare.com/safety-quality/pandemic-hampers-reopening-joint-replacement-gold-mine

Yakusheva, O., Rambur, P., & Buerhaus, P. (2020, August 10). Valued-informed nursing practice can reset the nurse-hospital relationship. *JAMA Health Forum, 1*(8), e200931. https://doi.org/10.1001/jamahealthforum.2020.0931

… CHAPTER 14

The Health Care Workforce: What Nurses Need to Know

Although the U.S. nursing workforce has been characterized by cycles of shortages and surpluses, the post–COVID-19 landscape reveals dramatic new dimensions. These dynamics existed before the pandemic, but they were largely submerged amidst power dynamics (Kearns et al., 2021) that silence nurses or were obscured by the kaleidoscope of change on the health care landscape. Now, COVID-19 has focused, illuminated, and amplified the central role of nurses in health care. As a result, the value of nurses is more visible to the public.

Early in the pandemic, nurses were lauded as heroes (Morin & Baptiste, 2020). COVID-19 and post–COVID-19 public appreciation of nurses is a widespread phenomenon. Studies across the globe—ranging from Korea (Kim & Lee, 2023) to Turkey (Uysal & Demirdağ, 2022) to Israel (Blau et al., 2023)—found enhanced, positive public perceptions of nurses amid the pandemic and its echo. At the same time, the hero motif may represent dangers to individual nurses and to the profession writ large. "Heroes" are selfless, are sacrificing, and demand nothing for themselves. Instead, "heroes" serve others at any and at all costs to themselves. This image sustains existing power structures and benefits that don't extend to nurses. A post-structural discourse analysis on the nurse-as-hero motif, for example, concluded that it is a "... tool employed to accomplish multiple aims such as the normalization of nurses' exposure to risk, the enforcement of model citizenship, and the preservation of existing power relationships that limit the ability of front-line nurses to determine the conditions of their work" (Mohammed et al., 2021, para 6).

Ironically, TikTok presented a similar perspective. In a short clip the nurse, initially lured by the seductive call of the hero, complies with an exhausting schedule, only to realize administrators were willing to compensate travel nurses at a generous rate they were not willing to compensate him . . . until, of course, he became a travel nurse. Still others have suggested that a broader understanding of these dynamics brought a needed end to nurses' "virtue script" of serving others without a two-way street for that giving (Pulcini & Rambur, 2022). Growing union activism provides at least some confirming evidence that the prototype of a nurse as martyr or hero has run its course. Labor activity has increased as nurses demand safe and effective working conditions and compensation that reflects their contributions (Anderson & Young, 2024).

So, if not to be a hero, what attracts people to nursing? Can a more practical and realistic orientation be the magnet that draws people to the profession? And once a nurse, why do nurses stay in their jobs? Their careers? Why do nurses leave? Each of these will now be reviewed in turn.

RECRUITING PEOPLE TO BECOME NURSES

Fussell's classic book titled *Class* posits that nursing was an educational vehicle to the middle class for women just as engineering was for men. Similarly, medicine offered a route to the upper class. He also posits that degree of supervision is "often a more eloquent class indicator than mere income" (Fussell, 1983, p. 48), possibly adding yet another nuance to the American Medical Association's (AMA's) insistence that NPs should not have independent practice. More recently, the Robert Wood Johnson Foundation's campaign lists nine reasons to become a nurse, including that it offers meaningful work in a growing profession that is comparatively well compensated and flexible (Robert Wood Johnson Foundation [RWJF], n.d.). But what does the research literature say?

Hoff et al. explored adolescents' response to the question: "If you could have any job you wanted when you grow up, what job would you really like to have?" In early adolescence, the top response was *doctor*, but by late adolescence, *nurse* rose above *doctor*, at number three, with *teacher* and *vet* (presumably veterinarian) landing in first and second rank, respectively. This study also found a preference for careers that can't be automated (discussed in Chapter 6, under the rubric of artificial intelligence). Finally, results also suggested that older adolescents were less likely than younger to be influenced by gendered stereotypes (Hoff et al., 2022). This has relevance for recruitment to nursing. Although the proportion of nurses who are men is increasing, men remain decidedly underrepresented in nursing (Munday, 2023); evidence suggests that recruitment of men to the profession is hampered by a lack of understanding of what nurses actually do (Guy et al., 2022).

A pre–COVID-19 integrative review of young people's view of nursing found that they perceive nurses' work as one with limited autonomy, poor working conditions, and shift work; nurses' work was also perceived as inferior to physician work. Nurses were perceived as kind, hardworking, and less intellectual than physicians (Glerean et al., 2017). Such perceptions have international parallels. Neumbe et al. (2023), for example, found that undergraduate nursing students in Uganda had positive *attitudes* toward the profession but negative *perceptions*. Respondents viewed nursing as an unpopular, inadequately compensated profession that offers hectic work in unsafe settings. Given the growing workplace violence, many in the United States would likely echo this concern. Nevertheless, the competition for enrollment in a nursing program remains high in the United States, and second-degree and master's entry programs abound. This suggests that—at least for the time being—nursing is viewed as an attractive career option.

At the present time, the number of RNs in the United States is at a record high of 5.2 million. Of these, roughly 4.6 million are working in a nursing role. Which leads to the second question: Why do nurses stay in their jobs? Their careers? Why do nurses leave? The job versus career distinction is important. Do nurses leave their *jobs* or the nursing profession entirely?

What About Nurses Themselves?—Intention to Stay . . . and to Leave!

In exploring the research literature, it is important to discern the operational definitions related to turnover and retention. *Intention to leave* a position differs from *intention to stay*, and—although both are sound measures of *intention*—neither is uniformly linked to the action of consistently staying or actually leaving a position. Moreover, job turnover differs from leaving the profession entirely, with the latter sometimes termed career turnover.

A nurse may leave a position for positive reasons such as better compensation, pleasant working conditions, or a lifestyle deemed a better fit yet remain in the overall pool of nurses. Leaving the profession entirely creates workforce gaps, yet at least some of the exodus is for retirement. Thus, overall predictive models of workforce adequacy are complex, shaped by measurement issues, and interact with many other variables.

Nevertheless, studies from around the globe have found consistent evidence supporting the importance of working conditions and job satisfaction as key to retention. Im and Koh (2023), for example, found job satisfaction to be the primary mediator of intention to leave among nurses in South Korea. They call for further analysis of the work environment of frontline nurses as a step toward reconstructing the workplace to enhance satisfaction. Closer to home, a study of nurses in U.S. Army hospitals found that 49% of nurses intended to leave, 44% for preventable reasons, specifically dissatisfaction with management and the nursing environment (Taylor-Clark et al., 2022). Rutledge et al. (2022) found a potentially related phenomenon, chronic fatigue, to predict hospital nurse turnover intentions. They note that although chronic fatigue is associated with two elements of burnout—emotional exhaustion and depersonalization—burnout itself did not predict turnover intention in this study. Conversely, other studies have found burnout to predict turnover (Aiken et al., 2023).

Pandemic-related stress, fatigue, and burnout certainly have impacted work satisfaction, intention to leave, and turnover. Sanchez (2023) reports a near doubling of nurses' intention to leave their position within a year compared to the immediate prepandemic era and nearly four times increase above the "typical" rate, with the planned departures highest among younger nurses: 59% for age 25 or younger and 53% for those 25 to 35 years old (Sanchez, 2023).

Returning to the question that opened this section: Does intention to leave turn into actual resignations? The data suggest not necessarily. A January 2023 survey found that 85% of hospital-based nurses said they planned to quit within 12 months, with 90% offering increased support staff as a strategy to decrease the negative workplace experiences that lead to resignation. Nearly 90% of respondents also cited the following as strategies to reduce turnover: lower patient-to-nurse ratios, increased salaries, safer work environments, and input into organizational decision-making (Hollowell, 2023). Indeed, some organizations that focused on nurse compensation and staffing have had retention success. One California system, for example, offered $100,000 sign-on bonuses to new nurses and $100,000 retention bonuses for existing nurse employees and has been able to fully staff the intended units with minimal use of travel nurses (Kayser, 2024).

Clearly, working conditions and job satisfaction are linked and represent a multifaceted confluence of phenomena. A systematic review by Stemmer et al. (2023), for example, found *unfinished nursing care* to be associated with intention to leave, burnout, and reduced job satisfaction. Similar to many other studies, they further suggest that creation of a positive work environment is critical to nurse retention, including a focus on strategies to decrease unfinished care. Papathanasiou et al. (2024) further explored this key contributor to nurse dissatisfaction in their investigation of *missed care*. Their umbrella review of articles found that care is "missed" due to organizational problems, the workplace climate, staffing levels, organizational problems, and the working climate. These elements are under the control of administrators and can be addressed with financial and human resources, yet these investments are inconsistently executed. Wang and Anderson (2022), for example, found that more generous commercial insurance rates did not result in more expenditures that directly impacted patients, for example, they found fewer than one additional registered nurse per 100 patient beds. Instead, these revenues resulted in contributions to reserves and administrative expenditures. Taken as a whole, these findings suggest an undervaluing of nursing care with a corollary underinvestment in the nursing workforce and optimizing nurse working conditions.

Finally, Aiken et al. (2023) found that nurse burnout was associated with not only nurse turnover but with physician turnover as well. This latter finding may be useful to nurses because of the potential for creating public awareness that consequences are broader than nursing itself. Recall from Chapter 2 that employer-based health insurance in the United States was designed to ensure payment to *physicians* and *hospitals*. To underscore, the U.S. health care payment system was built on an explicit (but publicly obscured) concern about payment to physicians and hospitals. Medicare and Medicaid were built on that conceptual foundation, and federal entities continue to examine *physician* payment adequacy. Yet downstream problems from this narrow orientation are evident and growing. But how did we get here? What follows next are some of the payment antecedents that shape current woes.

How Did Organized Medicine Become So Powerful?

As noted in Chapter 2, the Flexner Report of 1910 began to lay the foundation toward the powerful position organized medicine has held in recent history. The now-formidable AMA that represents physicians' interests had a rocky start. This was, in part, because physicians themselves were not held in high regard during the 19th century. Johnson notes that "the medical profession was unreliable and physicians had a difficult time treating even simple ailments" (Johnson, 2017, p. 16). They were commonly denounced in newspapers. The development of the AMA in 1847 represents one effort toward professionalism, as did the Flexner Report of 1910.

The AMA initially had difficulty gaining organizational traction and chose criminalizing abortion as a strategy toward legitimacy. Abortion, viewed as returning women to menses, historically had not been a controversial issue. Instead, it was a fairly common practice in the early years of the United States, representing a decision that was made privately by women and assisted by midwives (Abdelfata, 2022; Pfeiffer, cited in Arablouei & Abdelfata). A small group of physicians led by Horatio Robinson Storer set out to change this. Their prime concern was the role of female midwives in the care of women and the exclusion of male MDs who were beginning to specialize in gynecology and obstetrics. Race was also a concern. Specifically, Storer was concerned about the dropping birth rate among White Protestant women and unabashedly asked them to reproduce, using somewhat graphic language, to ensure White racial dominance (Goodwin, cited in Arablouei & Abdelfata, 2022). Arablouei notes that although Storer was concerned with racial dominance, he also saw the criminalization of abortion as a way to remove midwives as market competitors in the work of caring for women. Haugeber (cited in Arablouei & Abdelfatah, 2022) concludes that the AMA's stance was strategic and financially oriented. It aimed to direct the potentially lucrative care of women away from female providers and instead to male, university-educated physicians as they began to specialize in the fields of gynecology and obstetrics.

The power of the AMA grew exponentially, as did that of the American Hospital Association (AHA). Today, they are consistently among the top spending lobby groups in the United States, along with Pharmaceutical Research and Manufacturers of America and Blue Cross and Blue Shield of America (Robertson, 2021). Nursing is not represented in the top 20, despite being by far the largest group of health professionals. In 2023, the AMA spent over $23 million on lobbying, the American Nurses Association (ANA) slightly over $1 million (Open Secrets, 2024). Other health care trade organizations that spend a substantial amount of lobbying money per year include the AHA ($30,198,230), Blue Cross and Blue Shield ($28,589,340), and Pharmaceutical Researchers and Manufacturers of America ($27,628,000), with another $15,434,955 spent by the Pharmaceutical Care Management Association (cited expenditures occurred in 2023). Individual drug manufacturers also spend substantial amounts on lobbying, with Pfizer at $14,360,000 and Amgen at $1,429,000 (again, all 2023 sums; Open Secrets, 2024). Although disconcerting, given these figures, perhaps it shouldn't be surprising that nursing has not had an optimal policy imprint. Can we change that? What lessons can we learn from the past? If not the major political force, was there a time when nurses had more autonomy and were entrepreneurs?

Early Nurse Entrepreneurs

Indeed, there was. In the early part of the last century, nurses were entrepreneurs. Whelan notes that "Most [roughly 80%] early 20th century nurses were independent contractors, working for and receiving pay from private patients who required nursing care when ill" (Whelan, 2012, para 5). Few nurses worked in hospitals, in part because hospitals had a fleet of free labor in the form of students. For these hospital-based "training schools," graduation of nurses was a side effect, not the main intention. Ervin (2023) notes that their training was directed by physicians and their education was consistently interrupted to care for patients. She states: "From the institution's standpoint, graduates were a byproduct rather than the purpose of the training school" (p. 7). Similarly, Whelan notes: "Hospitals found the use of cheaper, *more easily controlled student workers* as staff preferable to one composed of nurse graduates" (para 10, emphasis added). Thus, attention to the hospital working environment for nurses and nurse career mobility was not part of the foundational culture of the U.S. health care system. Nor was nurse autonomy. Care delivery was predicated on the assumption that there would be plenty of free labor; when one nurse cohort graduated, there would be a new cast of students who demanded little but gave much.

The dynamic began to change somewhat when hospitals started to hire nurses. The date of the transition from entrepreneur to employee varies by source but is in the 1930 to 1940 range (Whelan). Hospitals hired private-duty nurses as temporary staff during and beyond WWII, but also started to view entrepreneurial nurses as competition. The response was to hire nurses directly and roll their work into the hospital room charge, more like a maid than a professional service. This creates a perverse incentive in fee-for-service reimbursement, namely to keep the volume of services and patient numbers high and the number of nurses low. This workforce dynamic continues to this day and is only partly offset by mandatory nurse–patient staffing ratios, which represents a regulatory response to a market imperfection (Yakusheva & Rambur, 2023).

Medicare was built within the parameters set by commercial insurance, namely ensuring reimbursement for hospitals and physicians. This retains the perverse incentives named earlier. Medicare, however, added a further barrier to nurse autonomy. Registered nurses could not be reimbursed. Specifically, Part A included, and continues to include, *places* the nurse may be employed (hospitals, skilled nursing facilities) *but not registered nurses themselves*. Part B precludes nurses from being directly reimbursed. "Incident to" billing allows a work-around (see Box 14.1) that brings its own problems. For example, incident to billing obscures the work of the nurse and does not easily allow for cost and outcome accountability for either the physician or the nurse. It is also expensive. Patel et al. (2022) found that the elimination of incident to billing (termed indirect billing in their study) would have saved Medicare roughly $194 million in 2018. Notably, for technical reasons, this study could only estimate visits in which there was a prescription, as incident to billing renders all visits without them invisible. Much like a black hole, it can only be perceived by the movement around it. Those visits that include a prescription are only visible through the sort of complex analytics used in this study.

Yet most incident to billers are anything but "ancillary." Many nurse practitioners, although functioning collaboratively, work independently yet bill via incident to billing. Volpe (2022) reported that 56% of the NPs and PAs in the practices surveyed used incident to billing, even when these providers were working independently. Why? There may be power dynamics at play, but these are more difficult to quantify than the financial incentives. And the financial incentives are clear. NPs and PAs who bill under their own National Provider Identifier (NPI) number are reimbursed at 85%. Incident to billing, instead, returns 100% revenue. The American Association of Nurse Practitioners (AANP) has advocated for the elimination of incident to billing,

 BOX 14.1

WHAT IS *INCIDENT TO* BILLING?

The federal legislation definition of incident to billing is defined as the provider billing of services and supplies that are performed by *auxiliary* personnel (Centers for Medicare and Medicaid Services [CMS], n.d., italics added).

as has the Medicare Payment Advisory Commission (MedPAC, 2019). Perhaps not surprisingly, the AMA opposed the elimination of incident to billing (American Medical Association [AMA] 2022). Incident to billing provides additional revenue that typically goes to the practice or physician, not the nurse practitioner or PA who is actually doing the work. Another Medicare policy that fuels the physician workforce and their revenue as well as that of some hospitals is the current graduate medical education (GME) model.

Graduate Medical Education

GME funding has been a staple of physician training since Medicare was enacted in 1965. Intended to be temporary (AMA, 2020, p. 4), this nearly $18 billion yearly subsidy ($17.8 billion in FY 21; Congressional Research Service, 2024) to physicians and hospitals has two elements. Direct medical education (DME) funds medical resident salaries and supervising physician stipends, and indirect medical education (IME) subsidizes the purported higher costs teaching hospitals incur because they educate residents. Health care lobbying organizations such as the AHA and the Association of American Medical Colleges have argued that these subsidies are essential to ensuring an adequate physician workforce. In the post–COVID-19 Congress, they lobbied for and received an additional 1,000 new Medicare-funded medical residencies (National Council of State Legislatures, 2024).

Yet if the past is prologue, the GME mechanism has performed poorly on its potential to meet the health workforce needs of the nation. Consider the pressing and growing primary care workforce gaps. Although rebounding somewhat in 2024, primary care physician residencies have gone unfilled, with these practice roles increasingly being filled by NPs and PAs. Roughly one-quarter of all care delivered to Medicare beneficiaries is delivered by NPs and PAs, and these providers are more likely to care for underserved populations (Patel et al., 2023). Yet their education is not similarly subsidized.

Trends in medical residencies are clear; physicians have chosen specialty care. For example, from 2003 to 2018, there was a 209% increase in the number of plastic surgery residencies, a 190% increase in neurosurgery, and a 153% in dermatology, to name but a few, even as "more primary care focused residents" such as psychiatry and family medicine languish (Royce, 2021, p. 586). Such selective fueling of the surgical side of the physician workforce at the expense of sorely needed primary care and mental health providers is particularly troubling given the mismatch between the financial investment and the nation's health outcomes. This has been disconcerting to at least some surgeons. Bamdad and Englesbe, for example, note: "The U.S. spends approximately 1/14th of its gross domestic product on surgical care ($9.4 trillion in 2017), which translates to nearly $4,000 per person in this country. When considering that healthcare overall has only a minimal impact on premature mortality and quality of life (likely less than 10%), we are left with a humbling assessment of our contribution as surgeons to health" (Bamdad & Englesbe, 2020, p. 799).

Medicare funds the majority of GME (AMA) and teaching hospitals, and their trade organizations argue that GME is essential to offset the cost of teaching residents. Others counter this view, suggesting that medical residents themselves bear the cost of their education (Chandra et al., 2014) and that their work contributes to the hospital's bottom line. They state: ". . . evidence is consistent with the view that residents bear the cost of their own training, which would mean that GME funds are treated as general monies going to their institutions; in fact, these funds are often used in ways that are difficult to trace, assess, and justify" (2014, p. 2360). Still others also note that GME is "lucrative" for hospitals (Grischkan et al., 2020, pp. 1035–1036).

Should this subsidy to hospitals be the financial responsibility of taxpayers and Medicare beneficiaries, particularly in an era when health care is projected to shift away from hospital settings? Although there have been recommendations to include outpatient settings in GME (Medicare Payment Advisory Commission, 2021), GME is hospital-centric and poorly aligned with the goals of value-based care that aims to decrease unnecessary use of health services (Grischkan et al., 2020, p. 2360). It also does not address a broader set of workforce needs.

In addition to Medicare, Medicaid also provides GME funding, as does the Department of Defense, Department of Veterans Affairs, Children's Hospitals GME, and Teaching Health Center GME (Congressional Research Service, 2024). Under Medicaid, individual states have the flexibility to mold that funding to state needs and policy priorities. At least 10 states have directed some Medicaid GME to the education of NPs and PAs (National Council of State Legislatures, 2024). This strategy has empirical support (via a Medicare pilot) as a cost-effective approach toward expanding the primary care workforce. The Medicare Graduate Nurse Education Demonstration found that residencies for nurse practitioners can be effectively executed at a fraction of the cost of physicians: $28,000 to 57,000 versus $157,602, respectively (Aiken et al., 2018; Government Accounting Office [GAO], 2019; Porat-Dahlerbruch et al., 2022). Serious consideration should also be given to Grischkan and team's suggestion that this massive investment move from being hospital- and specialty physician–centric to debt reduction and wage multipliers targeted to the physicians, nurses, and community health workers who actually work in underserved areas and practice in less lucrative areas like primary care.

Who funds the education of nurses? Well, for the most part, students and families. The $18 billion the nation spends on medical education in the form of GME has no even remote parallels on the nursing side. Most funding for nursing education is through Title 8, funded at $300 million in fiscal year 2023. Nursing students pay tuition, and practicing nurses serve as preceptors, typically without compensation to them or their organization. Ponder the tremendous investment the nation has made in the physician workforce compared to nursing. What is the role of gender? Educational class? Historical precedents? What can be done to better align workforce investment with societal need?

Workforce Challenges by Site

Recall that a shortage of health care workers means decreased access to the services that would be provided by these health professionals. Although workforce challenges abound, some segments of health care delivery face particular workforce challenges. This can be because of heightened demand for those services, too few providers of the service, or both. A few challenged sites will now be briefly reviewed.

Community-based care. As early as a decade ago, the U.S. Bureau of Labor Statistics raised attention to the increased demand for community-based services and the resulting workforce deficits. They described contributing factors as the aging population, lower cost for community-based care relative to nursing homes, and people's desire to stay in their own home (Bureau of Labor Statistics, U.S. Department of Labor, 2015). These issues have only accelerated as more Baby Boomers age into their senior years and virtual care, inclusive of remote monitoring and digitally supported care, evolves. Helpfully, they define three distinct yet overlapping industries that provide community care, as follows. Notably, each of these relies largely on different funding streams.

- *"Services for the elderly and persons with disabilities*, which provides for the social welfare of the elderly, people with intellectual and developmental disabilities, and people with disabilities, both in daycare settings and in the home.
- *Home healthcare services*, which provides skilled nursing services and a wide range of personal care and medical care services in the home.
- *Community care facilities for the elderly*, which provides residential care, personal care services, and, in some instances, skilled nursing care for the elderly and people who do not desire to live independently" (Bureau of Labor Statistics [BLS], 2015, para 5).

The development of the community-based workforce has not kept pace with the growth in this area, and the acute care hospital at home movement will also require an expanded pool of nurses and others who can deliver acute care in the home. Kreider and Werner (2023) detail the mismatch between growth of community-based care and the people who can deliver it. They also call for more focus on this segment of workforce as well as more funds.

Private equity has brought some such funding. This avenue has enabled venture capitalists to grow their footprint in some dimensions of community-based care, for example, home health, which Vollers calls "lucrative—and lightly regulated." Many nurses likely don't easily discern the role of private equity in health care, but its impact is huge. Consider this cautionary statement by Vollers:

> Private equity-owned healthcare companies are focused on generating robust profits for investors. Typically, they want to cut costs, increase cash flow, use debt to fund expansion and then sell within a few years for maximum profit. In healthcare, critics say, that business model can diminish the quality of care, increase costs and narrow access for patients—particularly in more lightly regulated industries such as home care and hospice care. (Vollers, 2024, para 9)

Private equity hospitals have been found to have a lower-risk pool of patients (less ill) but a 25% increase in hospital-acquired adverse events, suggesting poorer quality (Kannan et al., 2023). Other studies have found private equity acquisition of safety net hospitals resulted in worker layoffs or reduction of services, placing some patients in immediate jeopardy (Scruth et al, 2024). Terry recounts these and other perils in an article titled "Taming the Private Equity Beast by Shifting Its Focus to Value-Based Care," where he suggests encouraging private equity investment in independent primary care groups and accountable care organizations (ACOs) who need additional funds to shift from fee-for-service to value-based care (Terry, 2024).

It is important to be very clear-eyed on the private equity business model. Terry eloquently defines it as follows:

> The classic business model of private equity is not well matched to the needs of the healthcare industry. Following an acquisition, a PE firm will typically hold onto the acquired entity for four to seven years before trying to either sell it for a profit or take it public. In the meantime, the PE firm will cut costs and raise prices, frequently loading the acquired company with debt while taking exorbitant management fees. (Terry, 2024, para 12)

Reynold offers additional clarity: "The private equity model involves using investor money—and additional debt—to purchase an asset like a hospital. The firm typically then cuts operating costs, often sells the real estate portion, and attempts to re-sell the entity for a profit after several years" (Reynold, 2024, para 2).

Conversely, if you want to start your own nurse-run business, private equity may be the ideal way to finance your efforts. You also may be employed in a private equity–owned health care entity or work with individuals who are. One in three for-profit hospitals in the United States are owned by private equity investors (Vollers, 2024). Since 2020, private equity firms have also acquired 116 health care staffing companies and were involved in more than 60% of all clinical staffing transactions. Opponents of this model argue that equity-backed staffing companies will lead to lower provider pay and worse patient outcomes (Devereaux, 2024). As this text goes to print, the final verdict on this is not in, but ongoing scrutiny of private equity and investor-owned health care is expected. Why? One in every five dollars in the United States is spent on health care, and private equity will likely continue to follow the money to attempt to acquire a larger health care footprint. Ponder how to make that work for you and the community you serve.

Long-term care. Private equity also has a growing stake in long-term care, with evidence suggesting increased cost and lower quality, specifically increases in emergency department visits, hospitalizations, and Medicare costs (Braun et al., 2021). Although long-term care has faced staffing and quality challenges for decades, the COVID-19 pandemic provided broad public information about the pervasive nature of these challenges. A *New York Times* article, for example, poignantly explicated the disconnection between quality ratings and actual quality in an article titled "Maggots, Rape and Yet Five Stars: How U.S. Ratings of Nursing Homes Mislead the Public" (Silver-Greenberg & Gebeloff, 2021).

Perhaps because of such public scrutiny, Centers for Medicare and Medicid Services (CMS) promulgated a staffing ratio rule for RNs and certified nursing assistants (CNAs) but not licensed practical nurses (LPNs). This has been highly controversial, as many nursing homes are staffed far below the ratios. Grabowski and Bowblis (2023) report that only 51% of nursing homes would be in legal compliance with the RN ratio and 28% with the CNA ratio, although the proportions vary widely by state. In Texas, for example, 72% of nursing homes would need to increase their staffing levels, while in Delaware and Oregon, just 2% of the settings would need to increase their ratios. These authors also note that the nursing home industry is concerned about mandated ratios, given the workforce shortages as well as the cost, while advocates argue that this rule doesn't go far enough. Despite nursing home industry complaints about such rules, private equity acquisition of nursing homes has continued to increase, suggesting there is ample financial room for such requirements. In November 2023, a new administrative rule required nursing homes that receive Medicare or Medicaid funds (which is nearly all) to disclose additional information on owners, operators, and management, including entities with financial control, a move that enjoyed rare bipartisan support.

In addition to federal efforts, some states have mandatory staffing ratios for skilled nursing facilities, and these may vary dramatically between states. Is yours one of them? (see https://theconsumervoice.org/uploads/files/issues/CV_StaffingReport_AppB_Chart.pdf). If so, what do you think of their adequacy?

Hospitals. Mensik (2023) notes that for the second year in a row, hospital CEOs' greatest concern is workforce challenges. Financial challenges had been the greatest concern in the previous 16 years, marking a decisive shift in the zeitgeist. Shortages of RNs, technicians, and therapists were the top concerns, along with burnout. Financial concerns included a related issue: increasing labor costs (American College of Healthcare Executives, 2024).

Public health. Perhaps because of widespread controversy about public health measures, the at one time seemingly uncontainable pandemic, and backlash against public health workers, the public health workforce shrunk by half in 5 years; nearly half of all employees in state and local public health agencies left between 2017 and 2021. Similar to hospitals, this exodus was higher in young and new public health workers, at 75% for those with short tenures or under age 35 (Leider et al., 2023). The National Advisory Council on Nurse Education and Practice 18th Report to the Secretary of Health and Human Services and the U.S. Congress notes that "the pandemic revealed a lack of investment in the public health infrastructure in general and public health nurses in particular" (National Advisory Council on Nurse Education and Practice, 2023, p. 8). Long-term corrective action is essential.

Mental health. The nation is facing an epidemic of substance abuse and mental health challenges, particularly among our youth and our older persons. Access to providers, however, lags far behind the need. Moreover, although evidence suggests that people who are not professionals can provide needed services and alleviate, for example, depression among new mothers (Surkan et al., 2024), the U.S. payment and delivery system is not designed to meet these needs and opportunities. Tele–mental health services have expanded, in part to meet demand but also in response to new payment rules. Need for mental health and substance abuse care still dramatically outstrips the number of available providers.

Taken as a whole, fresh approaches to health care workforce development are sorely needed. Martin et al. (2023) summarize the issue, with particular note of the additional challenges faced by new, less experienced nurses, stating:

> "High workloads and unprecedented levels of burnout during the COVID-19 pandemic have stressed the U.S. nursing workforce, particularly younger, less experienced RNs. These factors have already resulted in high levels of turnover with the potential for further declines. Coupled with disruptions to prelicensure nursing education and comparable declines among nursing support staff . . . significant policy interventions [are needed] to foster a more resilient and safe U.S. nursing workforce moving forward" (p. 4).

Buerhaus and colleagues (2023) have developed a comprehensive approach to create a stronger post-COVID nursing workforce. It includes inflows, the hospital work environment, outflows, and interactions among those domains (https://pubmed.ncbi.nlm.nih.gov/37458259/).

Moving Beyond Nurse—The Physician Workforce

A great deal of public attention has been directed toward a physician shortage, particularly in primary care. And, as previously mentioned, physicians are not choosing primary care as nurse practitioners instead do. Although many alarms have been raised about the impending physician shortage, Kerns and Willis (2020) offer a counterview. Writing for the *Harvard Business Review*, they argue that there isn't a shortage of physicians and, using data from a previous *JAMA* study, found that the nation has the capacity to treat nearly twice the U.S. population. They relate the disconnection between the data and the rhetoric to the following phenomenon:

- A mismatch between supply of physicians and demand for care due to misaligned distribution of physicians, for example, not enough physicians in impoverished areas and rural areas
- Inadequate insurance coverage, meaning a substantial number of people can't afford care
- Delivery based on providers' convenience, not patients' needs and realities, for example, no coverage on nights and weekends
- Care models that are inflexible, relying on MDs when PAs and NPs can "delivery much primary care at a lower cost and equality high quality" (para 9)
- MD unwillingness to take on patients with "unprofitable" payers (para 10), for example, Medicaid, Medicare, and other public payers, which they term "payer aversion" (para 10)
- Care delivery designs that result in inefficient use of physician labor

OTHER CONTEMPORARY ISSUES CHALLENGING THE HEALTH CARE WORKFORCE

Additional troubling events have marred nurses' sense of workplace efficacy and safety, specifically, the criminalization of errors and workplace violence. These will now be discussed in turn.

The Criminalization of Errors

RaDonda Vaught, a former registered nurse, was convicted of gross neglect and negligent homicide following a fatal medication error. Although system issues were clearly also at play, Vaught paid the price. She lost her license, was convicted of negligent homicide, and then sentenced to 3 years of supervised probation (Townley et al., 2022). Dickinson, writing for the American Bar Association, states: "While some may argue that criminal prosecution for causing patient harm is appropriate, in actuality the prosecution of well-meaning clinicians for inadvertent errors does not protect the public" (Dickinson, 2022, para 1). Instead, she states that the long-term consequences of "criminally prosecuting healthcare providers leads to more, not fewer, error[s] and patient harm" through the mechanism illustrated in Figure 14.1.

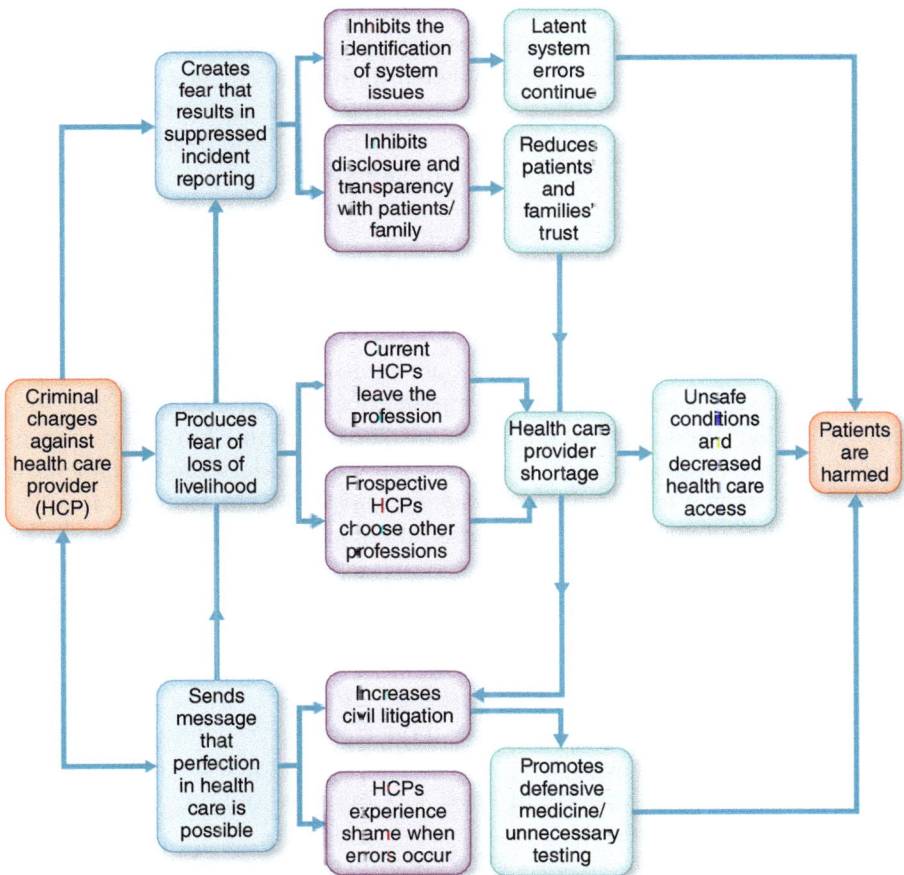

FIGURE 14.1: The long-term sequelae of criminally prosecuting health care providers lead to more, not fewer, errors and patient harm.
Source: Adapted from Dickinson, J. (2022, July 27). *The criminalization of human errors in healthcare*. American Bar Association. https://www.americanbar.org/groups/health_law/publications/aba_health_esource/2021-2022/july-2022/criminalization-of-human-errors-in-healthcare/

An emphasis on a culture of safety has been an aim of a wide array of organizations, ranging from the U.S. Agency for Health Research and Quality (n.d.) to the World Health Organization (WHO, 2019), with the latter noting that perceived high-risk industries, for example, nuclear and aviation, hold a far better safety record than health care. But it is not only patients who can be harmed in health care settings. Nurses and other health care workers are increasingly facing workplace violence.

Workplace Violence

In 1995, the Institute of Medicine (now called the National Academy of Medicine) published a report that called nursing a "uniquely hazardous occupation" (Pope et al., 1995, para 1). They listed four broad categories of hazards: chemical (e.g., toxic substance or radiation exposure), biological (e.g., infectious disease), physical (e.g., back injuries, shift work), and psychosocial (e.g., stress). Violence, of course, represents both a physical and psychological hazard. They identified high-risk settings for patient violence as mental health facilities, emergency departments, pediatric units, medical-surgical units, and long-term care facilities. They also stated that inexperienced workers and nursing students are at increased risk for assault (Pope et al., 1995). Fast-forward 30 years to the post–COVID-19 era; things have changed, but not for the better. Health care workplace violence has dramatically increased, so much so that it receives national media attention, for example, Yang and Mufson (2023) and Glatter and Papadakos (2023), to name but a few. Even as the author drafts this chapter, this harsh reality is underscored by breaking news of a person with a chainsaw attacking four health care workers in a Vermont hospital (Ashley, 2024) and a report that violence against nurses is at an all-time high (Carbajal, 2024).

The U.S. federal government identifies four categories of workplace violence (CDC, n.d.). These are criminal intent (e.g., a robber), customer/client (e.g., patient-on-nurse), worker-on-worker (e.g., physician-on-nurse), and personal relationship (e.g., a domestic issue that manifests in the workplace). Crimando (n.d.) adds another that may be more common in politically polarized times: ideological, for example, a pro-life zealot who targets a women's health facility or pro-Palestinian and pro-Israel supporters whose public demonstration escalates into violence.

The Bureau of Labor Statistics (2022) reports that nonfatal injuries and illnesses resulting in missed workdays was up an astonishing 291% in 2020. Huckenpahler and Gold (2022) note that the data on work-related violent fatalities are scarce, with 64 deaths reported in 2020. In that same year nearly 500,000 nonfatal assaults were reported, a figure near that of all other industries combined. These authors also note that workplace violence is underreported and that nurses are "far more susceptible to workplace violence than physicians" (p. 515).

Jones et al. also detail nurses' challenges with worker-on-worker violence, also termed horizontal violence, as follows:

> In addition to violence that healthcare workers may experience from patients, families, or visitors, horizontal violence is also prevalent in healthcare. Horizontal violence can be defined as hostile, aggressive, and harmful behaviors toward coworkers via attitudes, actions, words, or other behaviors such as bullying, incivility, or hazing. While this can occur across all healthcare professions, nurses are especially impacted, with one study estimating that 22% to 44% of nurses experience bullying at some point in their professional careers. (Jones et al., 2023, para 3)

Strategies to address workplace violence. Suggestions to address workplace violence abound. Virkstis et al. (2024), for example, have proposed a strategy that integrates digital advancements. Courses on active shooter preparedness abound. Oversight organizations offer parameters, for example, The Joint Commission promulgated Workplace Violence Prevention Standards, effective January 1, 2022 (2021).

Still others call for broad-scale policy-oriented solutions. Beeber et al., for example, call for comprehensive federal legislation, which has been introduced in each Congress since 2019 without action. They also underscore the critical nature of reporting, stating: "When nurses and nursing staff underreport acts of aggression, it sets the stage for that aggression to escalate. Within a female-identified nursing culture, values such as caring and conflict avoidance can perpetuate an unhelpful silence about the nature and frequency of aggressive acts. In some organizations, institutional management and policies may implicitly reinforce such silence and prevent the kind of essential collaboration that is necessary to reduce violence" (Beeber et al., 2023, para 16).

And what can you do? The first essential strategy is to always report and never tolerate workplace aggression or violence, regardless of who the perpetrator is. "What you permit, you promote. What you allow, you encourage" (the origin of the quote is uncertain). Push for a safe workplace culture and climate—safe for you, your colleagues, and your patients.

The Changing Nature of Work

The changing nature of work—robots, artificial intelligence (AI), virtual reality—has been explored for years, as just one example, West's 2018 book titled *The Future of Work: Robots, AI and Automation*. The introduction of large language learning models such as ChatGPT further accelerated the shift. Despite the resistance of some nurses, AI is here to stay. So, too, are new delivery models such as the acute care hospital at home described in Chapter 13. Besser and Jones (2020) offer a schematic of trends for the decade (Figure 14.2).

All of these will impact nurses' roles, opportunities, and challenges. How do you prepare?

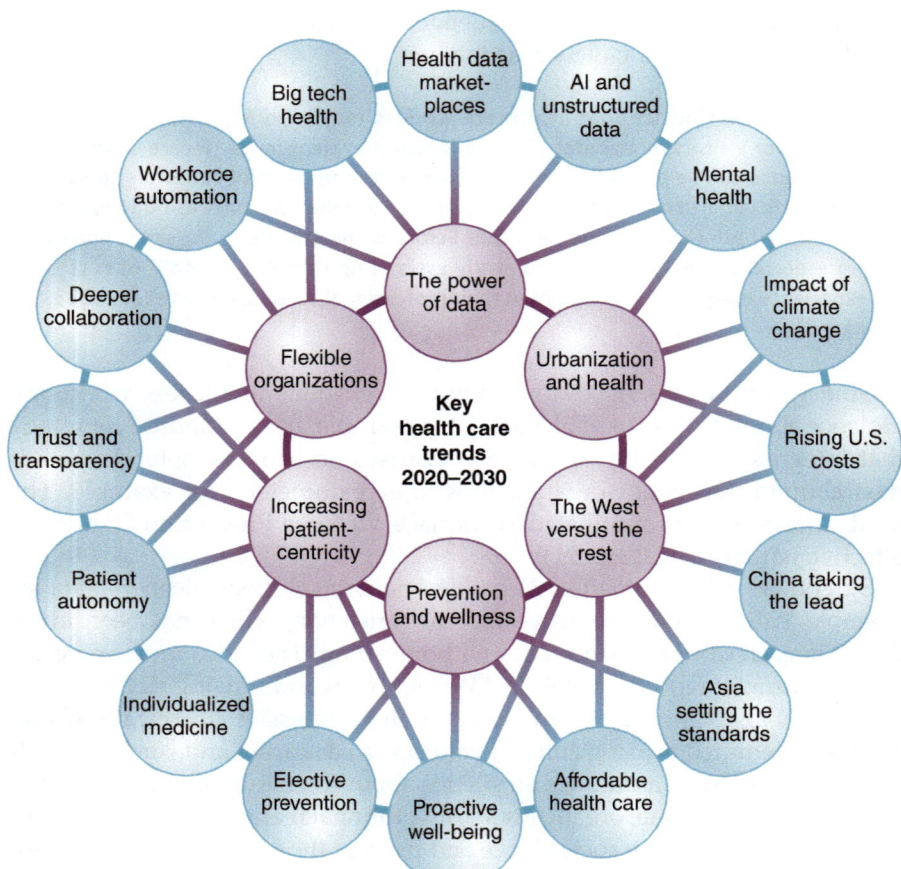

FIGURE 14.2: Key healthcare trends 2020 to 2030.
Source: Adapted from Besser, J. & Jones. T. (2020). *The future of health care*. Duke Corporate Education. https://www.dukece.com/insights/the-future-of-healthcare/

End-of-Chapter Resources

THOUGHT QUESTIONS

1. Now that you are aware of the health workforce challenges facing the United States and the spotty and irregular way health care is funded, what corrective actions do you suggest? Who are the winners and losers in the model you propose? How would it be funded? How do you get stakeholders and supporters on board?
2. Why has the nation invested far more money into educating physicians than nurses?

3. Who should fund the education of nurses? Defend your answer.
4. What is nurses' role in creating a comprehensive policy approach to ensure high quality in all skilled nursing facilities, places you would be happy to work as well as to live as a resident?
5. Define the following terms:
   Criminalization of errors
   Graduate medical education
   Horizontal violence
   Private equity

EXERCISES

1. Review the figures in this chapter and consider the content of the entire text. Develop a short-term (6 months) learning plan for yourself as well as a 2-year plan. Exchange notes with a colleague who has done the same. What did you miss? Be sure to revisit and revise the plan in 2 years.
2. Prepare a presentation on private equity, with an emphasis on its impact on health care access, safety, quality, and costs as well as innovation. Consider what the proper role of private equity in health care should be. Include parameters, boundaries, or limits, if any.

QUIZ

True and False

1. Graduate medical education, funded federally through Medicare, now offers similar funding for graduate nurse education.
2. Criminalization of medical errors is well established as a mechanism to decrease future errors.
3. There is substantial and consistent agreement that there is a physician shortage in the United States.
4. Incident to billing returns more revenue to practices than nurse practitioners billing under their own NPI.
5. The AMA and AANP both oppose incident to billing.
6. Nursing trade organizations are consistently among the highest-spending lobbying groups.
7. Private equity investment has a limited and uniformly positive reach in health care.
8. The United States has limited health care workplace violence through legislation.

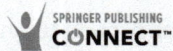

A robust set of instructor resources designed to supplement this text is located at http://connect.springerpub.com/content/book/978-0-8261-7236-5. Qualifying instructors may request access by emailing textbook@springerpub.com.

REFERENCES

Abdelfatah, R. (2022, May 19). *Before Roe: The physicians' crusade*. National Public Radio. https://www.npr.org/transcripts/1099795225

Agency for Health Research and Quality. (n.d.). *What is patient safety culture?* Author. https://www.ahrq.gov/sops/about/patient-safety-culture.html

Aiken, L. H., Lasater, K. B., Sloane, D. M., Pogue, C. A., Fitzpatrick Rosenbaum, K. E., Muir, K. J., McHugh, M. D., & US Clinician Wellbeing Study Consortium. (2023). Physician and nurse well-being and preferred interventions to address burnout in hospital practice: Factors associated with turnover, outcomes, and patient safety. *JAMA Health Forum, 4*(7), e231809. https://doi.org/10.1001/jamahealthforum.2023.1809

Aiken, L., Dahlerbruch, J., Todd, B., & Bai, G. (2018). The graduate nurse education demonstration—implications for Medicare policy. *New England Journal of Medicine, 378*(25), 2360–2363. https://doi.org/10.1056/NEJMp1800567

American College of Healthcare Executives. (2024). *Survey: Workforce challenges again cited by CEOs as top issue confrontiung hopsitals in 2023*.https://www.ache.org/about-ache/news-and-awards/news-releases/top-issues-confronting-hospitals-2023

American Medical Association. (2020). *Compendium of medical education*. https://www.ama-assn.org/education/improve-gme/compendium-graduate-medical-education-initiatives

American Medical Association. (2022). *Opposition to elimination of "incident-to" billing for non-physician practitioners*. Author. https://policysearch.ama-assn.org/policyfinder/detail/Opposition%20to%20Elimination%20of%20%E2%80%9CIncident-To%E2%80%9D%20Billing%20for%20Non-Physician%20Practitioners?uri=%2FAMADoc%2Fdirectives.xml-D-160.915.xml

Anderson, M., & Young, S. (2024, January 5). *Rise in healthcare worker strikes expected to continue in 2024*. Healthcare Brew. https://www.healthcare-brew.com/stories/2024/01/05/rise-in-healthcare-worker-strikes-expected-to-continue-in-2024

Arablouei, R., & Abdelfatah, R. (2022, June 6). *Abortion was once common practice in America: A small group of doctors changed that*. National Public Radio. https://www.npr.org/2022/06/06/1103372543/abortion-was-once-common-practice-in-america-a-small-group-of-doctors-changed-th

Ashley, M. (2024, April 1). *Man with chainsaw assaults Vermont hospital worker, destroys property: Police*. Becker's Hospital News. https://www.beckershospitalreview.com/legal-regulatory-issues/man-with-chainsaw-harms-vermont-hospital-workers-destroys-property.html

Bamdad, M. C., & Englesbe, M. J. (2020). Surgery and population health-redesigning surgical quality for greater impact. *JAMA Surgery, 155*(9), 799–800. https://doi.org/10.1001/jamasurg.2020.0808

Beeber, L., Delaney, K., Hauenstein, E., Iennaco, J., Schimmels, J., Sharp, D., & Shattell, M. (2023, August 23). Five urgent steps to address violence against nurses in the workplace. *Health Affairs Forefront*. https://doi.org/10.1377/forefront.20230822.174151

Besser, J., & Jones, T. (2020). *The future of health care*. Duke Corporate Education. https://www.dukece.com/insights/the-future-of-healthcare/

Blau, A., Sela, Y., & Grinberg, K. (2023). Public perceptions and attitudes on the image of nursing in the wake of COVID-19. *International Journal of Environmental Research and Public Health, 20*(6), 4717. https://doi.org/10.3390/ijerph20064717

Braun, R. T., Jung, H. Y., Casalino, L. P., Myslinski, Z., & Unruh, M. A. (2021). Association of private equity investment in US nursing homes with the quality and cost of care for long-stay residents. *JAMA Health Forum, 2*(11), e213817. https://doi.org/10.1001/jamahealthforum.2021 3817

Buerhaus, P., Fraher, E., Frogner, B., Buntin, M., O'Reilly-Jacob, M., & Clarke, S. (2023). Toward a stronger post-pandemic nursing workforce. *The New England Journal of Medicine, 389*(3), 200–202. https://doi.org/10.1056/NEJMp2303652

Bureau of Labor Statistics, U.S. Department of Labor. (2015, December). *Workforce growth in community-based care: Meeting the needs of an aging population*. https://www.bls.gov/opub/mlr/2016/article/workforce-growth-in-community-based-care.htm

Bureau of Labor Statistics, U.S. Department of Labor (2022, May). *The economics daily: Nonfatal injuries and illnesses resulting in days off work among nurses up 291 percent in 2020*. https://www.bls.gov/opub/ted/2022/nonfatal-injuries-and-illnesses-resulting-in-days-off-work-among-nurses-up-291-percent-in-2020.htm

Carbajal, E. (2024, April 6). *Violence against nurses hit an all-time high: 2 new reports*. Becker's Hospital Report. https://www.beckershospitalreview.com/nursing/violence-against-nurses-hits-all-time-high-2-new-reports

Centers for Disease Control and Prevention. (n.d.). *Types of workplace violence*. The National Institute for Occupational Safety and Health. https://wwwn.cdc.gov/WPVHC/Nurses/Course/Slide/Unit1_5

Centers for Medicare and Medicaid Services. (n.d.). *Medicare benefit policy manuel*. Author. https://www.cms.gov/Regulations-and-Guidance/Guidance/Manuals/downloads/bp102c15.pdf

Chandra, A., Khullar, D., & Wilensky, G. (2014). The economics of graduate medical education. *New England Journal of Medicine, 370*(25), 2357–2360. https://doi.org/10.1056/NEJMp1402468

Congressional Research Service. (2024). *Medicare graduate medical education, 2024*. https://crsreports.congress.gov/product/pdf/IF/IF12583

Crimando, S. (n.d.). *Five types of workplace violence incidents*. Everbridge. https://www.everbridge.com/blog/five-types-workplace-violence/

Devereaux, M. (2024, March 27). *How private equity-backed staffing companies impact providers*. Modern Healthcare. https://www.modernhealthcare.com/providers/private-equity-staffing-firms-hospitals?utm_source=modern-healthcare-alert&utm_medium=email&utm_campaign=20240327&utm_content=hero-readmore

Dickinson, J. (2022, July 27). *The criminalization of human errors in healthcare*. American Bar Association. https://www.americanbar.org/groups/health_law/publications/aba_health_esource/2021-2022/july-2022/criminalization-of-human-errors-in-healthcare/

Ervin, S. (2023). History of nursing education in the United States. In S. Stimac Deboor (Ed.), *Keating's curriculum development and evaluation in nursing education* (5th ed.). Springer Publishing.

Fussell, P. (1983). *Class: A guide through the American status system.* Touchstone Press.

Glatter, R. & Papadakos, P. (2023). T*he epidemic of violence in American hospitals.* Time. https://time.com/6337450/the-epidemic-of-violence-in-american-hospitals/

Glerean, N., Hupli, M., Talman, K., & Haavisto, E. (2017). Young peoples' perceptions of the nursing profession: An integrative review. *Nurse Education Today, 57,* 95–102. https://doi.org/10.1016/j.nedt.2017.07.008

Government Accounting Office. (2019). *Health care workforce: Views on expanding Medicare Graduate Medical Education funding to nurse practitioners and physician assistant.* Author. https://www.gao.gov/products/gao-20-162

Grabowski, D. C., & Bowblis, J. R. (2023). Minimum-staffing rules for U.S. nursing homes: Opportunities and challenges. *The New England Journal of Medicine, 389*(18), 1637–1640. https://doi.org/10.1056/NEJMp2310544

Grischkan, J., Friednman, A., & Chandra, A. (2020). Moving the financing of graduate medical education into the 21st century. *Journal of the American Medical Association, 324*(11), 1035–1036. https://doi.org/10.1001/jama.2020.15480

Guy, M., Hughes, K. A., & Ferris-Day, P. (2022). Lack of awareness of nursing as a career choice for men: A qualitative descriptive study. *Journal of Advanced Nursing, 78*(12), 4190–4198. https://doi.org/10.1111/jan.15402

Hollowell, A. (2023, Mary 1). *85% of nurse plan to leave hospital roles 1 year from now: Survey.* Becker's Hospital News. https://www.beckershospitalreview.com/nursing/85-of-nurses-plan-to-leave-hospital-roles-1-year-from-now-survey.html

Hoff, K., Van Egdom, D., Napolitano, C., Hanna, A., & Rounds, J. (2022). Dream jobs and employment realities: How adolescents' career aspirations compare to labor demands and automation risks. *Journal of Career Assessment, 30*(1), 134–156. https://doi.org/10.1177/10690727211026183

Huckenpahler, A. L., & Gold, J. A. (2022). Risky business: Violence in healthcare. *Missouri Medicine, 119*(6), 514–518. https://www.ncbi.nlm.nih.gov/pmc/articles/PMC9762232/

Im, A., & Koh, C. K. (2023). Effect of COVID-19 Frontline nurses' profession perception on their intention to stay: The mediating role of job satisfaction. *SAGE Open Nursing, 9,* 23779608231186043. https://doi.org/10.1177/23779608231186043

Johnson, R. (2017). A movement for change: Horatio Robinson Storer and physician's crusade against abortion. *James Madison Undergraduate Research Journal, 4*(1), 13–23. https://commons.lib.jmu.edu/jmurj/vol4/iss1/2

Jones, C., Sousane, Z., & Mossburg, S. (2023, October 31). *Addressing workplace violence and creating a safer workplace.* Patient Safety Network, AHRQ. https://psnet.ahrq.gov/perspective/addressing-workplace-violence-and-creating-safer-workplace

Kannan, S., Bruch, J. D., & Song, Z. (2023). Changes in hospital adverse events and patient outcomes associated with private equity acquisition. *Journal of the American Medical Association, 330*(24), 2365–2375. https://doi.org/10.1001/jama.2023.23147

Kayser, A. (2024, March 13). *85% of hospital nurses said they'd quite by 2024. Did they?* https://www.beckershospitalreview.com/workforce/85-of-hospital-nurses-said-theyd-quit-by-2024-did-they.html

Kearns, E., Khurshid, Z., Anjara, S., De Brún, A., Rowan, B., & McAuliffe, E. (2021). P92 Power dynamics in healthcare teams—a barrier to team effectiveness and patient safety: A systematic review. *BJS Open, 5*(Suppl. 1), zrab032.091. https://doi.org/10.1093/bjsopen/zrab032.091

Kerns, C., & Willis, D. (2020, March 16). *The problem with U.S. health care isn't a shortage of doctors.* Harvard Business Review. https://hbr.org/2020/03/the-problem-with-u-s-health-care-isnt-a-shortage-of-doctors

Kim, D. R., & Lee, G. R. (2023). Keyword network analysis of changes in the image of nurses pre- and post-COVID-19 in the media environment. *Journal of Clinical Nursing, 32*(21–22), 7883–7890. https://doi.org/10.1111/jocn.16860

Kreider, A. R., & Werner, R. M. (2023). The home care workforce has not kept pace with growth in home and community-based services. *Health affairs (Project Hope), 42*(5), 650–657. https://doi.org/10.1377/hlthaff.2022.01351

Leider, J. P., Castrucci, B. C., Robins, M., Hare Bork, R., Fraser, M. R., Savoia, E., Piltch-Loeb, R., & Koh, H. K. (2023). The exodus of state and local public health employees: Separations started before and continued throughout COVID-19. *Health affairs (Project Hope), 42*(3), 338–348. https://doi.org/10.1377/hlthaff.2022.01251

Martin, B., Kaminski-Ozturk, N., O'Hara, C., & Smiley, R. (2023). Examining the impact of the COVID-19 pandemic on burnout and stress among U.S. nurses. *Journal of Nursing Regulation, 14*(1), 4–12. https://doi.org/10.1016/S2155-8256(23)00063-7

Medicare Payment Advisory Commission. (2019, June). *Report to congress: Medicare and the payment delivery system.* https://www.medpac.gov/document/http-www-medpac-gov-docs-default-source-reports-jun19_medpac_reporttocongress_sec-pdf/

Medicare Payment Advisory Commission. (2021, June) *Report to congress: Medicare and the health care delivery system.* https://www.medpac.gov/wp-content/uploads/import_data/scrape_files/docs/default-source/reports/jun21_medpac_report_to_congress_sec.pdf

Mensik, H. (2023, February 13). *Workforce challenges top concern for hospital CEPs for a second year in a row, survey finds.* Healthcaredive. https://www.healthcaredive.com/news/hospital-CEOs-staffing-workforce-top-concern-2023/642615/

Mohammed, S., Peter, E., Killackey, T., & Maciver, J. (2021). The "nurse as hero" discourse in the COVID-19 pandemic: A poststructural discourse analysis. *International Journal of Nursing Studies, 117*, 103887. https://doi.org/10.1016/j.ijnurstu.2021.103887

Morin, K. H., & Baptiste, D. (2020). Nurses as heroes, warriors and political activists. *Journal of Clinical Nursing, 29*(15–16), 2733. https://doi.org/10.1111/jocn.15353

Munday, R. (2023). *Male nurse statistics: A look at the numbers. Nurse Journal.* https://nursejournal.org/articles/male-nurse-statistics/

National Advisory Council on Nurse Education and Practice. (2023, January). *Preparing the nursing workforce for future public health challenges.* Author. https://www.hrsa.gov/sites/default/files/hrsa/advisory-committees/nursing/reports/nacnep-18th-report.pdf

National Council of State Legislatures. (2024, January 9). *Graduate medical education.* Author. https://www.ncsl.org/health/graduate-medical-education-funding

Neumbe, I. M., Ssenyonga, L., Soita, D. J., Iramiot, J. S., & Nekaka, R. (2023). Attitudes and perceptions of undergraduate nursing students towards the nursing profession. *PloS One, 18*(7), e0280700. https://doi.org/10.1371/journal.pone.0280700

Open Secrets. (2024, February 21). *Federal lobbying*. Author. https://www.opensecrets.org/federal-lobbying/clients/summary?id=D000000173

Papathanasiou, I., Tzenetidis, V., Tsaras, K., Zyga, S., & Malliarou, M. (2024). Missed nursing care; prioritizing the patient's needs: An umbrella review. *Healthcare (Basel, Switzerland)*, *12*(2), 224. https://doi.org/10.3390/healthcare12020224

Patel, S. Y., Huskamp, H. A., Frakt, A. B., Auerbach, D. I., Neprash, H. T., Barnett, M. L., James, H. O., & Mehrotra, A. (2022). Frequency of indirect billing to Medicare for nurse practitioner and physician assistant office visits. *Health Affairs (Project Hope)*, *41*(6), 805–813. https://doi.org/10.1377/hlthaff.2021.01968

Patel, S. Y., Auerbach, D., Huskamp, H. A., Frakt, A., Neprash, H., Barnett, M. L., James, H. O., Smith, L. B., & Mehrotra, A. (2023). Provision of evaluation and management visits by nurse practitioners and physician assistants in the USA from 2013 to 2019: Cross-sectional time series study. *BMJ (Clinical Research Ed.)*, *382*, e073933. https://doi.org/10.1136/bmj-2022-073933

Pope, A. M., Snyder, M. A., & Mood, L. H. (Eds.). (1995). *Nursing health, & environment: Strengthening the relationship to improve the public's health*. National Academies Press (US). https://www.ncbi.nlm.nih.gov/books/NBK232400/

Porat-Dahlerbruch, J., Aiken, L. H., Todd, B., Cunningham, R., Brom, H., Peele, M. E., & McHugh, M. D. (2022). Policy evaluation of the Affordable Care Act graduate nurse education demonstration. *Health Affairs (Project Hope)*, *41*(1), 86–95. https://doi.org/10.1377/hlthaff.2021.01328

Pulcini, J., & Rambur, B. (2022). Travel nursing and the demise of the virtue-script: Steps to a new beginning. *Policy, Politics & Nursing Practice*, *23*(4), 211–214. https://doi.org/10.1177/15271544221130623

Reynold, S. (2024, January 23). *Infections and falls increased in private equity-owned hospitals*. NIH Research Matters. https://www.nih.gov/news-events/nih-research-matters/infections-falls-increased-private-equity-owned-hospitals

Royce, T. (2021). Financing of US graduate medical education. *Journal of the American Medical Association*, *325*(6), 585–586. https://doi.org/10.1001/jama.2020.23979

Robert Wood Johnson Foundation. (n.d.). *Why be a nurse?* Author. https://nursing.jnj.com/why-be-a-nurse

Robertson, M. (2021, August 25). *Top 20 healthcare lobbyists by 2021 spending through June*. Modern Healthcare. https://www.beckershospitalreview.com/finance/top-20-healthcare-lobbyists-by-2021-spending-through-june.html

Rutledge, D., Douville, S., & Winokur, E. (2022). Chronic fatigue predicts hospital nurse turnover intentions. *The Journal of Nursing Administration*, *52*(4), 241–247. https://doi.org/10.1097/NNA.0000000000001139

Sanchez, M. (2023, April 7). *Nearly 40% of Michigan hospital nurses want to quit within a year: Survey*. Modern Healthcare. https://www.modernhealthcare.com/nursing/michigan-hospital-nurses-want-quit-survey

Scruth, E., Martinez, V., & Worth, K. (2024). Private equity ownership in healthcare: Quality and patient safety are in jeopardy. *Clinical Nurse Specialist* 38(3):p 116-118, 5/6 2024. https://doi.org.10.1097/NUR.0000000000000814

Silver-Greenberg, J., & Gebeloff, R. (2021, August 4). *Maggots, rape and yet five stars: How U.S. ratings of nursing homes mislead the public*. New York Times. https://www.nytimes.com/2021/03/13/business/nursing-homes-ratings-medicare-covid.html

Stemmer, R., Bassi, E., Ezra, S., Harvey, C., Jojo, N., Meyer, G., Özsaban, A., Paterson, C., Shifaza, F., Turner, M. B., & Bail, K. (2022). A systematic review: Unfinished nursing care and the impact on the nurse outcomes of job satisfaction, burnout, intention-to-leave and turnover. *Journal of Advanced Nursing, 78*(8). 2290–2303. https://doi.org/10.1111/jan.15286

Surkan, P. J., Malik, A., Perin, J., Najia, A., Rowther, A., Zaidi, A., & Rahman, A. (2024). Anxiety-focused cognitive behavioral therapy delivered by nonspecialists to prevent postnatal depression: A randomized, phase 3 trial. *Nature Medicine, 30*, 675–682. https://doi.org/10.1038/s41591-024-02809-x

Taylor-Clark, T. M., Swiger, P. A., Anusiewicz, C. V., Loan, L. A., Olds, D. M., Breckenridge-Sproat, S. T., Raju, D., & Patrician, P. A. (2022). Identifying potentially preventable reasons nurses intend to leave a job. *The Journal of Nursing Administration, 52*(2), 73–80. https://doi.org/10.1097/NNA.0000000000001106

The Joint Commission. (2021, June 18). *Workplace violence prevention standards.* Author. https://www.jointcommission.org/-/media/tjc/documents/standards/r3-reports/wpvp-r3-30_revised_06302021.pdf

Terry, K. (2024, May 8). *Taming the private equity beast by shifting its focus to value-based care.* Health Affairs Forefront. https://www.healthaffairs.org/do/10.1377/foregront.20240506.635591/

Townley, J. N., Pogue, C. A., & McHugh, M. D. (2022). Criminal prosecution of clinician errors: A setback to the progress toward safe hospital work environments. *Journal of Hospital Medicine, 17*(10), 850–853. https://doi.org/10.1002/jhm.12952

Uysal, N., & Demirdağ, H. (2022). The image of nursing perceived by the society in the COVID-19 pandemic: A cross-sectional study. *Nursing Forum, 57*(6), 1339–1345. https://doi.org/10.1111/nuf.12813

Virkstis, K., Balá, L., Taylor, J., & Forester, R. (2024). The AWARE Framework: A technology-driven approach to creating a safer care environment. *The Journal of Nursing Administration, 54*(3), 139–141. https://doi.org/10.1097/NNA.0000000000001397

Vollers, A. C. (2024, January 31). *Private equity's growing footprint in home health care draws scrutiny.* Stateline. https://stateline.org/2024/01/31/private-equitys-growing-footprint-in-home-health-care-draws-scrutiny/

Volpe, K. D. (2022, September 8). *Medicare indirect billing: NPs and PAs speak out.* Clinical Advisor. https://www.clinicaladvisor.com/home/topics/practice-management-information-center/medicare-indirect-billing-nps-pas-speak-out/

Wang, Y., & Anderson, G. (2022). Hospital resource allocation decisions when market prices exceed Medicare prices. *Health Services Research, 57*(2), 237–247. https://doi.org/10.1111/1475-6773.13914

Whelan, J. (May 31, 2012). When the business of nursing was the nursing business: The private duty registry system, 1900–1940. *The Online Journal of Issues in Nursing, 17*(2), 6. https://doi.org/10.3912/OJIN.Vol17No02Man06

World Health Organization. (2019, March 9). *Patient safety.* Author. https://www.who.int/news-room/facts-in-pictures/detail/patient-safety

Yakusheva, O., & Rmbur, B. (2023, May 30). *How the hospital reimbursement model harms nurses and what to do about it.* Health Affairs Forefront. https://www.healthaffairs.org/content/forefront/hospital-reimbursement-model-harms-nursing-quality-and-do

Yang, J., & Mufson, C. (2023, September 23). *What's behind an alarming rise in violent incidents in health care facilities?* PBS Newshour. https://www.pbs.org/newshour/show/whats-behind-an-alarming-rise-in-violent-incidents-in-health-care-facilities

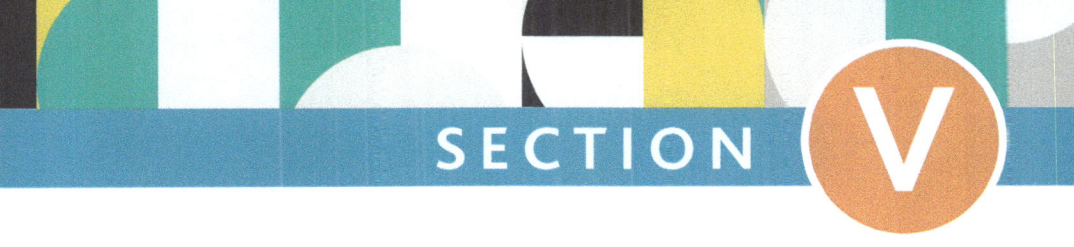

Epilogue

Epilogue

CHAPTER 15

Reflections on Living and Leading in a Changing Nursing World

TELL ME ONE MORE TIME: WHAT DOES ALL THIS FINANCING, ECONOMICS, AND POLICY HAVE TO DO WITH NURSING?

Throughout this text, we have navigated complex terrain that at one time was the domain of physicians, financial officers, chief executive officers, and a very few nurse leaders and graduate students in nursing. We have explored policy and boardrooms, individual and population ethics, and health and payment reform, to name but a few tours on our journey to an expanded sense of professional self. This stretch can create an ache, yet it is necessary. The image of what it means to be a nurse is being rewritten because society needs what nurses know, yet too often what nurses know has been bound by stereotypical roles and images.

The very metaphor of nursing is that of a personal relationship, with one meaning of the term literally referring to a mother nourishing a child. These personal, intimate images create a confining narrative of what it means to be a nurse in our contemporary culture. A focus on care of an individual patient is valuable in some instances, but it is not enough to fully serve society. More is needed of nurses, of each and every one of us. Society needs nursing intelligence, and finance, economics, and policy are tools with particular impact when in the hands of a nurse. A traditional story illustrates this well.

> *Imagine you are sitting on a beach, sunning. You hear shouts from the water and realize that someone has gone under! Hero that you are, you leap into the water, pull the person ashore, and revive the person to then receive eternal thanks. "Ah, what a good day," you muse, "I saved a life." Tired, you fall asleep on the shore.*
>
> *But wait, could it be? Now you are startled to hear not one, but two shouts! Drained but undaunted, you hold one person in each arm as you swim with your feet and torso. You perform serial resuscitation, and miraculously, both are fine, thanking you profusely.*
>
> *Exhausted but pleased with your superhuman day's work, you fall asleep, only to hear shouts from the water yet again. Now there are four people in trouble! So weary, but always a nurse of ingenuity, you leap into the water, make a human chain of each of the individuals, pull them to shore, and again resuscitate*

> *all four. Wow! What a day! Now, completely spent, you are lulled asleep in the warm summer sun, content in your virtue and skill.*
>
> *But no! You are stunned to hear a cacophony of shouts and splashes, and look to see the enormous bay full of people, all drowning, all screaming for help. Appalled, you know you will not be able to help them and will certainly drown trying. You instead decide a new approach is needed. "That's it," you declare. "I'm going upstream to see why people fall into the water in the first place."*

Health policy is about going upstream. And just like backhoes and forklifts in river engineering, finance and economics are simple tools that can help you do complex things. You can redesign the health care river and keep people from falling in.

It can feel very gratifying to care for individual patients, one by one. It can feel heroic. Indeed, it is why many of us became nurses. At the same time, there are only so many lives we can touch one by one. Policy is one tool to shape the top of the river, change the course, so people do not fall in. And finance and policy are key tools in the engineering redesign. It feels virtuous and certain to help individuals one by one, just like the nurse in the beach scenario. The work of policy and politics can feel less immediately gratifying—we cannot even see the lives we are touching—and less staunchly certain. It requires speaking up and speaking out, even when we cannot be sure that our policy change will be the right one. It requires a tolerance for ambiguity.

HOW TO RETAIN AND EXPAND ON WHAT YOU HAVE LEARNED

Now that you have the basics down, you have the canvas to create a deep and rich professional landscape. There is no better way to continue to grow than by applying these materials in everyday life. Board or political experience is one way, but so, also, is teaching. By teaching others, you, yourself, will also learn. Questions from others cause us to pause and question ourselves, and in so doing, we grow. As Einstein famously stated, "If you can't explain it simply, you don't understand it well enough." Struggling to make things clear to others will help you to clarify them for yourself. Mentoring others is also a great way to learn. Let us imagine each of us hanging on to a steady hand above us, while we simultaneously provide a steady hand to another.

Some high-quality journals are dedicated to health policy, for example, *Health Affairs, Health Affairs Forefront,* and *JAMA Health Forum.* They are written in a style that is understandable to an interdisciplinary audience. There are also nursing journals with a policy and economic focus, for example, *Policy, Politics and Nursing Practice; Nursing Economics;* and *Nursing Outlook.* Major U.S. newspapers regularly highlight health, health care, and health policy.

Consistent readership can help keep you abreast of thoughts and concerns your patients might be having.

Another important vehicle for staying current is your professional nursing organization. There are many nursing groups in which you might find meaningful membership. The American Nurses Association and its local state chapters typically also have student groups for undergraduates, and state associations are always on the lookout for nursing talent. This is a good place to begin practicing your leadership skills. There are also specialty organizations that may be of particular interest to the practicing nurse. Take the time to check out the options, read their mission statements, and then join those that feel like the best fit for you. And yes, joining costs money. That contribution to health, health care, and nursing is part of the obligation of being a professional. Even if you do not always have time to be involved directly, your financial support of these groups can help ensure that your cause is articulated in policy and political arenas.

Finally, lifelong learning is an essential element of the previously discussed ethical principle of role fidelity. To be faithful to the role of the nurse—and the responsibility we have to the public—we must continue to grow and learn. Usually, this is a bit uncomfortable because it feels safer to stay in the solid spot of what we know well, or think we know well, rather than alighting on the shifting ground of new learning. It can also be difficult to learn new things because they conflict with what we think we already knew. The idea that *learning is fun* just does not always hold. Learning is a struggle; *knowing is fun*. To be the nurse who can see new ways of doing things and enact change: *This* is fun. To midwife a sound policy change that impacts hundreds, thousands, or even millions of people is delicate but gratifying work: Having an impact is fun! Both formal education in graduate school and informal education through conferences and webinars are part of lifelong learning. Ongoing, continuous learning is part of your future.

So, what will health care look like in a year? A decade? A century? This is not fully clear, but one thing is clear. It will not look as it is today, and you can—and should—be part of the transformative process.

CHAPTER 16

Quiz Answers

Chapter 1

1. F
2. T
3. F
4. F
5. F
6. T
7. F
8. F
9. T
10. T
11. D
12. A*
13. D
14. B
15. A

Chapter 2

1. F
2. F
3. F
4. T
5. T
6. T
7. T
8. T
9. T
10. F
11. B
12. B
13. D
14. C: Note regarding choice B, services other than nursing care were unbundled, which is further discussed in Chapter 14
15. A* (As noted in * above)
16. 3
17. D

Chapter 3

1. F
2. F (They must select a silver plan)
3. T
4. F
5. F
6. D
7. D
8. A, C, D—Note, the first part of B is true, but not the latter. Children can stay on their parent's health insurance until age 26, even if they are married and no longer listed as dependents on their parent's income tax returns.
9. A
10. D

---

*Various strategies are used to finance the different parts of Medicare, that is, Medicare Part A, Medicare Part B, Medicare Part C (Medicare Advantage), and Medicare Part D. Review Appendix A.

337

Chapter 4

1. F
2. F
3. T
4. T
5. F
6. T
7. T
8. T
9. T
10. T
11. B
12. C
13. C
14. C
15. C
16. D
17. D

Chapter 5

1. T
2. T
3. T
4. F
5. T
6. T
7. F
8. F—In some cases it MAY be true for some individuals with complex chronic conditions.
9. T
10. F
11. C
12. A
13. A
14. C
15. C
16. C

Chapter 6

1. T
2. T
3. F
4. F
5. F—That is the intention; however, it is not always accomplished.
6. F
7. T
8. F
9. T
10. T
11. A
12. C
13. B
14. A
15. C

Chapter 7

1. F—It is provided to those who treat a defined proportion of Medicare and/or Medicaid patients.
2. T
3. T
4. T
5. T
6. T
7. F
8. T
9. A
10. D
11. C
12. C
13. A

Chapter 8

1. F
2. F
3. T
4. F
5. T
6. T
7. T
8. T
9. F
10. T
11. C
12. C
13. B
14. B
15. A

Chapter 9

1. T
2. T
3. F
4. T
5. T
6. F
7. T
8. T
9. T
10. F
11. A
12. B
13. C
14. A
15. B

Chapter 10
1. F
2. F
3. T
4. F
5. T
6. T
7. F
8. F
9. F
10. F
11. C
12. A
13. D
14. C
15. C

Chapter 11
1. T
2. F
3. T
4. F
5. T
6. T
7. T
8. F
9. T
10. T
11. C
12. D
13. B
14. B
15. C

Chapter 12
1. F
2. F
3. F
4. F
5. T
6. F
7. T
8. F
9. F
10. T
11. C
12. D
13. C
14. C

Chapter 13

1. F
2. F
3. T
4. T
5. T
6. T

Chapter 14

1. F
2. F
3. F
4. T
5. F
6. F
7. F
8. F

Appendix A: Medicare Eligibility

1. Part A—Hospital
   A. Premium free eligibility
      (1) Age 65 or older
         (a) Individual or spouse worked and paid Medicare taxes for at least 10 years
      (2) Under 65
         (a) Eligible for or are receiving Social Security or Railroad benefits
         (b) Entitled to Social Security or Rail Road Retirement Board disability for at least 24 months
         (c) Have amyotrophic lateral sclerosis (ALS) diagnosis, with eligibility beginning the first month of disability benefits
         (d) End-stage renal disease (ESRD)—kidney dialysis or kidney transplant patient
   B. If not eligible for premium free, may be able to purchase if:
      (a) A U.S. citizen
      (b) A U.S. permanent resident
2. Part B (Medical)—Not premium free. Cost deducted monthly from:
   A. Social Security check
   B. Railroad Retirement check
   C. Civil Service Retirement check
   D. Or direct billed every quarter for those who do not receive the previous benefits
3. Part C—Medicare Advantage (MA) Plans
   A. Replaces Part A and B for those who choose it
   B. Must cover all services covered by original Medicare A and B with the exception of hospice, which is covered by Part A
   C. Until 2021, excluded those with ESRD
   D. Includes a variety of plan types:
      (1) Health maintenance organization (HMO) plans
      (2) Preferred provider organization (PFO) plans
      (3) Private fee-for service plans
      (4) Special needs plans
      (5) Health maintenance organization (HMO) point-of-service plans
      (6) Medical savings account plans
4. Part D—Prescription drug coverage
   A. Available to all with Medicare, regardless of mechanism (i.e., traditional Part A and B or C)
   B. Some forms of Medicare Advantage such as HMO or PPO plans may offer preferable prescription drug coverage

C. Other forms of coverage that may be preferable to Part D for those who are eligible:
   (1) Federal Employees Health Benefits Program
   (2) Veterans Benefits
   (3) TRICARE (military health benefits)
   (4) Indian Health Services

NOTE: Traditional Medicare requires deductibles. It does not provide "first dollar coverage." Medicare Part B includes co-insurance of 20% after the deductible has been met. There is also no maximum out of pocket for either Part A or B; therefore, many on traditional Medicare obtain a supplemental policy from a commercial insurance company. These plans are often termed Medigap plans.

Adapted from:

Centers for Medicare & Medicaid Services. *Original Medicare (Part A and B) eligibility and enrollment.* https://www.cms.gov/medicare/enrollment-renewal/health-plans/original-part-a-b

Medicare.gov. *Drug coverage (Part D).* https://www.medicare.gov/drug-coverage-part-d

Medicare.gov. *Compare original Medicare & Medicare advantage.* https://www.medicare.gov/basics/get-started-with-medicare/get-more-coverage/your-coverage-options/compare-original-medicare-medicare-advantage

Appendix B: Key Concepts in Health Finance, Economics, Policy, and Ethics: Level Setting Pre-Survey

Please answer the following questions by providing the response that best describes your current situation. Note: Don't worry if you don't know too much about many of these. That is what you are here to learn! We just want to ensure that we are giving you new or renewed knowledge, not repeating what you already know.

1. I understand actuarial value and the "metal levels" in the health insurance exchange well enough that I could describe it to my peers. *True/False/Unsure*
2. I understand how health care markets differ from classic free markets and could detail the basic tenets of health care economics. *True/False/Unsure*
3. I understand the difference between national health insurance and "socialized medicine." *True/False/Unsure*
4. I am familiar with the basic tenets as well as limitations of classical health care ethics and ethical decision frameworks such as deontology, Rawls's theory of justice, virtue ethics, utilitarianism, feminist ethics, etc. *True/False/Unsure*
5. I understand how a bill becomes a law. *True/False/Unsure*
6. I know how to follow a bill through the legislative process. *True/False/Unsure*
7. I have testified before a legislative committee. *True/False/Unsure*
8. I understand the reach and limits of administrative rules. *True/False/Unsure*
9. I understand the reach and limits of executive orders. *True/False/Unsure*
10. I have written to policy makers. *True/False/Unsure*
11. I have called or emailed policy makers. *True/False/Unsure*
12. I vote. *True/False*
13. Please identify any of the following that you could describe in detail to a colleague:
    a. Direct democracy
    b. Cost shifting
    c. Cost sharing
    d. Moral hazard
    e. Payer mix
    f. Differences between bad debt and charity care

g. Impact of bad debt and charity care on commercial insurance prices
h. Bond covenants
i. Significance of days cash on hand
j. Telehealth payment changes
k. How commercial insurance rates are determined
l. Types of hospitals
m. Ways hospitals are reimbursed
n. History of Medicare
o. Types of Medicare, including inclusion categories
p. Funding of Medicare
q. Medicaid—Similarities and differences across states
r. Nature and impact of Medicaid 1115 and 1915 waivers
s. Certificate of Need legislation
t. Antitrust law's relationship to health care mergers and acquisitions
u. Impact of health care mergers and acquisitions on health care prices and costs
v. Affordable Care Act strategies toward universal insurance coverage
w. Affordable Care Act payment innovations
x. Affordable Care Act transparency initiatives
y. Fee-for-service reimbursement
z. Value-based care
aa. Financial risk sharing
ba. Financial risk bearing
ca. Patient-centered medical homes
da. Bundled payments
ea. Medicare Access and CHIPS Reauthorization Act (MACRA) and Merit-based Incentive Payment System (MIPS)
fa. Accountable care organizations

List policy issues that you are particularly interested in learning more about.*

_____

_____

_____

_____

Please list areas of expertise or any experience in health care finance, economics, policy, ethics, and organizational leadership you can share with the class. Thank you!

_____

_____

_____

_____

*Note: In the author's experience, some graduate students are interested in learning more about a micro issue related to their clinical practice. Although this may be of interest to them, it doesn't help broaden their focus. Occasionally, I have given students the opportunity to explore these areas in an assignment of their choosing.

Students may also be muddled on the levels of policy: organizational, state, federal, and international. Clarifying the "levers" by which to impact policy at the different levels is helpful.

Appendix C: The Policy Analysis Process

Will Durant, in his 1926 classic *The Story of Philosophy*, which launched Simon & Schuster Publishing Company, defines philosophy as inclusive of five fields of study and discourse. These are logic, aesthetics, ethics, politics, and metaphysics. He further states: "*Politics* is the study of ideal social organization (it is not, as one might suppose, the art and science of capturing and keeping of office)" (1961 edition, p. xxvii, italics and parentheses in the original). Much media attention and public rhetoric swirl around the latter, the art and science of capturing and keeping of office, and nurses may—and arguably should—be involved in political campaigns in meaningful and important ways. This is a strategy toward the higher-order responsibility, the creation of a just and salubrious society. This responsibility requires further skills inclusive of policy analysis.

Specifically, the study and creation of the ideal social organization is well aligned with nurses' social contract. (Nurses' social contract was outlined in the opening of this text in *A Note From the Author*.) Nursing programs typically strive to ensure that their students engage in health policy and advocate for their patients. Yet this first requires that students understand the details of the issue. Nuanced understanding can be complicated, and the right path is often obscured by interacting details, unexpected effects, and strident, polarized rhetoric. Do you, for example, support the 1:3 insurance rating bands that create moderately lower insurance cost for those approaching Medicare age but are not yet eligible? Or, instead, do you support 1:5 insurance rating bands that create moderately lower insurance costs for younger people? In the same vein, do you support offering health services without patient cost sharing ("first dollar coverage") to enhance access to care? Or are you instead concerned about moral hazard, with resulting increased use of unnecessary care and explosive health care costs that shackle future generations? How do you assess if a proposed policy action is a good idea, or if negative unintended consequences outweigh any possible good? Finally, if you deem an idea to be sound, is it a *good idea* or a *good idea that should become law*? Regarding the latter, what are the cost and impact of regulation? Who will regulate and how? What are the consequences?

Fortunately, there are tools to aid this discernment: the policy analysis process. There are many approaches, but perhaps one of the most accessible is offered by the Centers for Disease Control and Prevention (CDC, n.d.). Although the CDC model names public health, it is useful for other policy considerations, including health policy and health care policy. Take a moment to sort out the difference among these three terms to discern the overlaps and distinctions among health policy, public health policy, and health care policy.

The CDC model consists of five domains, with two overarching domains that permeate all five (see Figure C.1). The five domains are (I) *problem identification*, (II) *policy analysis*, (III) *strategy and policy development*, (IV) *policy enactment*, and (V) *policy implementation*. Throughout all, two overarching domains infuse and inform. These are (a) *stakeholder engagement and education* and (b) e*valuation*. The latter two are essential to reinforce or modify efforts as needed and will shape and reshape all five domains.

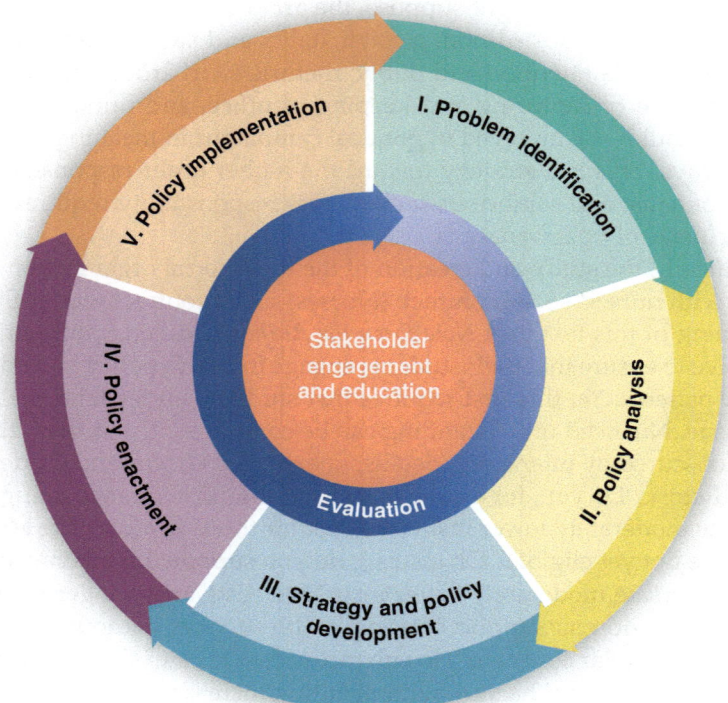

FIGURE C.1: U.S. Centers for Disease Control and Prevention's *Policy Analysis Process*.

Source: Centers for Disease Control and Prevention. (n.d.). *Policy analysis process*. https://ww.cdc.gov/policy/analysis/process/index.html.

Each of these steps in the process includes details that can guide you as you undertake the policy analysis process. These may be found at https://www.cdc.gov/polaris/php/policy-resources-trainings/policy-analytical.html

REFERENCES

Centers for Disease Control and Prevention. (n.d.). *Policy analysis process*. https://ww.cdc.gov/policy/analysis/process/index.html

Durant, W. (1961). *The story of philosophy*. Simon & Schuster.

Glossary

Accountable care organization (ACO)   Emerging from a provision of the Affordable Care Act, an ACO is a voluntary coalition of health care providers who accept health care and financial responsibility for a group of patients, with the latter also referred to as *attributed lives* (see *attribution*).

Ad hoc   Concerned or dealing with a specific, time-limited purpose or issue.

Administrative rule   Guidelines developed by an administrative agency that elaborate the requirement of a law. Once promulgated, administrative rules have the power of laws.

Agenda   An outline or plan of items to be discussed and possibly voted on at a meeting.

All payer   Inclusive of commercial insurance, Medicare, and Medicaid.

Antitrust   Legislation to prevent monopolies, with the intention of fostering competition.

Asymmetry   A lack of equivalence or equality among parts.

Attribution   The assignment of a provider who is responsible for the cost and quality of care for a patient, whether the patient sees that provider or not.

Audit   A formal examination of accounts or records for the purpose of verification.

Autonomy   Independence or freedom to choose and self-determine.

Beneficence   The act of doing good.

Bundled payment   In health care, bundling refers to reimbursement for a set of services or episodes of care rather than each unit of care provided.

Capitation   From the Latin word *caput*, meaning *head*; capitation means "by head," referring to a fixed payment for each person, regardless of the amount of services used.

Certificate of Need (CON)   State program to control the growth of health care facilities or services and the associated cost of such growth.

Co-insurance   A percentage of the costs of care a patient contributes when using services after the deductible is met.

Commodity   An article of trade, such as grain or special metals, in contrast to a service.

Consumer price index (CPI)   Measure of the prices paid by typical consumers for a representative set of services and goods.

Copayment   A fixed amount a patient contributes each time any health services are used, often at the initial time of each health care service encounter. Copayments are waived for some preventive and early detection health services.

Cost sharing   In health care, a contractual requirement that the patient bears at least some cost when seeking and using health care services. Examples include copayments, co-insurance, and deductibles (see *copayment*; *co-insurance*; *deductible*).

Covenant   A contract, agreement, or commitment.

Deductible   An amount of money determined by an insurance contract that must be expended by an individual or family before the insurance company provides reimbursement for health care services obtained.

Dehumanize   To remove or deprive of human qualities or characteristics.

Deontology   The branch of ethics that considers moral obligations and the duty to create right action.

Determinant   A determining factor.

Digitize   The conversion of information, images, or sounds into a digital form that can be processed by a computer.

Dilemma   A situation that demands a choice between equally undesirable alternatives.

Disparity   A difference rooted in inequality or injustice.

Economics   A science with many branches that is concerned with the production, distribution, and consumption of services and material goods.

Electronic health record (EHR)   Digitized health and clinical data replacing paper charts, which allow information to be shared more easily among providers of patient care (see *digitize*).

Entitlement   The right to a set of guaranteed benefits or compensation.

Ethics   A system of principles to guide moral action.

Ethinomics   The intersection of ethics and economics, particularly as it relates to policy formation.

Everyday ethics   Ethical challenges encountered in unremarkable or ordinary, daily events or circumstances.

Ex officio   By virtue of a position, role, or office.

Expenditure The act of expending or using something, particularly financial resources.

Federally qualified health center (FQHC) Community-based health care providers that receive federal funds to provide primary care services in underserved areas.

Fee-for-service Health care reimbursement schema in which each element of service is unbundled from the whole into individual units of procedure and charged for separately (in contrast, see *bundled payment*).

Fidelity Loyalty, faithfulness, and strict observance.

Financing The act, process, or mechanism to obtain money.

Fringe benefits Benefits received by an employee that are provided in addition to regular pay.

Gatekeeper A health care provider, typically primary care, who is the first line of access to the health care system and who also controls referral to a specialist for that patient.

In network In health care, a group of providers who have contracted with the patient's insurance company for reimbursement at a negotiated, typically lower, reimbursement rate (contrast with *out of network*).

Intergenerational Between different generations or age cohorts.

Knowledge worker Employee whose responsibilities are largely the creation, distribution, or application of knowledge.

Laissez-faire The system or practice of noninterference, derived from the French term for *let (them) act*.

Legislative crossover A designated date when a bill introduced in one chamber of the state legislature passes to the other for review, for example, a House bill "crosses over" to the Senate.

Liability The situation of being accountable for something, especially legal responsibility. May also refer to financial accountability.

Lobbyist An individual hired for a cause or business to persuade policy makers to support that cause or business.

Mandate A command, requirement, or authoritative order.

Market basket index The measure of how much more or less it costs to buy a set of goods and services in comparison to the amount in a base period.

Mentor A knowledgeable, experienced advisor and guide.

Monopoly Exclusive control of a product, supply, or trade of a service or commodity.

Moral Concerned with the distinction between right and wrong conduct and goodness or badness of human character.

Nonmaleficence Avoidance of harm.

Out of network In health care, providers who have not contracted with an individual's insurance company for a lower negotiated rate.

Pay for performance (P4P) Reimbursement in addition to traditional fee-for-service that is received for reaching defined quality metrics.

Per diem By the day, or, for each day.

Per member per month (PMPM) Reimbursement strategy in which the provider organization receives a fixed sum of money each month for each patient enrollee, regardless of the amount of services used or unused.

Philanthropy Charitable giving for a particular cause or organization.

Political action committee (PAC) An issues-oriented group that raises money and contributes to political campaigns and candidates who support its issues.

Premium In insurance, an amount to be paid for coverage under a contract, typically in monthly increments.

Quaternary Fourth in order.

Quorum The required number of group members needed to conduct group business.

Reimbursement Payment for services provided.

Reserve Financial resources held aside to be used for future financial demands, both expected and unexpected.

Risk adjusted An approach that accounts for differing severity of patients' conditions to enable fair cost, utilization, and quality comparisons among organizations and other providers.

Self-rationing Self-imposed restrictions on purchasing goods or using services.

Statute A law enacted by a legislative body and expressed in a formal document.

Subsidy Financial assistance provided by a governmental entity.

Superutilizer Individual, typically with complex health and social issues, who uses disproportionately high levels of health care, including emergency departments and hospitals.

Surplus The amount of money that remains above what is needed or used.

Sustainability The ability to be continued and ongoing.

Tertiary Third in order.

Throughput Derived from the phrase "put through"; the amount of material or number of individuals who can be moved through a process in a given time.

Transparent Undisguised or unconcealed, easy to perceive.

Universal Characteristic of or applicable to all.

Upcoding To inaccurately assign a medical billing code to increase or maximize the amount of reimbursement received.

Utilitarianism The branch of ethics that considers utility, promoting the greatest amount of good or happiness for the greatest number of people.

Virtue Behavior that shows moral excellence (see *moral*).

Index

academic medical center, 234
ACA. *See* Affordable Care Act
accountable care iterations, 88–91
   Medicare Shared Savings Program (MSSP), 89
   performance-based contract, 89
   sharing savings, 89–91
Accountable Care Organizations (ACOs), 81, 87–88, 313
   value of service, 87
   volume of service, 87
   health services for addiction treatment, 86
   structure, 88
acontextual actions or cherry picking, 83
ACO REACH. *See* ACO Realizing Equity, Access, and Community Health
ACO Realizing Equity, Access, and Community Health (ACO REACH), 58
ACOs. *See* Accountable Care Organizations
action items, 260
action meetings, 260
actuarial value, 62
ad hoc committees, 241–242
administrative rule making, 275–277
administrative rules, 255
advanced primary care, 81
advisory boards, 254
Affordable Care Act (ACA), 11, 25, 84, 115, 170, 236, 270
   employer mandate, 38
   in financial access to health care, 37–39
   individual mandate, 38
   and new (and renewed) payment models, 37
AHA. *See* American Hospital Association
All-Payer Claims Database (APCD), 60
AMA. *See* American Medical Association
American Association of Nurse Practitioners (AANP), 311
American Hospital Association (AHA), 138, 309
American Medical Association (AMA), 306
American Nurses Association (ANA), 205, 310
ANA. *See* American Nurses Association
antitrust law, 174–181
   consolidation, 175
   facility fees, 177
   horizontal integration, 175
   integration, 175
   M and A activity, 175
   market concentration measurement, 176
   mechanisms negatively impact nurses, 179–181
   merge, consolidate, or stand alone, 174–181
   monopoly versus monopsony, 178
   noncompete clause, 180
   relevant history, 176–177
   site-neutral billing, 177
   vertical integration, 175
APCD. *See* All-Payer Claims Database
appointed boards, 253
artificial intelligence (AI), 147, 151–152, 321
Artiga, 118
asymmetry of information, 135–136
at-hand mentors, learning from, 285–286
authority, 238

bad debt, 14, 264
   charity care versus, 264
balance billing surprise billing, 139
behavioral economics, 4
benchmarking, 82
beneficence, 84, 189
benefit package, 119
benefit period, 116
bid rigging, 179

big data, 148–152
  Artificial Intelligence (AI), 151–152
  data mining, 151
  data visualization, 150
  value, 150
  veracity, 150
bill becoming a law, 274
bill crossover deadline approach, 273
bill draft, 272
biomedical model, 33
blockchain, 147, 153–155
Blue Cross, 310
Blue Shield, 33, 310
blue states, 48
board appointments, 253
  appointed boards, 253
  elected boards, 253
  self-perpetuating boards, 253
  types, 253
board committees role, 241–244
board membership, building skills for, 251–265. *See also* financial operations and reports, understanding; meetings, understanding
  administrative rules, 255
  advisory boards, 254
  board of nursing, 255
  board skill mix, 252
  constituency boards, 254–255
  executive director, 255
  governing board, 254
  organizational fit, 251–252
  philanthropy, 251–252
  public speaking skills and visual appearance, 260–261
    ways to improve, 260
    appropriate professional attire, 261
  regulatory authority, 255
  regulatory boards, 255
  regulatory boards, 255
  regulatory body, 255
  zeal, 251–252
board of nursing, 255
board of trustees (BOT), 229
  role of, 230–231
board performance improvement, 244–245

bond covenants, 262
bond rating and covenants, 262
BOT. *See* board of trustees
budget surplus, 232
budget to actual liabilities, 263
budget to actual revenues, 263
budget variances, circumstances creating, 264
bundled payments, 58, 81, 91–95
  nursing skills in the value-based virtual world, 92–93
buprenorphine for opioid use disorder, 68–69
Bush, George W., 65, 278

CAA. *See* Consolidated Appropriations Act
call the question, 259
capitation payments, 34
care delivery improvement, 79–101. *See also* accountable care iterations; bundled payments; Pay for Performance (P4P)
  Accountable Care Organizations (ACOs), 87–88
  comprehensive primary care (CPC), 86–87
  decision-support tools, 98
  global budgets, 95–97
  making care primary, 87
  moving away from fee-for-service reimbursement, 81
    advanced primary care, 81
    patient-centered medical home (PCMH), 81
    accountable care organizations (ACOs), 81
    bundled payments, 81
  nursing roles within emerging payment models, 97–99
  patient-centered medical homes (PCMHs), 84–86
  real-time data, 98
  by reimbursement receiver change, 79–101
  superutilizers, 98
  from volume to value, 81
  web-based provider portals, 98

Index 359

CARES. *See* Coronavirus Aid, Relief, and Economic Security
catastrophic plans, 63
categorical imperative, 207
CARA. *See* Comprehensive Addiction and Recovery Act
Centers for Medicare and Medicaid (CMS), 86, 316
CEO's report, 258
Certificate of Need (CON), 167, 171–173
   and payment reform, 173
   state laws, 172
certified nursing assistants (CNAs), 316
chair's report, 258
charity care, 14, 264
   bad debt versus, 264
CHART. *See* Community Health Access and Rural Transformation model
chased revenue, 295
cherry picking, 112
Chevron deference. *See* Chevron Doctrine
Chevron Doctrine, 277
Children's Health Insurance Program (CHIP), 12
CHIPS, 14
CHIP. *See* Children's Health Insurance Program
circuit, 270
classic free market, 4
Clayton Antitrust Act of 1914, 175
clinical decision-making, models to guide, 208–211
CMS. *See* Centers for Medicare and Medicaid
Code of Ethics for Nurses (2015), 205
colluding, 179
collusion, 179
comentoring/collaborative mentoring, 287
commercial insurance, 10–11
committee charters, 241–242
committee reports, 258
community benefit, 170, 233
Community Health Access and Rural Transformation (CHART) model, 97
community health teams, 84
community hospitals, 234
community rating, 19
community-based care, 314
competition, 175
Comprehensive Addiction and Recovery Act (CARA), 68
comprehensive primary care (CPC), 58, 86–87
Comprehensive Primary Care Plus (CPC+), 86
CON. *See* Certificate of Need
consent agendas, 259–260
consequence-based decision-making, 205–206
   nurses and, 206
Consolidated Appropriations Act (CAA)
   of 2021, 234
   of 2023, 45, 49, 68, 69–71
consolidation, 175
constituency boards, 254–255
cooperation, 175
Coronavirus Aid, Relief, and Economic Security (CARES) Act, 296
cost containment, ethics of reform and, 215–217
cost sharing, 62, 115
   consequences, 117–118
cost-sharing reductions (CSRs), 62
cost-sharing subsidies, 62
cost-sharing surprise, 139
cost shifting, 14–16
COVID-19 pandemic, 4, 16, 39, 47, 49, 145, 153, 170, 174, 196, 278, 285, 293–299
   counterproductive competition, 294
   elective procedures, 295
   employer-based insurance, challenges with, 297
   ethics and clinical decision-making during, 212–215
   ethics, economics and, 214–215
   fee-for-service reimbursement, 295
   hospital at home, 298–299
   hospital financial downturn during, 80
   insurance lessons from, 66
   lessons from, 293–299
   look to the future, 293–299
   personal protective equipment (PPE), 293
   supply chain, 293–294

COVID-19 pandemic (*continued*)
  telehealth, 297–298
  traunch, 296
  value-based care, 296–299
  virtual care, 297–298
CPC. *See* comprehensive primary care
CPC+. *See* Comprehensive Primary Care Plus
credit worthiness, 262
criminal prosecution, 319
critical access, 234
CSRs. *See* cost-sharing reductions
cultural mentoring, 287
customer allocation, 179

DACA. *See* Deferred Action for Childhood Arrivals
data on quality, 145–147
data science, 147–155. *See also* big data
  blockchain, 153–155
  deep learning, 152
  digital transformation of health care, 148–151
  future of, 155
  Internet of Medical Things (IoMT), 148–149
  Internet of Things (IoT), 148
  machine learning, 152
  natural language processing, 152–153
data visualization, 150
days cash on hand, 262
debt to total capital, 263
debt-to-cap or D/C ratio, 263
deductibles, 116
  versus copayments, 118–123
deep learning, 147, 152
deep neural learning, 152
Deferred Action for Childhood Arrivals (DACA), 278
demand, 135
denied coverage, 49
deontology, rule-based decision-making, 207
diagnostic-related groups (DRGs), 34–37, 137
  financial incentives in, 35–36
  impact of, 36–37
  prospective payment and, 34–37

die in committee bills, 272
digital transformation of health care, 148–152. *See also* big data
  Internet of Medical Things (IoMT), 148
  Internet of Things (IoT), 148
direct democracy, 275–276
direct lobbying, 281
Direct medical education (DME) funds, 312
"dish" payment, 265
disproportional share hospitals (DSH), 169, 265
disproportionate share subsidies, 169
distributional equity concept, 219
diverse mentoring, 287
DME. *See* Direct medical education fund
downside risk, 81, 90, 112
DRGs *See* diagnostic-related groups
DSH. *See* disproportional share hospitals
duty, 207

early nurse entrepreneurs, 310–312
economic and policy solutions, challenges due to, 25–43. *See also* diagnostic-related groups (DRGs)
  Affordable Care Act (ACA), 37
  commercial insurance, 32
  early hospitals, 29
  employer-based health insurance, 30–31
  financial incentives to contain costs, 34
  Flexner Report influence, 27–28
  health maintenance organizations, 34
  nurses, 28–29
  public funding for health industry growth, 31–33
educational meetings, 260
EHRs. *See* electronic health records
elected boards, 253
elective procedure in health care, 295
  reliance on, 295
electronic health records (EHRs), 149
electronic mentoring, 287
emerging payment models, nursing roles within, 97–99
employer based system, 48–49
Employer Income Security Act (ERISA), 60

employer mandates, 48–50, 52
Employer Retirement Income Security Act (ERISA), 45
employer-based health insurance, 30–31, 114
  challenges with, 297
  social reform addressing, 30–31
end-stage renal disease (ESRD), 95
entitlement funding, 192
essential health benefits, 60
ERISA. *See* Employer Income Security Act
ERISA. *See* Employer Retirement Income Security Act
ESRD. *See* end-stage renal disease
ethic of caring, 208
ethical decision-making, models to guide, 205–219
  clinical decision-making, 208–211
  consequence-based decision-making, 205–206
  cost containment and, 215–217
  deontology, rule-based decision-making, 207
  In a Different Voice, 208
  during pandemics, 212–215
  ethic of caring, 208
  moral distress, 211–212
  nurses on boards and in politics, 219
  pandemics, ethics, and economics, 214–215
  Rawls's theory of justice, 207
  sustainability as an ethical issue, 218–219
  virtue ethics, 207–208
  waste in the U.S. System, 216–217
ethinomics, 84, 189–202
  emerging ethical systems, 198
  ethics and nurse role, 199–200
  health care learning system, 198
  intrinsically reflect moral choices, 190
  moral conduct of nurses in contemporary complexity, 197–200
  possibility, question of, 189–192
  public trust in groups to improve, 190
eudaimonia, 208
evaluated need, 123

everyday ethics, 208
ex officio board member. 240
executive director, 255
executive orders, 277–279
  in nursing and health care, 278
  presidents and governors using, 278
experience rating, 19

facility fees, 177
Family First Coronavirus Response Act (FFCRA), 49
federal judicial appeals process, 271
Federal legislation and judicial action, health care shaped by, 45–74
Federal Poverty Level (FPL) Guidelines, 15
Federal Trade Commission (FTC), 174–175
federally qualified health centers (FQHCs), 169
fee-for-service models, 80, 90, 95–97
fee-for-service, 33, 46
  reimbursement, 25, 33, 81, 264, 295
FFCRA. *See* Family First Coronavirus Response Act
fiduciary responsibility, 235
financial access to health care
  Affordable Care Act (ACA) in, 37–39
financial decision-making, consequences, 109–123. *See also* Medicare Advantage
  chronic illness patients, 118
  cost sharing, consequences, 117–118
  deductibles versus copayments, 118–123
  less immediate cost, 110–111
  self-limiting health events, 117
  third-party payers, 111
  patients and financial consequences of treatment, 115–117
  deductibles, 116
  cost sharing pros and cons, 116
  providers assuming financial risk, 112
financial incentives
  to contain costs, 34
  in diagnosis-related groups, 35–36

362 Index

financial operations and reports, understanding, 261–265
  bond rating and covenants, 262
  budget to actual, 263–264
    revenues, 263
    liabilities, 263
  budget variances, circumstances creating, 264
  days cash on hand, 262
  financial statements, 262
  payer mix, 264–265
  salaries and fringe benefits, 262
  variance, 263
financial risk terms, 112
  one-sided risk, 112
  two-sided risk, 112
financing, health care, 3–23
  agent, 9
  payer, 9
  economics versus, 8–9
  reimbursement versus, 8–9
  in the United States, 9
Flexner Report, 27–28, 33
Flexner, Abraham, 27
formal mentoring, 287
for-profit institutions, 232–234
FPL. *See* Federal Poverty Level Guidelines
FQHCs. *See* federally qualified health centers
friendly amendment, 258
fringe benefits, 30, 262
full cost accounting, 219
full risk, 81, 112
fundraising, 239–240
Future of Nursing, The, 240
Future of Work: Robots, AI and Automation, The, 321
FTC. *See* Federal Trade Commission

gaming, 83
Garfield, James A., 277
get-out-the-vote effort, 281
global budgets, 95–97
GME. *See* graduate medical education model
golden mean, 208
governance and organizational type, 229–247
  ad hoc committees, 241–242
  advisory committees, 242
  authority, 238
  board audit committee, 243–244
  board committees role, 241–242
  board of trustees (BOT), 229–231
  board performance improvement and quality committee, 244–245
  committee charters, 241–242
  directors and operators liability insurance, 230
  ex officio board member, 240
  for-profit institutions, 232–234
  fundraising, 239–240
  governance–management boundaries, navigating, 236–240
  hospitals and health systems, types, 231–236
  mission, hospital type, and reimbursement, 234–237
  nonprofit institutions, 232–234
  organizational structure and values, relationship, 240–241
  organizational type impact, 231
  reporting lines, importance, 237–239
  responsibility, 238
  senior leadership team, 237
    chief information officer (CIO), 239
    chief quality officer (CQO), 239
    health care change and, 239
governance–management boundaries, navigating, 236–237
governmental or tax-funded insurance coverage, 11–14. *See also* insurance coverage
governmental payers, in reimbursement, 10
governmental, 232
government branches, in health care improvement, 270–272
graduate medical education (GME) model, 312–314
grassroots lobbying, 282
Great Society, 31
green tree canopies, 6
group mentoring, 287

GUIDE. *See* Guiding an Improved Dementia Experience model
Guiding an Improved Dementia Experience (GUIDE) model, 58, 94

HaH. *See* hospital at home
Haley, Nikki, 285
health care, 193
 as a vulnerable purchase, 112–113
 ethics, 218–219
 less immediate cost consequences in, 110–111
 public trust in groups to improve, 190
health care exchange, 51, 60–65
 health insurance plans, comparison, 62–63
 low-cost plans in exchange, 63–65
 maximum out-of-pocket (MOOP) and ACA, 63
 required by Affordable Care Act, 61
health care laws post ACA, 66–71
 21st Century Cures Act, 67
 Consolidated Appropriations Act (CAA) of 2023, 68, 69–71
 health care workforce shortages, 70
 Mental Health Parity and Addiction Equity Act (MHPAEA), 70
 No Surprises Act, 69
 omnibus spending legislation, 69–70
 Opioid Crisis Response Act of 2018, 68–69
 prescription drug price reporting, 70
 provider network, 70
 telehealth and digital care, 70
 U.S. Food and Drug Administration (USFDA), 67
health care learning system, 198
 ethical framework elements, 198–199
 fundamental obligations, 198
health care markets, significance, 109–129. *See also* financial decision-making, consequences
health care organizations, 165–171
 market status of, 169–171
 tax-exempt status, 170
 volume-based payment, challenges with, 170–171

Health Care PRICE Transparency Act 2.0, 111
health care workforce, 318–322
 contemporary issues challenging, 318–322
 changing nature of work, 321–322
 criminal prosecution, 319
 criminalization of errors, 318–322
 workplace violence, 320–321
 health care trends 2020 to 2030, 322
 nurses in, 305–322
 changing nursing world, 333–335
 early nurse entrepreneurs, 310–312
 graduate medical education (GME) model, 312–314
 incident to billing, 311
 nurses intention, 307
 organized medicine, power of, 309–310
 recruiting people to become nurses, 306–318
 workforce challenges by site, 314–318
 shortages, 70
health coaches, 84
health economics, 3–23
 behavioral economics, 4
 classic free market, 4
 economists thinking, 5–6
 financing versus, 8–9
 health economics, 5
 laissez-faire economics, 4
 reimbursement versus, 8–9
 studying, importance, 5
 theoretical approaches, 4–5
health economics in health care improvement, 269–288. *See also* policy makers role in health care
 at-hand mentors, 285–286
 bill draft, 272
 contemporary mentoring relationships, 287. *See also* mentoring relationships
 federal judicial appeals process, 271
 government branches, 270–272
 influencing at the committee level, 273
 influencing ways, 280–282
 law making, 271
 learning from distant others, 285–286

health economics in health care improvement (*continued*)
  legislative committees, 272
  public ambassador for nursing, 285
  through federal and state policy formation, 269–288
  timing, importance, 273–275
    get-out-the-vote effort, 281
    lobbying, 281–282. *See also individual entry*
    political action committees, 281
    political campaigns, 280
    voting, 280
  overcoming impediments to involvement, 284–285
    stereotypical images of nurses and policy, 284–285
    tensions with powerful others, 284
health equity, 6
  green tree canopies in, 6
health industry growth, public funding for, 31–33
  allied health roles, 32
  biomedical model, 33
  commercial insurance, 32
  fee-for-service system, 33
health insurance
  marketplace, 51
  nurse assistance in navigating, 65–66
Health Internet of Things (HIoT), 148
health maintenance organizations (HMOs), 25, 34, 87, 116
health services for addiction treatment, 86
Herfindahl–Hirschman Index (HHI), 175
HHI. *See* Herfindahl–Hirschman Index
high-margin procedures, 295
HIoT. *See* Health Internet of Things
historical revenue, 95
HMOs. *See* health maintenance organizations
home health care services, 314
horizontal integration, 175
hospital at home (HaH), 297–299
Hospital Readmission Reduction Program, 36
hospital-readmission reduction program, 57

hospitals and health systems, types, 231–236
hybrid financing model, 50

IME. *See* indirect medical education
indirect medical education (IME), 312
  individual mandates, 50–52
  individuals who cannot afford, 51–60
Inflation Reduction Act, 71
informal mentoring, 287
information role in health care, 133–159. *See also* data science; surprise billing
  asymmetry of information and supplier-induced demand, 135–136
  buying power and vulnerability, 135
  data on quality, 145–147
  domain weights and measures, 146
  information science, quality science, and data, 155–156
  outcomes, cost, safety, and value, 133–159
  patient choice role, 142–145
    informed patient choice, 142
  price transparency legislation and administrative rules, 141–142
  price transparency, 136
  price variability, 136–139
Informed Medical Decisions Foundation, 143
informed patient choice, 142
insurance access, 48–49
insurance coverage, 11–16
  commercial insurance, 11
  cost shifting, 14–16
  for-profit, 11
  insurance pool, 17
  monthly premium, 18
  negative margin, 11
  non-profit, 11
  payer mix, 14–16
  positive margin, 11
  risk sharing, 17
  term premium, 18
insurance eligibility reforms
  Affordable Care Act in, 49–50
insurance pool, 17

integration, 175
Internet of Medical Things (IoMT), 148–149
Internet of Things (IoT), 148
investor owned hospitals, 232
IoMT. *See* Internet of Medical Things
IoT. *See* Internet of Things

Johns Hopkins, 27
Johns Hopkins model of medical education, 28
judicial review and case law, 279–280
Justice as Fairness, 207

Kaiser Family Foundation [KFF], 48
Kant, Immanuel, 207
Kennedy, John F., 277
KFF. *See* Kaiser Family Foundation

labor cost, 97
laissez-faire economics, 4
law making, 271
legislative committees, 272
licensed practical nurses (LPNs), 316
licensing laws, 173
lifetime caps, 49
Lincoln, Abraham, 277
lobbying, 281–282
  direct lobbying, 281
  as official authority, 282
  grassroots lobbying, 282
long-term care, 316
long-term debt, 263
Lower Costs, More Transparency Act of 2023, 111
Lower Prices More Transparency Act, 141
lower-than-expected volumes, 264
LPNs. *See* licensed practical nurses

machine learning, 152
MACRA. *See* Medicare Access and CHIPS Reauthorization Act of 2015
main motion as amended, 259
making care primary, 87
making payroll, 262
MA. *See* Medicare Advantage

market competition, 175
market concentration measurement, 176
market entry, exit, and antitrust law, 167–183
  freedom to enter the market, 171–173
  health care organizations, 169–171
  importance to nurses, 167–183
  licensing laws, 173
  monopolistic market power, 173
  nurses and medical licenses, 173–174
MA special need plans (SNP), 120
Mathews, Merrill, 191
MAT. *See* Medication-Assisted Treatment
maximum out-of-pocket (MOOP), 52, 116
measure fixation, 83
Medicaid expansion, 48–49
Medicaid, 11, 14, 31, 32, 37, 48, 50, 52, 98, 264
medical licenses, nurses and, 173–174
Medicare, 11–12, 14, 31, 32, 34, 37, 50, 95, 114, 120–121, 264, 311
  reimbursement, 15
  types of, 12
Medicare Access and CHIPS Reauthorization Act of 2015 (MACRA), 45, 66–67
Medicare Advantage (MA), 116, 119–123, 296
Medicare for All" campaign, 115
Medicare "Medigap" supplement, 121
Medicare Part C, 118
Medicare Shared Savings Program (MSSP), 89
medication-assisted treatment (MAT), 68
meetings, understanding, 256–260
  action items, 260
  action meetings, 260
  approval of minutes, 258
  call to order, 256
  CEO's report, 258
  chair's report, 258
  committee reports, 258
  consent agendas, 259–260
  convening chair, 256
  educational meetings, 260
  meeting agenda, 256
  open meeting laws, 258

meetings, understanding (*continued*)
  permanent chair, 256
  quorum establishment, 256
  standing reports, old business, and new business, 259
  voting process, 258–259
mental health, 317
Mental Health Parity and Addiction Equity Act (MHPAEA), 70
mentoring relationships, 287
  comentoring/collaborative mentoring, 287
  contemporary, 287
  cultural mentoring, 287
  diverse mentoring, 287
  electronic mentoring, 287
  formal mentoring, 287
  group mentoring, 287
  informal mentoring, 287
  multilevel mentoring, 287
  peer mentoring, 287
Merit-Incentive Payment System (MIPS), 66–67
Merkel, Angela, 285
metal or metal levels, 62
metric-driven unintended consequences, 83
MHPAEA. *See* Mental Health Parity and Addiction Equity Act
MIPS. *See* Merit-Incentive Payment System
misrepresentation, 83
missed care, 308
Modern Rules of Order, 256–260
monopolistic power of medical licenses, 173–174
monopoly versus monopsony, 178
monopsony, 178
monthly premium, 18
MOOP. *See* maximum out-of-pocket
moral conduct of nurses in contemporary complexity, 197–200
moral distress, 211–212
moral eustress, 212
moral hazard, 32, 111
motion, 259
MSSP. *See* Medicare Shared Savings Program

multilevel mentoring, 287
myopia, 83

National Provider Identifier (NPI), 311
natural language processing (NLP), 147, 152–153
Nightingale, Florence, 284
1974 Health Planning Resources Development Act, 171
Nixon. Richard, 46
NLP. *See* natural language processing
no poaching agreements, 179
No Surprises Act, 69
noncompete clause, 180
nonmaleficence, 189
nonprofit institutions, 232–234
  for-profit hospitals, differences between, 233
NPI. *See* National Provider Identifier
nurses in health care, 3–23, 28–29, 305–322. *See also* health care workforce
  on boards and in politics, 219
  contemporary, 4
  nurse-sensitive indicators, 145
  roles within emerging payment models, 97–99
  skills in the value-based virtual world, 92–93

Obama, Barack, 278
one-sided risk, 81
open meeting laws, 258
operating margin, 232
Opioid Crisis Response Act of 2018, 68–69
organizational fit, skill for board membership, 251–252
organized medicine, power of, 309–310
ossification, 83
out-of-pocket cost sharing, 62
overtreatment, 123–126
  regional differences in, 126
  small-area variation and supplier-induced demand, 123–126
  traditional markets oversupply decreasing demand, 125–126

P4P. *See* pay for performance
patient choice role, 142–145
Patient Protection, 21, 25
Patient Protection and Affordable Care Act of 2010, 45–48
  ACO realizing equity, access, and community health, 58
  as a hybrid model, 47–48
  bundled payments, 58
  CLASS Plan, 59
  community benefit, 55
  comprehensive primary care, 58
  employer mandates, 48–49, 52
  enhanced access to health insurance, 52–54
  essential health benefits required by, 61
  Guiding an Improved Dementia Experience Model (GUIDE), 58
  health care laws post ACA, 66–71. *See also individual entry*
  health insurance, nurse assistance in navigating, 65–66
  hospital value-based purchasing, 56
  hospital-acquired condition reduction program, 56–57
  hospital-readmission reduction program, 57
  individuals not covered by insurance, 50–60
    individual mandates, 50–52
    individuals who cannot afford to, 51–60
  insurance access, 48–49
  in insurance eligibility reforms, 49–50
    preexisting health condition exclusions, 49
    lifetime caps, 49
    maximum out-of-pocket (MOOP) and, 63–64
    maximum out-of-pocket (MOOP) limits, 52
  Medicaid expansion, 48–49, 52
  medical loss ratio, 55
  Medicare Shared Savings Program, 56
  metal levels and essential benefits, 55
  noteworthy aspects of, 64–65
    "three Rs", 64
  not socialized medicine, 46–47

patient-centered medical homes, 57
premium tax credit, 54
public and private configurations in health care, 47
quality improvement and cost reduction testing, 57
quality-focused initiatives, 56–58
shared decision-making, 55
state innovation model, 57
subsidies, 54
Sunshine Act, 54
transparency/accountability, 54–56
patient-centered medical homes (PCMHs), 57, 81, 84–86
pay for performance (P4P), 80, 82–84
  metric-driven unintended consequences, 83
payer mix, 10–11, 14–16, 264–265
payers of reimbursement, 10
payment reform, 37, 79–101, 113–114. *See also* care delivery improvement
  Certificate of Need (CON) and, 173
  employer-based insurance scenario, 114
  provider accountability, 113
PCMHs. *See* patient-centered medical homes
peer mentoring, 287
per member per month (PMPM) method, 95
perceived need, 123
personal protective equipment (PPE), 293
perverse incentive, 35
philanthropy, skill for board membership, 251–252
PMPM. *See* per member per month method
policy makers role in health care, 275–280
  administrative rule making, 275–277
    significance, 276
  beyond legislative process, 275
  contacting, 282–284
  emails to, 283
  executive orders, 277–279
  executive orders in nursing and health care, 278
  health staff to, 283–234
  judicial review and case law, 279–280
    supreme court in, 279
  phone calls to, 283

political action committees, 281
political campaigns, 280
politics, 270
PPE. *See* personal protective equipment
PPO. *See* preferred provider organization MA
pre–COVID-19 analysis, 14
predictions, 264
preferred provider organization (PPO) MA, 116, 121
premium subsidies, 62
prescription drug price reporting, 70
price fixing, 179
price transparency, 111, 136, 141–142
private configurations in health care, 47
private equity business model, 315
prospective payment, 35, 137
provider accountability, 113
provider network, 70
public configurations in health care, 47
public funding for health industry growth, 31–33
public health, 317
public health emergency (PHE), 49
public trust in groups to improve health care system, 190

Q-APM. *See* qualified advanced alternative payment model
qualified advanced alternative payment model (Q-APM), 66–67
quality committee, 244–245
quality metrics, 82
quaternary care, 234
quorum establishment, 256

rating bands, 50
Rawls, John, 207
Rawls's theory of justice, 207
red states, 48
referendum, 276
regulatory authority, 255
regulatory body, 255
REH. *See* Rural Emergency Hospital
reimbursement, 10–11. *See also* insurance coverage
  commercial insurance companies, 10
  economics versus, 8–9

fee-for-service reimbursement, 25
financing versus, 8–9
governmental payers, 10
Medicare reimbursement, 15
payer mix, 10–11
payers, 10
single-payer system, 10
reporting lines, importance, 237–239
rescission, 264
responsibility, 238
retrospective payment, 35, 95
revenue drivers, 97
reward-only payment models, 84
risk adjustment, 112
risk-sharing arrangement, 17
  community rating, 19
  experience rating, 19
  impacting factors cost, 18–20
Robert Wood Johnson Foundation, 306
Robert's Rules of Order, 256–260
robots, 321
role fidelity, 199–200, 217
Roosevelt, Franklin D., 31, 277
Rural Emergency Hospital (REH), 169–170

salaries, 262
Sarbanes–Oxley Act 242–245
science of sustainability, 219
SDHs. *See* social determinants of health
SDM. *See* shared decision-making
self-limiting health events, 117
self-perpetuating boards, 253
senior leadership team, 237
shared decision-making (SDM), 142
  barriers to, 144
  defining, 143
shared risk, 81
sharing savings, 89–91
SHIP. *See* State Health Insurance Assistant Program
Sherman Antitrust Act of 1880, 175
single-payer system, 10
site-neutral billing, 177
small-area variation, 123–126
social determinants of health (SDHs), 6–8, 193–197
  autonomy, justice and, 194–197
  ethics, economics and, 193–197

upstream, 7
WHO defining, 8
Social Security Act, 31
span of control, 237
standing committees, 241
State Health Insurance Assistant Program (SHIP), 66
state innovation model, 57
suboptimization, 83
subsidy, 51
Substance Use Disorder Prevention that Promotes Opioid Recovery and Treatment (SUPPORT) Act, 68
superutilizers, 98
supplier-induced demand, 123–126, 135–136
　description, 124
supply chain, 153, 293–294
SUPPORT. *See* Substance Use Disorder Prevention that Promotes Opioid Recovery and Treatment Act
surprise billing, 139–141
　balance billing surprise billing, 139
　cost-sharing surprise, 139
　out-of-network, 139
Surprise Medical Bills Act of 2019, 140

Tax Cuts and Jobs Act (TCJA), 45
TCJA. *See* Tax Cuts and Jobs Act
teamness, 86
TEAM *See* Transforming Episode Accountability Model
telehealth, 297–298
　and digital care, 70
tele–mental health services, 317
term premium, 18
tertiary care, 234
Theory of Justice, A, 207
third-party payers, 111
3Rs (reinsurance, risk corridors, and risk adjustment), 64
threshold trigger, 171
throughput, 36
timing, importance, 273–275
Transforming Episode Accountability Model (TEAM), 94
traunch, 296
TRICARE, 14

Trump, Donald, 278
tunnel vision, 83
21st Century Cures Act, 67
two-sided risk model, 81, 91, 112

USFDA. *See* U.S. Food and Drug Administration
Uncertainty and the Welfare Economics of Medical Care, 5
uncertainty, 113
　as an economic concept, 113–114
unfinished nursing care, 308
United States, 9
　budget allocation, 13
　health care financing in, 9
　out-of-pocket money, 9
　insurance premiums, 9
　taxes, 9
universal coverage, 46
universal principles of health care ethics, 191
universalizability, 207
upside only risk, 81
upside risk, 89, 112
U.S. Food and Drug Administration (USFDA), 67
utilitarianism, 206
utilities, 264

value-based care, 296–299
value-based payments (VBPs), 80
value-informed nursing practice, 296
variance, 263
VBPs. *See* value-based payments
veil of ignorance, 207
vertical integration, 175
virtual care, 297–298
virtual reality, 321
virtue ethics, 207–208
virtuous organization, 212
volume-based payment, challenges with, 170–171
voting process, 258–259
voting, 280
vulnerable purchase, 135

wage fixing, 179
Washington, George, 277

workforce challenges by site, 314–318
  community-based care, 314
  hospitals, 317
  home health care services, 314
    for the elderly, 314
  long-term care, 316
  mental health, 317
  physician workforce, 318
  public health, 317
workplace violence, 320–321

zeal, board membership skill, 251–252